**1990
YEAR BOOK OF
SURGERY®**

The 1990 Year Book® Series

Year Book of Anesthesia®: Drs. Miller, Kirby, Ostheimer, Roizen, and Stoelting

Year Book of Cardiology®: Drs. Schlant, Collins, Engle, Frye, Kaplan, and O'Rourke

Year Book of Critical Care Medicine®: Drs. Rogers and Parrillo

Year Book of Dentistry®: Drs. Meskin, Ackerman, Kennedy, Leinfelder, Matukas, and Rovin

Year Book of Dermatology®: Drs. Sober and Fitzpatrick

Year Book of Diagnostic Radiology®: Drs. Bragg, Hendee, Keats, Kirkpatrick, Miller, Osborn, and Thompson

Year Book of Digestive Diseases®: Drs. Greenberger and Moody

Year Book of Drug Therapy®: Drs. Hollister and Lasagna

Year Book of Emergency Medicine®: Dr. Wagner

Year Book of Endocrinology®: Drs. Bagdade, Braverman, Halter, Horton, Kannan, Korenman, Molitch, Morley, Odell, Rogol, Ryan, and Sherwin

Year Book of Family Practice®: Drs. Rakel, Avant, Driscoll, Prichard, and Smith

Year Book of Geriatrics and Gerontology®: Drs. Beck, Abrass, Burton, Cummings, Makinodan, and Small

Year Book of Hand Surgery®: Drs. Dobyns, Chase, and Amadio

Year Book of Hematology®: Drs. Spivak, Bell, Ness, Quesenberry, and Wiernik

Year Book of Infectious Diseases®: Drs. Wolff, Barza, Keusch, Klempner, and Snydman

Year Book of Infertility: Drs. Mishell, Paulsen, and Lobo

Year Book of Medicine®: Drs. Rogers, Des Prez, Cline, Braunwald, Greenberger, Wilson, Epstein, and Malawista

Year Book of Neonatal and Perinatal Medicine: Drs. Klaus and Fanaroff

Year Book of Neurology and Neurosurgery®: Drs. Currier and Crowell

Year Book of Nuclear Medicine®: Drs. Hoffer, Gore, Gottschalk, Sostman, Zaret, and Zubal

Year Book of Obstetrics and Gynecology®: Drs. Mishell, Kirschbaum, and Morrow

Year Book of Occupational and Environmental Medicine: Drs. Emmett, Brooks, Harris, and Schenker

Year Book of Oncology: Drs. Young, Longo, Ozols, Simone, Steele, and Weichselbaum

Year Book of Ophthalmology®: Drs. Laibson, Adams, Augsburger, Benson, Cohen, Eagle, Flanagan, Nelson, Reinecke, Sergott, and Wilson

Year Book of Orthopedics®: Drs. Sledge, Poss, Cofield, Frymoyer, Griffin, Hansen, Johnson, Springfield, and Weiland

Year Book of Otolaryngology—Head and Neck Surgery®: Drs. Bailey and Paparella

Year Book of Pathology and Clinical Pathology®: Drs. Brinkhous, Dalldorf, Grisham, Langdell, and McLendon

Year Book of Pediatrics®: Drs. Oski and Stockman

Year Book of Plastic, Reconstructive, and Aesthetic Surgery: Drs. Miller, Bennett, Haynes, Hoehn, McKinney, and Whitaker

Year Book of Podiatric Medicine and Surgery®: Dr. Jay

Year Book of Psychiatry and Applied Mental Health®: Drs. Talbott, Frances, Frances, Freedman, Meltzer, Schowalter, and Yudofsky

Year Book of Pulmonary Disease®: Drs. Green, Ball, Loughlin, Michael, Mulshine, Peters, Terry, Tockman, and Wise

Year Book of Speech, Language, and Hearing: Drs. Bernthal, Hall, and Tomblin

Year Book of Sports Medicine®: Drs. Shephard, Eichner, Sutton, and Torg, Col. Anderson, and Mr. George

Year Book of Surgery®: Drs. Schwartz, Jonasson, Peacock, Shires, Spencer, and Thompson

Year Book of Urology®: Drs. Gillenwater and Howards

Year Book of Vascular Surgery®: Drs. Bergan and Yao

1990

The Year Book of SURGERY®

Editor

Seymour I. Schwartz, M.D.
Professor and Chair, Department of Surgery, University of Rochester, School of Medicine and Dentistry

Associate Editors

Olga Jonasson, M.D.
Robert M. Zollinger Professor and Chair, Department of Surgery, The Ohio State University, Columbus

Erle E. Peacock, Jr., M.D.
Chapel Hill, North Carolina

G. Tom Shires, M.D.
Professor and Chairman, Department of Surgery, New York Hospital—Cornell Medical Center

Frank C. Spencer, M.D.
George David Stewart Professor of Surgery; Chairman, Department of Surgery, New York University; Director, Department of Surgery, New York University Medical Center and Bellevue Hospital

James C. Thompson, M.D.
John Woods Harris Professor and Chairman, Department of Surgery; Chief of Surgery, University Hospitals, The University of Texas Medical Branch, Galveston

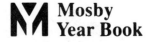

Mosby Year Book

St. Louis Baltimore Boston Chicago London Philadelphia Sydney Toronto

Editor-in-Chief, Year Book Publishing: Nancy Gorham
Sponsoring Editor: Sharon Tehan
Manager, Medical Information Services: Edith M. Podrazik
Senior Medical Information Specialist: Terri Strorigl
Assistant Director, Manuscript Services: Frances M. Perveiler
Associate Managing Editor, Year Book Editing Services: Elizabeth Fitch
Production Coordinator: Max F. Perez
Proofroom Supervisor: Barbara M. Kelly

Editorial Office:
Mosby-Year Book, Inc.
200 North LaSalle St.
Chicago IL 60601

International Standard Serial Number: 0090-3671
International Standard Book Number: 0-8151-7699-2

Table of Contents

The material covered in this volume represents literature reviewed up to November 1989.

Journals Represented

Year Book Medical Publishers subscribes to and surveys nearly 700 U.S. and foreign medical and allied health journals. From these journals, the Editors select the articles to be abstracted. Journals represented in this YEAR BOOK are listed below.

Acta Chirurgica Scandinavica
American Journal of Epidemiology
American Journal of Otolaryngology
American Journal of Physiology
American Journal of Surgery
American Journal of Surgical Pathology
American Surgeon
Annals of Emergency Medicine
Annals of Internal Medicine
Annals of Surgery
Annals of Thoracic Surgery
Annals of the Royal College of Surgeons of England
Archives of Internal Medicine
Archives of Otolaryngology—Head and Neck Surgery
Archives of Pathology and Laboratory Medicine
Archives of Surgery
British Journal of Plastic Surgery
British Journal of Surgery
Canadian Journal of Surgery
Cancer
Cancer Research
Circulation
Circulatory Shock
Contemporary Orthopaedics and Related Research
Clinical Science
Critical Care Medicine
Digestive Disease and Sciences
Gastroenterology
Gastrointestinal Radiology
Head and Neck Surgery
Infections in Surgery
International Journal of Cancer
International Journal of Pediatric Otorhinolaryngology
Journal of Burn Care Rehabilitation
Journal of Cardiovascular Surgery
Journal of Clinical Oncology
Journal of Experimental Medicine
Journal of Hand Surgery (American)
Journal of Investigative Dermatology
Journal of Laboratory and Clinical Medicine
Journal of Otolaryngology
Journal of Parenteral and Enteral Nutrition
Journal of Pediatric Surgery
Journal of Surgical Research
Journal of Thoracic and Cardiovascular Surgery
Journal of Trauma
Journal of Vascular Surgery

Journal of the American College of Cardiology
Journal of the American Medical Association
Journal of the National Cancer Institute
Journal of the Royal College of Surgeons of Edinburgh
Lancet
Laryngoscope
Mayo Clinic Proceedings
New England Journal of Medicine
Otolaryngology—Head and Neck Surgery
Pediatrics
Plastic and Reconstructive Surgery
Proceedings of the National Academy of Sciences of the United States of America
Radiology
Scandinavian Journal of Thoracic and Cardiovascular Surgery
Southern Medical Journal
Surgery
Surgery, Gynecology and Obstetrics
Surgical Research Communications
Thorax
Transplantation
Transplantation Proceedings
World Journal of Surgery
Yale Journal of Biology and Medicine

Publisher's Preface

Publication of the 1990 YEAR BOOK OF SURGERY marks the end of an outstanding era of YEAR BOOK editorship by Erle E. Peacock, Jr., M.D. During Dr. Peacock's 19 years of editorship, the volume's readers have been treated to perceptive commentary of the highest caliber. Dr. Peacock has fulfilled Dr. Schwartz' mission for the editorial board as set out in the preface of their first edition in 1971: "We regard our position as a responsibility to provide an important service to surgeons and interested physicians . . . . The conviction of the importance of our task inspires our efforts." On publication of the 1990 edition, we extend our deepest appreciation for this service and for Dr. Peacock's truly inspired efforts.

Annual Overview

General Considerations

The issue of intra-abdominal surgery in patients with immunodeficiency syndrome has become increasingly important. Although many patients with AIDS have abdominal symptoms, relatively few require an operation. Acalculous cholecystitis occurs relatively frequently; appendicitis and intestinal perforations are also on the list of indications for surgical intervention. von Willebrand's disease represents a potential risk for surgical procedures, but modern substitute therapy has minimized this risk. The appropriate prophylactic therapy with fresh plasma should negate the complication of excessive bleeding. Aspirin should be avoided for 10 days before an elective operation. It has been shown that combining clinical data and thallium studies optimizes the preoperative assessment of cardiac risk before major vascular surgery. In diabetic patients the combination of distal arterial reconstruction and microvascular free tissue transfer avoids limb loss.

Fluid, Electrolytes, and Nutrition

Emphasis on nutritional support and the means by which to deliver such support continues. The relationship of such nutritional support to the newly explained mediators is also under intensive investigation.

One clinical article this year extols the virtues of total parenteral nutrition (TPN) in the treatment of significant acute pancreatitis. The addition of glutamine to commercial TPN solutions appears to have real benefit, and this is to be expected. Although glutamine is not an essential amino acid, it is a primary nitrogen donor, and it stands to reason that this should be a useful addition to parenteral feeding. Investigators continue to look at the reason for acalculous cholecystitis developing after trauma; more evidence accumulates to indicate that the gallbladder does not empty following trauma and, furthermore, it appears not to respond to cholecystokinin at that time.

Hypertonic saline has been evaluated after standardized operative trauma and is useful as far as normal fluid and electrolyte maintenance is concerned. However, the associated hyperosmolality in one third of the patients, necessitating a change in the regimen, suggests that, as in the burn patient, this solution has to be so carefully monitored that its general utility is in serious doubt.

Several studies indicate that patients are more susceptible to infection if they are receiving TPN. Furthermore, it appears that when the bowel is totally at rest, there is an increase in translocation of either mediators or bacteria, which triggers mediators in response to sepsis at some other site. As more investigations continue it should become increasingly clear how and when one can manage the mediators either by reducing their activity with monoclonal blockers or antagonists, or suppressing their generation by not allowing bowel injury and increased permeability to affect the initiation of endogenous mediators, largely from macrophages.

Shock

The pathogenesis and better management of shock continue to be of major interest. Studies on pathogenesis are focused largely on the role of the various lipid mediators. Access, mode of administration, and type of fluids required for better resuscitation are areas of interest. Several papers evaluated the use of blood warming and fluid warming devices in the patient who needs massive transfusion and fluid replacement. Because hyperthermia is a serious problem interfering with platelet function, most trauma surgeons now avoid hypothermia by using blood warming devices. Of the several evaluated, it appears that countercurrent heat exchangers are the most valuable; they afford rapid thermal clearance and have been modified recently to afford large volumes of fluids and even packed red blood cells. These devices work with little damage to the red blood cells, as measured by a lack of hemolysis.

Central line placement is associated with high morbidity; better avenues for access for rapid resuscitation are sought. One large series reported excellent results using the common femoral vein with a large catheter for volume replacement.

Several more articles appeared this past year comparing crystalloid versus colloid resuscitation; crystalloid solutions were most desirable. One study specifically examined the effects of additional albumin on renal free water clearance, finding that albumin, in addition to resuscitative fluid, decreases sodium and free water excretion and leads to a higher incidence of renal failure.

Several groups are evaluating smaller volumes of hypertonic saline, particularly in conjunction with colloid, but one critical article appeared this past year indicating that in uncontrolled bleeding the use of hypertonic saline, a potent vasodilator, increased blood loss and early mortality. These authors warn that the use of hypertonic saline as an immediate resuscitative fluid should be monitored very carefully because of the potential hazards in its use.

The evaluation of several drugs for treatment of shock continues. It appears that naloxone has a pharmacologic effect in septic shock, and that the blood pressure can be elevated, but there is no increase in survival when this drug is administered. Other articles have evaluated the addition of triiodothyronine in hemorrhagic shock, with some encouraging results. The deleterious effects of morphine sulfate in the presence of shock have been documented again as promoting an increase in the low flow state.

The evaluation of crystalloid versus colloid solution in the presence of brain injury revealed that the intracranial pressure response to either solution was not significant in increasing the brain edema that inevitably occurs at the direct side of injury.

The role of the lipid and nonlipid mediators continues to undergo extensive evaluation in the pathogenesis of shock. It appears still that cachectin is a primary mediator turned on by lipopolysaccharide, but it is also activated by other forms of injury as well. Platelet-activating factor is also a proximal mediator and can reproduce the signs and symptoms of sepsis and septic shock with subsequent elevation of other leukotrienes. Further work on the role of lipopolysaccharide in activating bowel translocation of mediators in bacteria continues to indicate that this may be a potent source of infection in the patient who is stimulated by lipopolysaccharide in a remote site of infection. Further studies on the comparison of crystalloid versus colloid solutions in resuscitation from sepsis and septic shock indicate that crystalloid solution, while reducing osmotic pressure, does not increase pulmonary edema in the face of sepsis.

Trauma

It is encouraging to see the continuing accumulation of good sound control in clinical research studies in the specific area of management of the severely injured patient. Another carefully designed, prospective, randomized evaluation of military antishock trousers (MAST) has been carried out. This study indicated not only no benefit from the MAST device, but an increase in mortality in patients in whom it was used whose initial blood pressure was 90 mm Hg or less. These investigators have now banned the use of MAST in their urban transport system.

Another study found that the prehospital administration of fluids is preferably carried out during transport, with results similar to those when fluids are started at the scene. The disadvantage of fluid administration at the scene is the delay in transport time, and this can no longer be justified.

Prospective medical data on the use of seat belts in automobile injuries reveal what would be suspected—a far higher severity score index in patients who are unbelted at the time of accident, resulting in higher mortality, a longer hospital stay, and increased costs. A review of the use of helicopters for medical transport shows that even if the transport time is the same as with ground transport, morbidity and mortality are lower because of the availability of a team and a medically equipped helicopter for critical resuscitation en route.

Interesting studies on the current use of trauma severity scoring indicate that, although these scores predict outcome and give a sense of survival versus nonsurvival, they are not useful as predictors of the onset of sepsis. The addition of some measure of bacterial contamination and immunologic competence should be added to the trauma severity scoring system.

Many articles continue to evaluate the usefulness of abdominal sonography or CT scanning as opposed to peritoneal lavage in the diagnosis of intra-abdominal injury in the patient who sustains blunt trauma. The net result of these studies is the finding that although sonography is a decent screening procedure, its accuracy, specificity, and sensitivity are not as good as those of peritoneal lavage. The two procedures might be complementary. The CT scan is a complementary study in the hemodynamically stable patient for delineation of certain specific injuries. Once again, however, it does not have the specificity, sensitivity, or accuracy of diagnostic peritoneal lavage.

The usefulness of early, presumptive, single-drug antibiotic therapy in the patient with abdominal trauma continues to be described in the literature. This approach has now been advocated for several years and should become the standard therapy in the management of patients with significant abdominal injury.

Significant efforts continue in patients with splenic injury to avoid subsequent septic episodes. The techniques for splenorrhaphy are better detailed, and it appears that splenic autotransplantation into an omental pouch is successful as far as growing tissue is concerned. Whether this proves successful in terms of prevention of infection is yet to be shown.

The usefulness of percutaneous catheter drainage for abdominal abscess developing after trauma is documented with more proponents. One new modality of controlling massive bleeding from intra-abdominal injury is use of a femoral artery placed via intra-aortic balloon. This technique has proved successful and has avoided thoracotomy in many instances.

Wound Healing

One of the most interesting reports in the wound healing field in 1989 was that topically applied silicone gel reduces the size and modifies the appearance of hypertrophic scars in human beings. The mechanism of action is not clear, but the results are impressive and justify more widespread clinical trials as well as basic investigation. The old problem of a scar that becomes wider over time was restudied last year. The most recent data confirm earlier impressions that a permanent subcuticular suture can reduce the tendency of a tight scar to widen during secondary remodeling. Data refuting this fundamental concept in plastic surgery appear now to have been misinterpreted. Reports documenting that polypropylene mesh can be placed in infected abdominal wounds to prevent evisceration, and that wound closure is possible after granulation tissue grows through the mesh, still appear. Long-term problems remain significant, however; despite early success it does not appear advisable to place a synthetic material in a deeply infected wound.

More enthusiasm appeared in 1989 for no-tension repair of all sorts of abdominal hernias. Polypropylene mesh and Gore-Tex are being used most effectively to prevent tension during repair jof ventral and groin defects. Reconstitution of skin by combining cultured epithelial cells with cryopreserved allogeneic dermis still suffers at the basement membrane level. The unique juncture of epithelium and dermis in normal human skin has not been reproduced satisfactorily in artificial skin.

The search for a practical use for various growth factors continued in 1989. In a tightly controlled study, topical application of epidermal growth factor shortened the time of reepithelialization of human split-thickness skin graft donor sites. The reduction, although statistically significant, was not practically as dramatic as some think possible. Transforming growth factor-beta partially reversed Adriamycin-impaired healing. Much of the activity in this field seems to be directed toward correction of wound healing defects; little work is being done on acceleration of normal wound healing. Topical antimicrobial agents have been known for some time to interfere with skin healing; the mechanism was shown recently to be specific interference with fibroblast function and replication. Closure of a previously difficult wound—midline sacral decubitus ulcers—has been simplified by continued modification and refinement of V-Y advancement gluteus maximus flaps. A refreshing simplicity in technique for resurfacing lower extremity defects is the use of local fasciocutaneous turn-down flaps.

Infection

Local infusion of antibiotic solutions was again reported to be effective in preventing infection after closure of heavily contaminated wounds. It is not clear from these reports whether mechanical débridement was a confounding factor. In addition, preincisional, intraparietal injection of augmentin was compared in 1989 with intravenous administration of the same antibiotic. The investigators concluded that intraparietal injection was more effective than intravenous administration in preventing wound infection. The old concept that a "load of antibiotics should be on board" before abdominal surgery involving heavy contamination or infection was challenged by studies in 1989 which showed that intravenous administration of antibiotics at the time the need becomes apparent was just as effective as preoperative prophylactic administration.

The increased susceptibility to pneumococcal infection of patients who have had splenectomy may be reduced by administering pneumococcal vaccine. Protection apparently is the result of improved pulmonary clearance of live bacteria in the circulation. Serum elastase α_1-proteinase inhibitor was shown to be a sensitive indicator of sepsis; in patients with peritonitis, a persistent increase may be correlated with the necessity to reoperate because of undrained pus.

An encouraging report evaluating single-agent antibiotic treatment of intra-abdominal sepsis revealed that treatment with cefotetan alone was as effective as combinations of ampicillin, gentamicin, and metronidazole. The results were no different in patients with positive blood cultures.

Studies in 1989 emphasized the need to resect small bowel when multiple perforations occur during the treatment of peritonitis. The etiology of perforations often is not clear, but reluctance to resect bowel in the presence of active peritonitis is usually not good judgment. Although there remains controversy over the risk of performing splenectomy, more data were presented to support the conclusion that there is a life-long risk of severe infection and thromboembolism after removal of the spleen. Postoperative necrotizing fasciitis still goes unrecognized and undiagnosed early because the surgeon does not think of the condition and perform a biopsy on suspected tissue. The diagnosis of necrotizing fasciitis must be made by tissue biopsy to afford the optimum chance for control.

Burns

There was a timely reminder in 1989 that acute cholecystitis, often the result of pharmacologically induced spasm of the sphincter of Oddi, can complicate the early treatment of burned patients. Emergency cholecystectomy sometimes can be avoided by paralyzing the sphincter with an appropriate nerve block. The intravenous catheter remains a high-risk source of infection; *Pseudomonas* and coagulase-negative *Staphylococcus aureus* are the most common organisms recovered from intravenous catheters. Interestingly, the incidence of infection associated with catheters was reported to correlate inversely with distance from the site of catheter insertion.

A report that propranolol improves myocardial oxygenation in burned children yields some insight into why digitalization has never seemed to help cardiac function in burned children and young adults with heart failure. A report showing that fish oil is not a remedy for postburn metabolic defects, and that it does not improve immunologic function, should put that previously popular concept to rest.

Further scientific evidence was presented in 1989 to show that early excision of burned tissue is important from an immunologic as well as metabolic and wound healing view. Excision of eschar may partially mediate immune changes and prevents splenic hypertrophy and lymphocyte alteration. The search for plasma substitutes continued in 1989 with demonstration that pentastarch in relatively small amounts can be equal, or even superior, to albumin in burn resuscitation. Pentastarch, like albumin, however, results in increased bleeding and prolonged clotting times.

The need for whole-tissue biopsy specimens to evaluate infection accurately was emphasized; acridine orange staining was recommended along with fluorescent staining in quantitative culture techniques. Most of these techniques are available in the usual hospital setting.

Contour deformities developing tangential excision of burned tissue and grafting were shown to be preventable by altering the depth of excision of the edges of a burned wound and by careful consideration of the thickness and type of graft. Prolongation of skin allograft survival was accomplished by administering cyclosporine. None of the patients treated with cyclosporine had increase susceptibility to infection while creeping substitution of the allograft occurred. Glycerol-preserved nonviable cadaver skin combined with wide expanded autografts was shown to be effective in the treatment of very extensive third-degree burns.

Transplantation

Cyclosporine has proven to be a highly effective immunosuppressive drug. Although the drug is expensive, its use has resulted in considerable improvement in the outcome of all types of organ transplants, with substantial reduction in the costs of hospitalization. Nephrotoxicity, the principal complication of cyclosporine treatment, remains a problem. The report from UCLA (Abstract 8–26) of the long-term follow-up of children with successful liver transplants is especially disturbing, in that the children treated with cyclosporine demonstrated a progressive loss of renal function. The search for better immunosuppressive drugs, more specific and less toxic, continues.

One of the newest drugs, FK506, seems promising in that excellent graft survival and even "rescue" from progressively severe rejection resistant to other therapy, has been noted. Although phase I studies in animal models were complicated by severe toxicity, patients seem to tolerate the drug but nephrotoxicity did develop to some degree. Further clinical trials seem indicated. Monoclonal antibodies to the CD3 antigen of helper T cells, OKT3, have been most effective in treating rejections, although the usefulness of this agent is sharply limited when the host develops antibodies against the monoclonal antibody. A new type of monoclonal reagent, directed against the CD4 antigen of helper T cells, seems to suppress this troublesome humoral immune response and may even be immunosuppressive and tolerogenic.

Further studies of the mechanism of the immunosuppressive effects of blood transfusion have focused on prostaglandin production. The power of the transfusion effect has also been documented in attempts to induce tolerance through peritransplant infusion of nucleated stem cells from the donor; Barber et al. (Abstract 8–18) report a successful clinical trial using this strategy.

The role of the antigen-presenting cells in inducing allograft rejections remains of considerable interest. Modulation of the antigen-presenting cells, or their elimination from the allograft, is an effective means of delaying or averting rejection. Studies of fetal organs during phases of development in which proper antigen-presenting cells are absent corroborate the modulation experiments; when these cells are not present, rejection does not occur.

The graft-infiltrating lymphocytes include populations of macrophages. The importance of induction of class II antigen expression on the graft cells; the presence of lymphokines, including the products of the activated macrophages, and the interactions of the graft-infiltrating lymphocytes and the graft, are not entirely clear. The induction of intercellular-adhesion molecules by cytokines produced by activated infiltrating cells may be of considerable importance at the outset of graft destruction, and their inhibition by steroids may provide an explanation for some of the immunosuppressive effects of these drugs.

Much progress has been made in short-term liver preservation with the use of a perfusate developed after years of steady work by Belzer and his associates (Abstract 8–22). This agent, the "UW solution" has made it possible to transport livers over longer distances and provides hours to prepare the recipient and perform the operation under optimal conditions. The organ most in need of an effective short-term preservation method is the heart; no real progress has been made, although the report of Bando et al. (Abstract 8–29) concerning oxygen free radical scavenging and the use of perfluorocarbons is encouraging.

The major problem facing transplantation is the organ donor shortage. The significant problems associated with the use of anencephalic infants as heart donors have been thoroughly discussed but remain unresolved. Many patients, at least 25% on the waiting lists for liver and heart transplants, die before an organ becomes available, and only those most desperately ill receive transplants. The failure of the Routine Inquiry legislation to improve the rate of organ donation among patients who are brain dead, is most disappointing. The problem seems to be at the professional level, with lack of interest and involvement on the part of physicians caring for comatose patients with irreversible brain injury. A means to encourage organ donation must be found if the achievements of improved immunology, immunosuppression, and organ preservation are to be realized.

Oncology and Tumor Immunology

The more we learn about the peculiarities of the immune response to tumors, the more complex this system appears. The simple rules of classic immunity, wherein immunization with antigen results in a cytotoxic immune response mediated by cells or by specific antibody, do not seem to apply. For instance, in the first paper reviewed in this section, tumor-infiltrating lymphocytes were obtained from tumors, expanded with interleukin-2 infused into patients with advanced cancers. Those that responded to this treatment (patients with melanoma or renal cell cancer) did not have heavy infiltration of their tumors with lymphocytes but, rather, seemed to develop heightened cell-mediated immunity in general with resultant tumor control. The effects appeared to be systemic rather than local.

The relative inefficiency of the immune responses generated by tumor antigens have been studied by several investigators who seek to manipulate the antigens to create a more effective response. One of the most promising new approaches has been to create a mirror-image of the antigen by immunizing against monoclonal tumor-specific antibodies (anti-idiotypic antibodies). These newly generated antibodies reflect the tumor antigen, and when inoculated into the patient prove to be much stronger immunogens than the tumor itself. Clinical trials of this anti-idiotypic antibody treatment are underway, using a mouse system to generate the monoclonal antibodies for later injection into patients.

Lymphokines and other mediators continue to be of real interest. One of the areas newly identified are the cell surface adhesion molecules (CAMs), which may be activated by cytokines, and, in the case of endothelial cells, provide the sites for adhesion and penetration of tumor vessels by activated lymphocytes. Some of the effects of adoptive immunity may be to activate the CAMs and interfere with tumor blood supply. Activation of CAMs and cell adhesion may also be responsible for pulmonary toxicity during interleukin-2 infusion.

The adverse impact of blood transfusion on length of survival in patients with malignancies has been the subject of numerous studies reported during this past year. Although all studies to date have been retrospective and uncontrolled, circumstantial evidence is accumulating to show that blood transfusion diminishes host defenses and abbreviates survival time. One of the best studies to date has been that of Blumberg et al. (Abstract 9–5). Using sophisticated statistical methodology, blood transfusion was implicated in shortened survival time in patients with cervical cancer. Possible mechanisms for this effect include the "veto cell" concept of Martin and Miller (Abstract 9–9), production of prostaglandins that are immunosuppressive (and can be blocked by indomethacin), suppressor cell generation, and the induction of antibodies to block the immune response. Further clinical studies of a prospective nature are called for.

Growth factors such as epidermal growth factor, cholecystokinin, and bombesin are important in the establishment and proliferation of tumors. Receptors for the growth factors are found on many types of tumor cells, lending support to the possibility that receptor-related hormonal treatment schemes might be developed that are tumor- and receptor-specific.

Skin, Subcutaneous Tissue, and the Hand

A plea was made in 1989 for hand surgeons to use soft tissue reconstruction and synovial resection to treat metacarpophalangeal joint rheumatoid arthritis in some patients. The investigators do not think that all patients with metacarpophalangeal joint disease should have replacement arthroplasty. The major problem in rheumatoid surgery, however, still is the reluctance of rheumatologists to refer patients for early surgery. A report this past year implicated failure to eradicate proliferating synovial disease as the cause of late flexor tendon rupture. Removal of bone spurs as well as synovium can protect long tendons against rupture. Silastic joint arthroplasty apparently has not been used as much as it should be in the proximal interphalangeal joint area after intra-articular fractures.

Apparently, fear of joint degeneration and soft tissue coverage problems have caused hand surgeons to be more reluctant than they should be to repair traumatic destruction of proximal interphalangeal joints with Silastic as a primary procedure.

A new idea for the treatment of scaphoid malunion with necrosis of one fragment is replacement of the dead fragment with a free autogenous graft and screw fixation to the living fragment. Early results seem impressive; revascularization of the graft appears uniformly successful.

A classification for digital ring avulsion injuries was presented as a guide to which digits should be amputated primarily and which are worthy of reconstructive surgery. Key in the new classification is the presence or absence of bone and joint injuries.

The difficult differential diagnosis between suppurative tenosynovitis and surrounding cellulitis without tendon sheath infection is improved by the use of ultrasonography. A comparison of sonograms between the same digits on opposite hands makes it possible to demonstrate fluid within the digital sheath in a high percentage of patients with suppurative tenosynovitis. False positive results were not reported.

A new warning was issued that *Mycobacterium marinum* tenosynovitis, although rare, is still a problem, particularly among fish handlers, in whom it is often overlooked. Treatment with rifampin and ethambutal and radical synovectomy usually are necessary for cure.

Reports of reduction in the cost of replantation of amputated fingers at the level of the distal interphalangeal joint kept alive the possibility that such replantations can be cost effective in some centers. Reported costs are so far below the usual expense, however, that distal replantation in most hospitals probably is not justified in 1990. Dynamic splinting after repair of extensor tendons was advocated this past year, although the rationale is not overwhelming.

Breast

Serious evaluation of mammography as a practical technique for mass screening of women appeared in 1989. Some of the data raised profound questions strongly suggesting that serious problems are developing. Some studies showed no more than 7% positive biopsy results in lesions reported highly suspicious on mammograms. Only about 27% of biopsies are positive around the country. The combinatin of a relatively low rate of positive diagnosis, the time required for repeated mammograms and scheduling of preoperative needle placement and operative procedures, and the expense of surgical and radiologic procedures appear now to be formidable objections to mammography as a mass screening technique. Preoperative needle localizations particularly may be an area where time and expense can be reduced.

A recommendation that mammography be used to determined adequacy of local excision of carcinoma suggests that "lumpectomy" may not be as safe as originally conceived.

Another attempt to reduce the time and expense of needle placement and open biopsy was the use of mammography in performing fine-needle aspiration biopsy of non-palpable lesions. A 94% correlation was reported between fine-needle aspiration with mammographic guidance and conventional open biopsy through a surgical incision. The problem of removing the correct duct and lobule when nipple discharge can be localized was approached by injection of methylene blue dye to outline the structures drained by a duct. Results reported in 1989 support the idea that dye localization is a reasonable substitute for mammographic localization.

New reports in 1989 emphasize the importance of careful histologic examination of the specimen after local excision of breast cancer. Wide reexcision is indicated when residual cancer, found in 66% of patients in one series, is encountered. Patients with nipple discharge and comedo carcinoma are at particularly high risk for residual disease after local excision. A higher incidence of lymph node metastasis than previously expected suggests that in situ ductal carcinoma may be more generally invasive than believed previously. Some of the pathologic features reported in the past year as being associated with local recurrence are extensive necrosis, inflammatory infiltrate, and lack of elastosis.

The low possibility of finding metastasis, reported in 1989, confirms earlier suspicions that hepatic imaging as a preoperative study should be abandoned.

More data supporting immediate reconstruction at the time of mastectomy were reported. Most of the theoretical objections seem to have disappeared in 1989.

The Head and the Neck

Subglottic infantile hemangioma, a dangerous lesion because of respiratory obstruction, does not respond predictably to steroid administration. New techniques using CO_2 laser destruction also have been less than completely satisfactory. Midline cricotracheostomy to expose the lesion and meticulous dissection of the tumor mass, followed by reconstruction of remaining tissues, was reported in 1989 as being successful. It appears that open dissection should be done when steroid therapy does not produce dramatic improvement.

Reports of carotid artery resection and reconstruction during radical neck dissection revealed limited usefulness for the occasional patient with isolated artery involvement. Although technically more feasible than previously, carotid resection does not often extend the curative potential of a neck dissection. Studies on patients undergoing neck dissection after preoperative radiation therapy reveal that radiotherapy alone is not always as effective as some recent reports suggest, and that properly administered radiotherapy does not interfere significantly with wound healing in the cervical area.

Morbidity, speech, and swallowing functions, and survival data after transoral CO_2 laser ablation of cancer and some benign tumors support the continued use of multimodality treatment. Blood loss appears minimal during CO_2 laser ablation of cancer.

Cable grafting of the facial nerve after extirpative surgery can result in protection for the eye, some voluntary facial motion, prevention of drooling, and maintenance of facial muscle tone. Postoperative radiation does not appear to compromise neurologic regeneration following cable grafting or direct suture of the facial nerve.

Studies of the treatment of nasal vestibule squamous cell carinoma confirm earlier reports that radiation therapy can be so successful that surgical extirpation should be reserved for occasional recurrences. Bone invasion, however, is an exception; the high rate of recurrence when bone is involved supports wide surgical excision as the primary treatment for these potentially dangerous neoplasms. A combination of primary radiotherapy and surgical removal if recurrence develops can produce a 90% cure rate unless bone is involved.

Although sialography is still of dubious value in the preoperative evaluation of parotid masses, various other new imaging techniques, including CT and magnetic resonance, can add considerable information about the risk of malignancy. Such studies are not practical for small children; the use of magnetic resonance imaging provides the best soft tissue resolution in adults. A new classification of parotid fistula based on a sialographic findings is reported to clarify early which ducts should be operated on and which will heal spontaneously. Reoperation on the parotid gland after inadequate excision of tumor apparently is no more dangerous as far as protection of the facial nerve is concerned than primary surgery. A unique new free flap utilizing pleura for lining was introduced to reconstruct compound oral and oropharyngeal defects.

Thorax

The extensive data reported by Haller et al. (Abstract 13–2) describing experiences with more than 600 children treated for pectus excavatum document a very plausible approach. Operation at ages 4 to 6 years has negligible morbidity and produced excellent long-term results in about 95% of patients.

Progress is slight with pulmonary neoplasms. Faber and associates (Abstract 13–5) described early results with the preoperative use of both chemotherapy and irradiation for stage III tumors, apparently obtaining some benefit compared with preoperative radiation alone, previously demonstrated to be of no value. In small cell cancer the role of pulmonary resection is minor, but the fortunate few with stage I disease seemed to receive significant benefit if resection was performed after chemotherapy.

All 12 patients reported by DeMeester et al. (Abstract 13–8) had significant tumor involvement of the vertebral column, usually considered an unequivocal sign of inoperability. With en bloc removal of the involved bone, 6 of the 12 patients survived, 4 of them for more than 5 years after operation.

Excision of multiple pulmonary metastases from soft tissue sarcomas is described in a large report from the National Cancer Institute. The surgical approach was somewhat unusual, using a median sternotomy even for operations repeated two or three times. Wedge resections were performed. No operative deaths occurred.

Two reports describe experience with operations for emphysema. Surgical resection is beneficial only for that small group in whom the large bullae significantly compress adjacent functioning parenchyma. A key consideration is avoiding an air leak, the major cause of morbidity. A report by Venn et al. (Abstract 13–10) describes an unusually conservative approach from the Brompton Hospital in London. A large Foley catheter was brought through the chest wall to establish a bronchocutaneous fistula. The fistula closed in all patients within a short time after the catheter was removed.

A report from England by Sarsam and Moussali (Abstract 13–12) describes a series of 332 pneumonectomies by one group of surgeons performed over a period of 10 years; no bronchopleural fistula developed. These impressive results again raise the question of what, if any, is an acceptable percentage of bronchopleural fistulas after pneumonectomy. I discussed this in a short publication in 1972 (Bond AD, Spencer FC: *Ann Thorac Surg* 13:195, 1972). Staple closure of the bronchus has been widely adopted for its simplicity, but the question remains whether it produces a higher fistula rate than a precise suture closure.

A report by Ginsberg et al. (Abstract 13–13) of 10 patients describes a transsternal approach to the dread problem of postpneumonectomy bronchopleural fistula.

Cooper et al. (Abstract 13–1) document the safety of silicone stents in the tracheobronchial tree. These silicone tubes, developed by Montgomery in 1968, have now been left in place in some patients for longer than 5 years.

A report from my institution by Gouge and associates (Abstract 13–14), combined with an extensive review of publications by others, documents that suture closure of an esophageal perforation should be routinely buttressed with autogenous tissue. This report describes experiences with a pleural flap originally described by Grillo, although intercostal muscle may be even more effective. In this small series the buttress closure was uniformly effective even though 50% of the patients were treated more than 24 hours after perforation.

An important report by the late Robert Henderson and associates (Abstract 19–5) describes experiences with a selective group of 25 patients treated by cricopharyngeal myotomy. The authors indicate the importance of precise radiologic diagnosis and precise surgical technique in recognizing this uncommon condition, for only 25 such procedures were done in a series of more than 1,500 patients.

Congenital Heart Disease

An unusual alternative to the Fontan operation totally diverts the vena cava from the right heart, theoretically avoiding energy loss from turbulence in the right atrial chamber (Abstract 14–1).

With transportation, uncertainty remains about the performance of the classic atrial baffle operation or the corrective but more complicated arterial switch procedure. Turley et al. (Abstract 14–2) describe impressive 10-year results in a group of 36 infants operated on at an early age. Late survival was 97%, with 89% free from reoperation.

Current data from the 20-institution cooperative study evaluating the arterial switch operation describe experience with 466 neonates (Abstract 14–3). The importance of a precise technique seems indicated because 6 of the 20 institutions reported a much lower mortality than the others did. Bove described experiences in 81 patients in a period of 4 years, with only one death in the most recent 56 repairs (Abstract 14–4).

An unusual report from Scandinavia (Abstract 14–6) provides further data for the long-standing puzzle about the development of aortic insufficiency after operation for subaortic stenosis. In a group of 21 patients followed for up to 6 years, some insufficiency ultimately developed in 8, in some as long as 5 years postoperatively. The cause of this unusual event is unknown.

The aggressive surgical approach for a patent ductus in premature infants emphasizes the safety of surgical treatment (Abstract 14–7). All patients were operated on within 72 hours, without any significant surgical morbidity or mortality.

The report by Backer et al. (Abstract 14–8) describes an unusual experience in 204 patients with vascular rings: There have been no operative deaths in the past 28 years.

Valvular Heart Disease

The report of Magilligan et al. (Abstract 15–1) is one of the first to present a meaningful 15-year follow-up of experience with porcine prostheses, analyzing experiences with more than 1,000 valves implanted over a period of years with a 99% follow-up. The most sobering fact is the sharp increase in degeneration between 10 and 15 years after operation: only 31% of valves functioned at a late date. The report by Cohn et al. (Abstract 15–2) of experiences with 1,678 prostheses over 15 years found 57% functioning at 15 years. Unless recent improvements in preservation of such valves significantly affect durability, the long-term function of porcine valves seems limited to between 10 and 15 years in most patients.

Extensive data are now available concerning the St. Jude prosthesis, introduced in 1977. The experience of Arom et al. (Abstract 15–4) with 1,298 patients indicated that the major morbidity is from thromboembolism (1.5% per 100 patient years) and anticoagulant bleeding. Fortunately, endocarditis is rare. Similar findings were reported by Myers et al. (Abstract 15–5) from a series of 785 patients.

Because of the sobering late results with porcine prostheses, interest is again increasing in aortic homografts. The report by Bodnar and colleagues (Abstract 15–6) compared late results with freeze-dried, frozen, and antibiotic preservations. No long-term difference could be found, raising the question of the importance of viable fibroblasts in the aortic homografts on durability. In children, however, cryopreserved homografts have been adopted with increasing frequency, avoiding the need for anticoagulants in a growing child.

The report by Coselli and Crawford (Abstract 15–8) describes a technical modification of composite aortic root replacement using a 10-mm Dacron tube to reestablish flow to the coronary ostia. Experiences with 90 patients were reported.

Five-year results were compared among patients undergoing one of three types of mitral valve operations: mitral valve reconstruction, replacement with porcine prosthesis, or replacement with mechanical prosthesis. The virtual absence of thromboembolism in patients with mitral valve reconstruction was reaffirmed, as well as the virtual absence of endocarditis. In the group receiving mechanical protheses, selected because of their ability to take warfarin reliably, a similar low frequency of thromboembolism occurred. Two of the major causes of morbidity after mitral surgery—thromboembolism and endocarditis—are not present with mitral reconstruction; longevity should be significantly improved. Otherwise, operation should be performed earlier before some degree of irreversible left ventricular dysfunction develops. Good results were also reported by Scott and associates (Abstract 15–11) in Florida with 176 mitral valve reconstructions, reflecting the growing popularity of the reconstructive technique.

Two reports (Abstracts 15–12 and 15–13) from the National Heart Institute present data about obstructive hypertrophic cardiomyopathy. One report clearly demonstrates important improvement in myocardial metabolism after relief of the subaortic obstruction. The other report describes results with mitral valve replacement, long championed by Dr. Cooley, for patients in whom myomectomy did not seem feasible or had previously been unsatisfactory.

Coronary Heart Disease

Additional important data have appeared demonstrating the increased longevity after coronary bypass in selected groups. An extensive study of 5,800 patients from Duke University found the best results in those who had a significant decrease in ventricular function (Abstract 16–1). Similar conclusions were reached in the report by Myers et al. (Abstract 16–2), especially in patients who had severe angina. With severe left ventricular dysfunction and angina, the 63% long-term survival after operation was better than that in medically treated patients (30% long-term survival).

The role of angioplasty versus bypass continues to be evaluated with new data. In the report by Hochberg and associates (Abstract 16–3) concerning a matched series of 125 patients reported better results at 3 years in the surgically treated group, a finding that could be predicted considering the vast improvement in coronary blood flow with bypass grafts. Reports continue to accumulate demonstrating that the mortality rate after failed angioplasty is sobering despite the degree of planning beforehand. The report by Naunheim et al. (Abstract 16–4) found an 11% mortality and a 22% infarction rate. As discussed in last year's Overview, a similar report from the Mayo Clinic found a mortality rate 4 times higher for bypass performed after failed angioplasty than after elective bypass, even though an operating room was kept on a stand-by basis and operation started within 1 hour after angioplasty failed.

A study comparing transplantation to bypass in patients who have advanced left ventricular dysfunction and an ejection fraction near 20% reports that the 3-year survival after bypass was 83%; the main cause of death was arrhythmias. Progress in antiarrhythmic therapy could significantly decrease this late mortality.

Two articles by Mills and Everson (Abstracts 16–6 and 16–7) describe the use of the right gastroepiploic artery. This represents a continuing search for an artery as useful as the internal mammary. In 15 of the 39 patients reported it was significant that the gastroepiploic artery was detached and used as a free graft. If long-term results are satisfactory, a free graft would greatly enhance the usefulness of the gastroepiploic artery.

The problem of combined coronary and carotid artery disease is addressed again (Abstract 16–8). Among 71 simultaneous operations performed, the perioperative stroke rate ranged between 0.5% and 2%. The frequency of simultaneous operations seems to have decreased progressively in the United States because of a lack of significant data demonstrating substantial benefit.

Miscellaneous Cardiac Conditions and the Great Vessels

Retrograde coronary sinus cardioplegia is emerging as a valuable technique, especially when antegrade cardioplegia is cumbersome or ineffective. The reasons for its apparent efficacy are physiologically unclear. It produces more uniform cooling of the myocardium, avoiding the inevitable maldistribution of cardioplegia when injected antegrade for patients with coronary disease. Whether oxygen transport to the myocardium is equally effective is yet unknown.

Documentation is provided about the risk of phrenic nerve injury when iced slush is used for topical hypothermia (Abstract 17–7); the conclusions are similar to those reported from New York University in 1987. To my knowledge there are very few, if any, indications for the use of iced slush, because the potential benefit is small and the hazard of phrenic nerve injury is significant.

Rossi et al. (Abstract 17–2) found no differences between two techniques of hypothermic perfusion in 27 children; total arrest for 40 minutes versus perfusion at about 25% of normal. With improved oxygenators, as well as concern about the safety of circulatory arrest for 60 minutes or longer, there seems to be increasing use of low-flow perfusion.

What type of circulatory support is best for the patient who cannot be weaned from bypass remains unknown. My institution has long used the simple but crude roller pump. The report by Rose et al. (Abstract 17–9) summarizes total experience with more than 70 patients, 30% of whom survived. Pennington et al. (Abstract 17–8) describes experiences with the physiologically superior Pierce-Donachy pump, with a survival of about 35% in 30 patients. Clearly, the Pierce pump is superior as a bridge to transplantation, permitting effective perfusion for several days. The value of the roller pump is its simplicity of use in the operating room.

The problem of postoperative bleeding remains a common one after open-heart surgery. Fortunately, this has decreased progressively in recent years, probably because of improved oxygenators that minimize injury to the blood elements. The report by Gundry et al. (Abstract 17–10) documents that heparin rebound, a familiar hypothesis from bygone years, is extremely rare. Fibrin sealant is shown as effective in controlling localized bleeding after operation. Problems for which fibrin glue is effective are usually those characterized by moderate coagulopathy, resulting in oozing from needleholes in multiple suture lines.

The sternotomy incision and its complications remains significant causes of morbidity. Garrett and Matthews (Abstract 17–12) describe a technique for reoperative sternotomy, using previously inserted sternal wires to elevate the sternum away from the mediastinal structures. I strongly support the concept of using some form of *upward* traction on the sternum at the time it is divided with an oscillating saw, minimizing the hazard of injury to underlying cardiac structures.

The report by Nahai et al. (Abstract 17–13) from Emory is of land-mark status, summarizing 10 years of experience of sternal infections in 211 patients with muscle flaps. The 5% mortality rate is impressive, as is the performance of the entire procedure in a single operation in more than 70% of the patients and an average hospitalization of 15 days. These results are better than those reported by Grossi et al. in 1985 (*Ann Thorac Surg* 40:214, 1985). At New York University initial treatment with operative débridement, wound closure, and closed mediastinal anti-biotic irrigation has remained the procedure of choice.

An unusual report describes the use of omentum in 17 patients with a sternotomy infection (Abstract 17–14). Further experiences with omen-tum will be of particular interest. Providing significant morbidity does not occur as a result of mobilizing the omentum from the peritoneal cav-ity, the method seems simpler than the use of muscle flaps. Johnson et al. (Abstract 17–15) describe débridement and local wound treatment, fol-lowed by delayed primary closure, with good results.

The safety of delayed sternal closure in neonates is reinforced in the report by Odim and colleagues (Abstract 17–16). In nine patients sternal closure was delayed for an average of 5 days, with two patients recover-ing when the sternum was closed 11 days and 12 days postoperatively. The absence of infection was remarkable.

Two reports deal with the uncommon but serious problem of neuro-logic injury following bypass, a major cause of morbidity. Studies by Brusino et al. (Abstract 17–1) could not document impairment of blood flow autoregulation in elderly patients that might make them more vulnerable to hypotensive injury at the time of perfusion. The fact that the frequency of neurologic injuries increases with age and length of perfusion suggests a perfusion defect, but the mechanism remains un-known.

The dread but fortunately rare problem of permanent visual defects af-ter open-heart surgery is described in the report by Shahian and associ-ates (Abstract 17–17), finding four patients after 700 operations, a fre-quency of near 0.6%. Microemboli seem the most plausible cause, but this remains unproved.

Ergin et al. (Abstract 17–18) describe experiences with annular de-struction found in 15 patients with advanced endocarditis among a group of 82 treated in a period of 10 years. A number of reconstructive tech-niques were used. Despite the introduction of "foreign bodies," such as Teflon felt patches or graft replacement, a high success rate was obtained. This reaffirms the importance of adequate débridement of all infected tis-sue, even though it extends into adjacent structures. The prompt surgical treatment of endocarditis not responding to antibiotic therapy should make these complex problems rare.

Two reports (Abstracts 17–19 and 17–20) analyzed prognostic fac-tors with myocardial contusion, a frequent consideration in patients with multiple injuries following blunt trauma. The data from both reports in-dicate that monitoring with ECG and cardiac enzymes determination reg-ularly detect serious abnormalities within 24 hours. If serious cardiac injury has not been documented during that time, the likelihood of major cardiac problems evolving subsequently is small.

The Arteries, the Veins, and the Lymphatics

It is pointed out that anaphylactoid reactions to protamine are often lethal complications in insulin-dependent patients undergoing vascular procedures. Deficiencies of natural anticoagulants and disorders of the fibrinolytic system, as well as also the presence of lupus-like anticoagulants, may cause a hypercoagulable state and lead to limb ischemia in young adults. It may be appropriate to screen young adults with peripheral vascular disease for hypercoagulable situations.

Results in a large series addressing injuries to the ascending aortic arch and great vessels demonstrated that management has been refined to the extent that the mortality rate has been signficantly reduced. It is pointed out that inflammatory aortic aneurysms are generally atherosclerotic aneurysms with an unusual degree of inflammatory process. The results of operation are very good, and extensive dissection and lysis of the ureter and duodenum should be avoided. Because of the high incidence of ischemic colitis, routine flexible sigmoidoscopy within 48 hours of successful repair of a ruptured abdominal aneurysm is recommended.

A randomized study of vein patch versus primary closure for carotid endarterectomy shows equivalent results in *men*. The vein patch procedure is also associated with a higher incidence of early recurrence and longer operating time. The saphenous vein patch closure, however, is appropriate in selected patients. Bypass to the pedal arteries in patients with atherosclerotic disease yields a high rate of foot salvage and is comparable to more proximal bypass procedures. Wound complications are common and require special technical considerations. Surveillance by serial postoperative monitoring of the functional patency of saphenous vein bypasses can identify grafts with correctable lesions before thrombosis occurs, enabling elective revision.

Chronic compartment syndrome is described, and it has been shown that the syndrome will not improve without fasciotomy. Open fasciotomy has been associated with fewer complications than closed, subcutaneous fasciotomy. Comparative analysis of retroperitoneal and transperitoneal aortic replacement of aneurysms demonstrates that the retroperitoneal approach has distinct advantages, particularly in the obese patient, and should be preferentially considered unless there are circumstances that preclude the approach.

A review of extra-anatomical bypass procedures defines the fact that there is great variability in the results obtained. Carotid artery stenosis has been managed by resection of the common carotid and internal carotid placement by autogenous vein graft. This represents a safe alternative to a second endarterectomy with patch grafting.

A prospective randomized trial in patients with intermittent claudication has demonstrated that arterial reconstruction is clearly more effective than physical training alone, but that the addition of physical training to arterial reconstruction improves the symptom-free walking distance.

The role of sympathectomy in arterial surgery remains controversial, but one group suggests that it should be considered in selected patients. The management of spontaneous aortocaval fistula is reviewed, and it is pointed out that the operative mortality remains significant. It is emphasized that anticoagulants continue to play a significant role in the management of patients with peripheral arterial emboli. Mesenteric venous thrombosis should be suspected in patients with a history of thrombotic events and hypercoagulable states when there are acute abdominal symptoms. Infusion CT is useful in establishing the diagnosis.

Esophagus

It has been shown that primary repair without gastrostomy is suitable for most infants with esophageal atresia and tracheoesophageal fistula. The hospitalization period is shortened and the complication rate reduced. A significant mortality rate is indicative of the serious nature of spontaneous rupture of the esophagus. Surgical repair, even when delayed, offers the best chance of recovery. Diverticulopexy and cricopharyngeal myotomy are reported as reasonable alternatives for patients with a high risk of potential complications from diverticulectomy, but it is generally believed that diverticulectomy represents the treatment of choice for Zenker's diverticulum.

In many centers pneumatic dilatation has replaced the Heller myotomy as primary treatment for achalasia. Results are less effective than hoped, and surgery may well be used more often in the future. Assessment of the combined Collis-Nissen operation reveals a success rate of about 75%. With scleroderma, previous antireflux operations, and stricture, favorable results occur less frequently.

Total thoracic esophagectomy is a cervical esophagogastric anastomosis has been performed in patients with failed esophagomyotomy and has been associated with more favorable long-term results than cardioplasty or limited esophageal resection in this group of patients. The stomach is the preferred organ for esophageal replacement for benign diseases, and the results associated with esophagogastric anastomosis for a variety of benign diseases are very good.

Esophagogastrectomy without thoracotomy is an effective and safe method for restoring swallowing in patients who have adenocarcinoma of the esophagogastric juntion. Bypass procedures do not provide good palliation for patients with advanced esophageal carcinoma, considering the short postoperative time and frequent complications. Esophagectomy with reconstruction results in a longer survival time. The outcome after laser or photodynamic therapy is encouraging, and comparable palliation is achieved compared with more extensive surgical operations.

The Stomach and the Duodenum

Although the incidence of duodenal ulcer is increasing in third-world countries, the incidence and prevalence of duodenal ulcer in Western Europe and North America has fallen almost steadily in the past 30 years. Complications of hemorrhage and perforation, however, appear not to have changed greatly. Acid-reducing operations for intractability have, on the other hand, greatly diminished in frequency. Because perforations occur often after years of ulcer disease, and the mortality risk of perforations in elderly patients is high, we should consider surgical treatment with selective proximal vagotomy in patients with long-standing ulcer disease. When all information is subjected to multivariant analysis, the most important contribution to mortality in patients with perforated duodenal ulcer is increasing age. A strong case may be made that operative therapy is more cost effective than maintaining life-long drug treatment. Studies suggest that this is already the case in Great Britain.

Although somatostatin has proved to be effective in managing secretory diarrhea and small bowel fistulas, it does not seem to ameliorate bleeding from peptic ulcer. Several recent studies have given what appears to be definitive evidence of lack of effect.

Certain technical points in gastric surgery deserve mention. The technique for vagotomy can be greatly simplified so as to allow for rapid and secure identification or division of the vagal trunks. The routine use of gastrostomy for postoperative drainage of the stomach has led to serious complications. The putative ill effects of nasogastric suction have been exaggerated, and because patients die of leaking gastrostomies, there seems to be no comparison between the risk of the two methods. Why use a potentially lethal technique to accomplish a goal that is easily achieved otherwise? As soon as someone advocated use of Roux-en-Y drainage of the stomach for treatment of alkaline reflux gastritis, it was only a matter of time until someone else advocated it as a routine hookup after gastrectomy. This offers no advantage over gastroduodenostomy or gastroenterostomy and carries the very real threat of high rate of marginal ulceration because of the absence of neutralizing bicarbonate from bile and pancreatic secretions.

Gastric perforations are associated with a high risk of mortality and should always be managed by an acid-reducing procedure if at all possible. The best acid-reducing procedure in these patients is a distal gastric resection that encompasses the perforation.

Many fear that adoption of omeprazole therapy for the treatment of duodenal ulcer will achieve such success in promoting achlorhydria that a high incidence of formation of gastric carcinoid tumors will follow. Several have used this in arguments against the use of omeprazole for hypersecretion unless it is of a malignant (for example, from a gastrinoma) variety. A similar potential complication of long-term curtailment of acid secretion is seen in the development of gastric cancer in the remnant of the stomach after gastric resection for duodenal ulcer disease. Although controversial for many years, the concept gradually seems to have gained acceptance. The problem is that one must follow patients for more than 20 years to demonstrate the phenomenon. It certainly does raise the question of the possible carcinogenic effect of long-term acid suppression by highly effective drug therapy.

Analysis of nuclear DNA from human solid tumors has shown correlation between abnormal DNA content and a poor prognosis. The relationship between DNA ploidy and prognosis in human stomach cancers has been controversial, but recent careful analysis has confirmed the role of DNA ploidy as a major determinant in survival.

Widespread application of endoscopic biopsy has led to problems in management of duodenal villus adenomas. The high percentage of malignancy of these tumors and their excellent response to Whipple resection supports the use of radical pancreaticoduodenectomy as the initial operative procedure for villus adenoma. Probably the last thing one would want to do is to treat it by laser ablation because the tissue is vaporized, and there is no way in the world of knowing whether or not the tumor is malignant.

Every few years the matter of obstruction of the third part of the duodenum caused by vascular compression arises, and surgeons often become zealots advocating operative treatment. One can usually treat these patients successfully by getting them off their backs and having them lie on their stomachs and putting some fat on them. If an operation is needed, an anastomosis between the proximal obstructed duodenum and the jejunum is the procedure of choice.

The Small Intestine

Jejunal diverticula are uncommon and rarely symptomatic. They can bleed and they can perforate, and if they cause these complications, they should be excised. There appears to be no justification, however, for removing an asymptomatic jejunal diverticula found incidentally at operation.

Careful study of fetal distress has led to detection of important lesions, including bowel obstruction, in fetuses. In the fetus with discrepancy between size and date of gestation, the use of ultrasound can detect bowel obstruction and often localize it to the proximal or distal bowel (distal bowel obstruction has a worse prognosis). Prenatal diagnosis permits counseling of the parents and prompt resuscitation and operation.

Contrast radiography facilitates the diagnosis of bowel obstruction in patients in whom physical examination and plain abdominal films are inadequate to allow diagnosis. The technique of small bowel enteroclysis greatly facilitates separation of true mechanical obstruction in early postoperative patients from those who have prolonged ileus.

A common problem when operating on patients with small bowel obstruction finding a strangulated loop, the viability of which is unclear. All sorts of tricks and devices (fluorescent dyes, electrical stimulation, and Doppler ultrasound, among others) may be helpful. If in doubt, the safest thing to do is to close the abdomen and have another look in 24 hours.

High-output small bowel fistulas can tax the ingenuity of any surgeon. Many of them respond to long treatment with total parenteral nutrition, but recent studies suggest that enteral nutrition is safer than parenteral and leads to spontaneous closure in almost 40% of patients. The duration of hospitalization is long and the mortality risk is high, but enteral nutrition may prove to be safer than intravenous nutrition. Somatostatin is helpful in decreasing volume and in facilitating healing.

We are going to need to face several moral issues in dealing with neonatal conditions that affect gut length. We have learned to keep alive children who have only about 10% of the normal length of jejunoileum, but at extraordinary cost and average hospitalizations of more than 1 year. The results are marvelous, but the question is whether we are doing the right thing morally and economically. How can one tell?

A few years ago we learned that blood transfusions acted to protect renal allografts; recent studies show that blood transfusions appear to protect against recurrence of Crohn's disease, presumably by an immunologic mechanism. Blood transfusions have taken such a drumming for their role in transmitting disease, it is interesting to see that, in addition to their obvious role as replacement therapy, they can occasionally be of great help.

The Colon and the Rectum

Matters of cost containment conflict at times with good patient care, and mandatory efforts to secure second and third opinions and preadmission certification have introduced cumbersome bureaucracy. There is also evidence that these efforts may actually have interfered with good patient care, especially in causing delay of admission of patients with acute appendicitis. The fatality rate associated with acute appendicitis seems to be dropping all over the country except in patients older than 80 and in whom there is a delay in diagnosis and a high incidence of lethal perforation.

The risk of appendiceal carcinoids is apparently related to their size, and those less than 2 cm rarely metastasize. Studies in children with appendiceal carcinoids confirm this notion, because tumors rarely get above 2 cm and they appear to metastasize only rarely.

The matter of proper preoperative preparation of the colon occupies all gut surgeons, and recent studies indicate that the combination of neomycin plus erythromycin not only diminishes the colonic count of organism but, also, in experimental biopsy samples there is morphological evidence of eradication of colonic mucosal flora.

Colonic volvulus seems to be sex related; about 80% of patients with sigmoid volvulus are men and two thirds of patients with cecal volvulus are women. Endoscopic decompression of sigmoid volvulus often allows elective operation, which should be excision of all redundant sigmoid. Patients with cecal volvulus should probably be operated on right away because colonoscopic decompression is difficult and often unreliable and may lead to a dangerous delay in operation.

Ongoing experience with colonic injuries provides strong support for the notion that most all of these can be managed primarily, either by local suture or by resection and anastomosis, and that colostomy can usually be avoided.

Because there is no safe way to distinguish between a right paracolonic phlegmon that is caused by either a ruptured appendix, a perforated cecal diverticulum, or a perforated cecal carcinoma, the best approach is to excise the entire mass and do a primary ileocolostomy; if there is free pus, however, probably a diverting ileostomy and mucous fistula of the colon would be best.

We all know that obstruction or perforation of a colon cancer greatly diminishes the chance of survival. Recent studies show that colonic obstruction cuts 5-year survival in half.

How aggressive should we be in treating recurrent colon cancer? A report of survival of 20% of such patients certainly gives impetus to the adoption of an aggressive attitude. If there is distant spread, operation, as we all know, is futile. The only way we will greatly improve survival is by early diagnosis, yet large numbers of patients die of unsuspected colorectal cancer, many of whom had never sought help for any symptom related to the large bowel. Malignant neuroendocrine (carcinoid) tumors of the colon, particularly those with small and intermediate-sized cells, behave aggressively and often lead to curtailed survival. The tumors may elaborate one or more neuroendocrine markers but rarely give rise to recognizable syndromes of endocrinopathy.

Defunctionalized loops of bowel, especially the rectum, become narrow, shorter, and hypoplastic. Measurement of rates of crypt cell production confirms this hypoplasia by demonstrating a lower index of cell turnover.

The major problem in dealing with elderly patients who have massive colonic hemorrhage, of course, is finding the bleeding site. Angiography is potentially splendid but often fails because the patient stops bleeding when the dye is injected. Unless the bleeding site can be clearly identified by angiography or nuclear scan, total colectomy will usually avert the need for reoperation and will probably give the best survival rate.

The Liver and the Spleen

Computed tomography-guided sclerotherapy is safe and effective initial therapy for nonparasitic cysts, but long-term follow-ups are awaited. Surgical drainage and roentgenographically controlled drainage of hepatic abscesses both achieve success. In a small subset of patients hepatic resection represents the treatment of choice. Intraoperative ultrasound of the liver is an important addition to the armamentarium in evaluating the feasibility and extent of resection for primary and secondary malignancies. The clinical manifestations of hemangioma in infants are significantly different from those in adults; if the lesion fails to respond to steroid therapy, therapeutic embolization may be considered. Operation is recommended for solitary large hemangiomas and hemangiomas that have ruptured. A large series of patients with liver cell adenomas is reported; surgical excision is advocated when possible because this eliminates the patient's symptoms and removes the complications of hemorrhage and malignant transformation.

In the Oriental literature liver resection has been carried out for hepatocellular carcinoma in patients with severe cirrhosis. Preoperative transcatheter arterial embolization and portal vein embolization appear to improve the survival rate of patients. Reoperation for subclinical recurrence and solitary metastases remains an important strategy for prolonging survival. In an attempt to prevent recurrence, ultrasonically guided intraoperative portal venous embolization with starch microspheres has been performed. Total vascular occlusion, including occlusion of the supra- and infrahepatic cavas, is a useful technique in resection of hepatic lesions that involve the hepatic veins. It is essential that these patients be in a euvolemic state before caval occlusion. An incidence of 28% posthepatectomy intra-abdominal infection is reported. In most instances, percutaneous drainage is effective in managing this complication.

Endoscopic sclerotherapy has been associated with low mortality from variceal bleeding and a low rebleeding rate in the management of esophageal varices in children with biliary atresia. In an adult patient population staple transection of the esophagus as emergency treatment of bleeding varices is as safe as sclerotherapy and more effective than a single sclerotherapy procedure. Endoscopic elastic band ligation of varices is effective in the initial and long-term control of bleeding. The procedure is technically no more difficult than endoscopic sclerotherapy. A success rate of approximately 95% has been reported for an H-type shunt with venous graft used for treating young children with portal hypertension of extrahepatic origin.

In patients with alcoholic cirrhosis, improved results have been reported for distal splenorenal shunt, coupled with splenic pancreatic disconnection. In nonalcoholic patients there is no proved advantage. The technique, however, is associated with an increased rate of bleeding and does not improve the encephalopathy rate in other series.

Assessment of long-term results of treatment of the Budd-Chiari syndrome have shown the side-to-side portacaval shunt to be extremely effective. The mesoatrial shunt may be the procedure of choice in treating patients with Budd-Chiari syndrome associated with inferior vena caval obstruction.

Pediatric wandering spleen is the subject of a review, and it is suggested that splenopexy using a Dexon mesh is the treatment of choice. Intracranial hemorrhage remains the most serious manifestation of idiopathic thrombocytopenic purpura. Emergency splenectomy is indicated for these patients. Removal of a massively large spleen is associated with high mortality and morbidity rates. Benefit has been demonstrated for patients with myeloproliferative disease and non-Hodgkin's leukemia. In leukemic patients the procedure should be performed only for disease intractable to therapy, symptomatic splenomegaly, or hemorrhage.

The Biliary Tract

Assessment of a large series of patients with biliary atresia subjected to surgery concludes that, when possible, the Kasai procedure should be the initial operative approach; the best results are in infants operated on when younger than 3 years. In an interim report of the lithotripsy prospective study it was shown that shock-wave lithotripsy leads to fragmentation of bile duct stones and is safe. It is regarded as a valuable part of the multidisciplinary approach to biliary calculi. There is an apparent increase in the incidence of acalculous cholecystitis, and high morbidity and mortality figures persist. This is often related to the patient's underlying disease. Acute cholecystitis is reported to be a complication of percutaneous transhepatic drainage. Cholecystectomy should be performed if prospective transhepatic drainage is planned for unresectable conditions. A difference of opinion about the association of cholecystectomy and colorectal cancer persists, and an irrefutable conclusion cannot be reached at this time.

Selective endoscopic retrograde cholangiopancreatography (ERCP) and stone removal in bile duct surgery is proposed to reduce the incidence of choledochotomy. A review of the late results of immediate primary end-to-end repair in accidental transection of the common bile duct provides further evidence that a Roux-Y hepaticojejunostomy represents the procedure of choice unless there is a clean-cut transection and reanastomosis can be accomplished with no tension. Although balloon dilatation is an alternative in high-risk patients with benign postoperative biliary strictures, the results do not match those of surgical repair. A new technique that addresses proximal stenosis of the bile ducts, usually associated with tumors at the confluence, has been reported. It incorporates the use of a new surgical endoprosthesis that has long-term patency. A report on transduodenal sphincteroplasty and transampullary septotomy for primary sphincter of Oddi dysfunction indicates that there are poor outcomes in patients with sphincteric stenosis, and it is essential to evaluate the results postoperatively with ERCP.

Factors that suggest a more favorable result in patients with carcinoma of the biliary tract include the absence of serosal infiltration and the presence of a papillary lesion rather than a sclerosing lesion. In patients with biliary obstruction secondary to the pancreas, there is a role for both percutaneous biliary drainage and biliary enteric bypass, because both provide palliation.

The Pancreas

Studies on the isolated perfused human pancreas have confirmed many observations previously available only in experimental animals. The method will certainly provide important information regarding mechanisms for the release of insulin and glucagon.

Is there any way to improve the dismal outlook in patients with necrotizing pancreatitis? There seems to be no clear answer, but operations in desperately ill patients for removal of necrotic peripancreatic debris seems to offer the best chance. Peritoneal lavage and instillation of intraabdominal antibiotics do not appear to help. Pancreatic abscesses must be drained aggressively and, often, frequently.

Long-term steroid treatment seems to predispose to pancreatitis, and experimental evidence is available that blockage of cholecystokinin (CCK) receptors can prevent the lethal consequences of steroid-induced pancreatitis. Perhaps the two (CCK plus steroids) synergize to create havoc.

The debate continues on how best to treat patients with chronic relapsing alcoholic pancreatitis. If they have a dilated pancreatic duct, pancreaticojejunostomy (Puestow) seems to be the best. What do we do in patients with small ducts? Pancreatic resection does not seem to help unless you take the whole pancreas out; then, you often are faced with an unstable diabetic state. We are reluctant to do total pancreatectomy in any patient unless we can be sure that their alcoholism has been vanquished. Can you ever be sure? The diabetes after total pancreatectomy seems to be best managed by use of recombinant DNA human insulin, because it does not evoke anti-insulin antibodies and allows close control in patients who otherwise often experience wild swings of blood glucose levels.

Intraductal papillary cancers of the pancreas are uncommon tumors that appear not to spread to distant sites and respond unusually well to pancreatectomy. Although multiple foci have been reported, the vast majority of tumors are located within the small area of the pancreas. This is often in the head, so that a Whipple resection may be necessary. Involvement of the pancreas in a lymphoma, on the other hand, calls for a totally different response. The excellent results obtained so far with chemotherapy are encouraging.

Syndromes of acute respiratory distress are common in patients with severe pancreatitis and appear to be linked to decreased pulmonary surfactant. Recent experimental morphological studies have shown damage to type II pneumocytes after experimental pancreatitis, supporting the theory that reduction in surfactant causes the atelectasis. An unusual and potentially dangerous complication of pancreatitis may be an inflammatory injury to the left transverse colon and splenic flexure that may progress to colonic necrosis. In such cases the necrotic colon should be excised and the remaining two ends of the colon exteriorized.

Even though the clinical use of islet transplantation has been in abeyance for the past several years because of lack of clinical effectiveness, and even though pancreatic whole-organ allografts are successful, the great potential attractiveness of islet cell transplantation persists, and studies from several centers suggest improvement in the rate of recovery of isolated islets, which may portend resumption of clinical trials of islet transplantation within a few years.

Controversy continues over the proper application of fine-needle aspiration biopsy in thyroid nodules. The question revolves around the expertise of the cytologists who interpret the cells. Great cytologists get great results. Surgeons should not depend on the technique unless they get excellent correlation between preliminary needle aspiration results and results after removing the gland.

Large thyroids may compress the trachea, and the compressing tumors may range from absolutely lethal anoplastic carcinomas to huge benign goiters. Patients with respiratory distress should be treated by endotracheal intubation, with tracheostomy avoided at almost any cost.

Surgeons who operate nearly every day on the thyroid gland gain vast experience and are probably correct in the assumption that they can handle thyroid cancer best by total thyroidectomy. Usually, however, especially in patients with papillary cancer, there is little scientific indication for total thyroidectomy when one compares the advantages conferred by the operation to the risk incurred. Prognosis in papillary cancer of the thyroid does not seem to be influenced by extrathyroid extension of the tumor at the primary site that is surgically resectable.

Vasoactive intestinal polypeptide stimulates thyroid tissue, and it also stimulates cells from thyroid cancer, although in a less potent manner than does thyrotropin.

Long experience with islet cell carcinomas of the pancreas confirms a much more benign course than that associated with cancers from exocrine pancreatic tissue. Functioning endocrine carcinomas of the pancreas vary in rates of malignancy from 60% to 70% for gastrinomas to about 10% for insulinomas. Nearly half of the patients with pancreatis islet carcinomas have nonfunctioning tumors; of those that do function, gastrinomas are the most common.

Somatostatin is a potent suppressor of pancreatic secretion in animals and in man, and recent studies show that it is also useful in alleviating symptoms of the dumping syndrome.

The study of DNA ploidy has been applied to the adrenal, and experience confirms that aneuploid tumors have a worse prognosis than do diploid tumors. Further, DNA flow cytometry failed diagnostically to differentiate between benign and malignant tumors.

1 General Considerations

The Incidence of Intra-Abdominal Surgery in Acquired Immunodeficiency Syndrome: A Statistical Review of 904 Patients
LaRaja RD, Rothenberg RE, Odom JW, Mueller SC (Cabrini Med Ctr, New York)
Surgery 105:175–179, February 1989   1–1

Many patients with AIDS have abdominal symptoms, but relatively few require laparotomy. In the past few years an ever-increasing number of patients with AIDS have been seen at the Cabrini Medical Center. Between January 1985 and January 1988, 904 patients with documented AIDS were admitted to the hospital. Of the 904 patients, 36 (4.2%) underwent intra-abdominal surgery. The operations included 12 cholecystectomies, 7 splenectomies, 7 appendectomies, 6 laparotomies because of gastrointestinal perforations, and 6 laparotomies for miscellaneous conditions.

Acute acalculous cholecystitis was found in 9 of the 12 patients undergoing cholecystectomy, and the gallbladders in 3 patients contained calculi. Cultures of specimens taken from 5 patients showed cytomegalovirus, *Candida albicans, Enterobacter cloacae,* and coagulase-negative staphylococci. Four of the 12 patients died of overwhelming sepsis in the postoperative period. Pathologically enlarged spleens and pancytopenia refractory to the administration of steroids and blood products were found in all 7 patients who underwent splenectomy. All patients having splenectomy made an operative recovery. Of the 7 patients undergoing appendectomy, 3 had gangrenous lesions, 2 had suppurative appendicitis with rupture, and 1 had acute nonsuppurative appendicitis secondary to cytomegalovirus. Six of the 7 patients recovered; 1 died of acute adrenal insufficiency.

The high incidence of inflammatory involvement in the gallbladder, appendix, and intestines in patients with AIDS probably resulted from the nature of the blood supply to the organs. The high postoperative mortality rate of 22.2% was attributed to immunodeficiency rather than to complications of surgery. Of the 36 patients, 21 (58.3%) had documented pathologic conditions that were secondary to AIDS.

Surgical intervention was satisfactory in those patients with AIDS who had splenomegaly, appendicitis, and other lesions of the gastrointestinal tract, but not in those with cholecystitis.

► The demonstration of the great complication rate associated with cholecystectomy for acalculous cholecystitis in these patients is significant. Robinson et al. (1) reported on 21 patients with AIDS undergoing operations. After emergency procedures the 30-day operative mortality was 57%; for elective surgery the rate was 43%. Miller (2) reported 38 patients who underwent 49 operations related to thoracic disease for AIDS. Operative mortality was 26%.—S.I. Schwartz, M.D.

References

1. Robinson G, et al: *Arch Surg* 122:170, 1987.
2. Miller JI: *J Thorac Cardiovasc Surg* 92:977, 1986.

Surgery in Patients With Von Willebrand's Disease
Blombäck M, Johansson G, Johnsson H, Swedenborg J, Wabö E (Karolinska Hosp, Stockholm)
Br J Surg 76:398–400, April 1989
                                                                    1–2

The bleeding complications associated with Von Willebrand's disease represents a potential risk in surgical procedures, but modern substitution therapy has greatly minimized this risk. During a 15-year period, 51 patients with von Willebrand's disease underwent 64 major surgical procedures requiring a hospital stay of more than 24 hours. In 18 operations performed on 16 patients, the bleeding disorder was unknown at the time of operation. The mean age of these 5 men and 11 women was 32 years. Postoperative bleeding occurred in 12 of the 16 patients, 2 of whom required reoperation to control it. There was no mortality.

In the remaining 35 patients the diagnosis of von Willebrand's disease was known before operation. These 13 men and 22 women, (mean age, 35 years) underwent a total of 45 major operations. All 35 received prophylactic therapy preoperatively, including administration of factor concentrate, fresh plasma, desmopressin acetate, and tranexamic acid as needed. There were no deaths and none of the patients required reoperation for bleeding. Hemostatic complications occurred in 3 of the 45 operations (6.7%), but all were easily managed. Patients with von Willebrand's disease no longer are at increased operative risk, provided appropriate precautions are taken and the bleeding disorder is diagnosed before operation.

▶ The 67% reported incidence of bleeding complications in patients in whom the disorder was not recognized indicates the importance of assessing patients preoperatively. Cryoprecipitate is relatively effective. It can be administered every 12 hours in a dose of 10 to 40 units per kg. To correct the bleeding time, replacement therapy should begin 1 day before a surgical procedure. Aspirin should be avoided for 10 days or for the life of the platelet before an elective operation. The duration of therapy is the same as that applicable to a patient with classic hemophilia, i.e., it should be continued until all sutures are removed.—S.I. Schwartz, M.D.

2 Fluid, Electrolytes, and Nutrition

A Single Dose of Endotoxin Increases Intestinal Permeability in Healthy Humans
O'Dwyer ST, Michie HR, Ziegler TR, Revhaug A, Smith RJ, Wilmore DW
(Brigham and Women's Hosp, Boston; Joslin Diabetes Ctr, Boston)
Arch Surg 123:1459–1464, December 1988   2–1

Many of the host responses that follow trauma, burns, chemotherapy, and inflammatory bowel disease may be related to an increase in permeability of the bowel to gastrointestinal tract microorganisms and their endotoxins. To determine if the host responses that occur during endotoxemia are associated with an alteration in intestinal permeability, paired studies of intestinal permeability were performed in 21 healthy human beings, who were given *Escherichia coli* endotoxin, 4 ng/kg, or 0.9% saline solution intravenously. Two standard permeability markers, lactulose and mannitol, were given orally 30 minutes before and 120 after test injections. Intestinal permeability was quantitated using the 12-hour urinary excretion of these substances.

Systemic absorption and excretion of lactulose increased by almost twofold after endotoxin was administered. Changes in mannitol absorption and excretion after endotoxin injection were similar but less significant. When individual 12-hour lactulose excretions were related to the magnitude of systemic response, there was a significant association between lactulose excretion and elaboration of norepinephrine and between lactulose excretion and the minimum white blood cell count.

Increased permeability develops in individuals with a normal gastrointestinal tract after exposure to a bacterial toxin. Intestinal permeability changes can occur within hours of exposure to a provocative stimulus. These findings support the hypothesis that, in critically ill patients, prolonged or repeated exposure to systemic endotoxins or cytokines can significantly compromise the gastrointestinal tract mucosal barrier.

▶ This interesting article is following the emerging trend toward the concept that, after endotoxin exposure, there is an alteration in bowel function permitting translocation of either mediators, bacteria, or, as in the study here, permeability markers such as lactulose and mannitol. The permeability markers were given orally before and after these otherwise normal volunteers were challenged with an intravenous *E. coli* endotoxin. Intestinal permeability to these tracers was measured by the 12-hour urinary excretion of the substances after the endotoxin challenge. These data suggest that a brief exposure to circulating endotoxin increased by permeability of normal bowel.

These observations are consistent with the hypothesis that during critical illness and exposure to systemic endotoxin, or associated cytokines, there may well be a compromise in the integrity of the gastrointestinal mucosal barrier.— G.T. Shires, M.D.

Post-Traumatic Changes in, and Effect of Colloid Osmotic Pressure on the Distribution of Body Water
Böck JC, Barker BC, Clinton AG, Wilson MB, Lewis FR (Univ of California, San Francisco; San Francisco Gen Hosp)
Ann Surg 210:395–405, September 1989   2–2

To define the time course of posttraumatic changes in body water distribution and to assess the role of plasma colloid osmotic pressure in the partitioning of extracellular body water between the intracellular and interstitial fluid spaces, 8 severely injured patients and 2 with surgical sepsis, as well as 8 controls, were examined. Plasma volume was estimated using indocyanine green dye, extracellular volume was estimated using bromine, and total body water was estimated using deuterium.

Colloid osmotic pressures ranged from 10 mm Hg to 30 mm Hg in these patients. The interstitial volume was increased by 55% compared with controls, whereas intracellular volume decreased by 10%. Both intracellular and interstitial space volumes tended to decline over time, but not to a significant degree, and blood volume remained constant.

Posttraumatic peripheral edema secondary to hemodilution is located in the interstitial compartment. Interstitial, but not intracellular, volume is closely related to plasma colloid osmotic pressure. Body water distribution can be assessed reproducibly in the clinical setting using nonradioactive markers.

▶ These authors used a combination of nonradioactive tracers to measure body fluid distributions in the time period considerably following shock or the traumatic event. In this setting the increase in interstitial volume is expected after the necessary initial resuscitative efforts. Certainly, the use of slowly equilibrating and stable ions such as bromide are useful in this setting, which is not attempting to describe the initial complex interrelationship between cell water and interstitial water. The finding that in this posttraumatic stable state the interstitial volume is more responsive to plasma colloid osmotic pressure is also a fairly predictable result.

I think the major points to understand in this paper, as were expressed by the discussants at the time the paper was presented, relate to the time the patients were studied, which was well beyond the occurrence of acute cellular changes. It also is to be noted that patients who had normal diuresis of the initial loading fluid for resuscitation were removed from the study, so that those who remained were the ones who persistently required intensive care unit care, such as those with sepsis. In addition, it should be pointed out that these studies included patients receiving packed red blood cells rather than whole blood; thus, in this case, even the several-day posttraumatic measurements will be reflective of more volume replacement without colloid than would be seen if whole blood had been used. With these caveats, these are certainly elegant baseline studies.—G.T. Shires, M.D.

The Effects of Hypoproteinemia and Volume Expansion on Lung and Soft Tissue Transvascular Fluid Filtration
Harms BA, Pahl AC, Radosevich DG, Starling JR (Univ of Washington, William S Middleton Mem VA Hosp, Madison, Wis)
Surgery 105:605–614, May 1989   2–3

Protein depletion and plasma volume expansion frequently occur during resuscitation from major trauma and surgery if major blood loss takes place. Hypoproteinemia by itself is a major factor in lung and soft tissue edema. Changes in lung and soft tissue fluid filtration and protein transport were quantified in sheep in the normal and protein-depleted states. Lymph flow rates were estimated in animals with chronic lung and soft tissue lymph fistulas. Ringer's lactate or fresh frozen plasma was administered after plasmapheresis-induced protein depletion of 30% to 35%.

Volume expansion with plasma limited the increase in soft tissue lymph flow compared with expansion with Ringer's lactate. There was, however, no apparent advantage to plasma in limiting lung lymph flow.

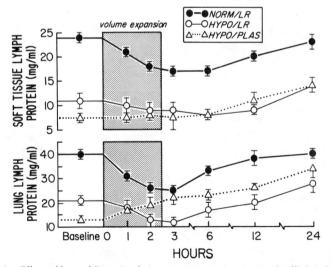

Fig 2–1.—Effects of lactated Ringer's solution on normoproteinemic animals *(filled circles)*, of lactated Ringer's solution after plasmapheresis-induced protein depletion *(open circles)*, and of fresh frozen plasma after protein depletion *(open triangles)* on volume expansions of lung and soft tissue lymph protein concentrations. (Courtesy of Harms BA, Pahl AC, Radosevich DG, et al: *Surgery* 105:605–614, May 1989.)

During plasma infusion protein transport into the interstitium of soft tissue, but not lung, was delayed by 10–12 hours. Significant widening of the oncotic gradient in soft tissue resulted. The effects of various volume expansion regimens on protein levels in lung and soft tissue are shown in Figure 2–1.

Plasma protein infusion was not superior to Ringer's lactate in limiting pulmonary transvascular fluid filtration. It was, however, helpful in limiting soft tissue edema because of delayed protein transport to the soft tissue interstitium.

▶ This interesting experimental study in sheep examined the effects of protein depletion and plasma volume expansion that commonly occur during resuscitation after multisystem trauma and major operative procedures in which blood loss occurs. The specific question addressed was what happens to lung lymph flow and the development of pulmonary edema after resuscitation. The study showed that, insofar as limiting pulmonary transvascular fluid filtration, the outcome of volume expansion was not different whether lactated Ringer's infusion or plasma protein infusion was given. This occurred in this experimental study because prompt transport of protein into the pulmonary interstitial space restored deficits, limited significant widening of the oncotic gradient, and corrected any increase in plasma of lymph fluid conductivity produced by protein dilution or depletion.

This study once again indicates that the pulmonary response to trauma, shock, and resuscitation does not follow the predictable Starling equations insofar as reduction in colloid osmotic pressure is concerned, probably because of the movement of protein across the capillary membrane.—G.T. Shires, M.D.

Hypertonic Saline Fluid Therapy Following Surgery: A Prospective Study
Cross JS, Gruber DP, Burchard KW, Singh AK, Moran JM, Gann DS (Brown Univ; Rhode Island Hosp, Providence)
J Trauma 29:817–826, June 1989   2–4

Successfully resuscitating injured patients may be done faster and with less fluid using hypertonic crystalloid solutions than isotonic solutions. A randomized, double-blind study was done to compare 0.9% normal saline with 1.8% hypertonic saline in 20 postoperative coronary artery bypass patients with uniform injury.

Solutions were administered to maintain the physiologic end points of heart rate, blood pressure, and pulmonary capillary wedge pressure. Patients given hypertonic saline needed 30% less fluid than patients given normal saline and were in negative fluid balance during the study period. Patients given normal saline were in positive fluid balance after 8 hours and required more chest tube drainage than the other group. The 2 groups were similar with regard to systemic and pulmonary hemodynamic measures, oxygen delivery, oxygen consumption, and shunt fraction. The serum level of sodium and osmolality rose in patients given hypertonic saline, peaking at 12 hours, and were correlated with the volume of hypertonic saline given. None of the patients died, and no complication was attributed to the hypertonicity of the solution.

Hypertonic saline, 1.8%, is a safe alternative to isotonic crystalloid treatment in the fluid management of patients after surgery. Reduced third-space losses might occur with hypertonic saline, as suggested by the lower thoracic losses observed in patients given this fluid. When excess free water administration is not desired, and when interstitial edema is detrimental to function or survival, 1.8% sodium chloride may be preferred.

▶ This study was done in patients immediately after coronary artery bypass to compare the use of a smaller volume of hypertonic saline with the usual volume of normal saline. The 2 groups were similar in systemic and pulmonary hemodynamic measures, oxygen delivery, oxygen consumption, and shunt fraction. The significant difference between them was that less fluid was used in the group given hypertonic saline and that serum sodium and osmolality rose; in fact, the concentration of sodium had to be reduced in a third of the patients.

This study is not dissimilar to the study of Monafo et al. (1) in burn patients. That is, hypertonic saline can produce satisfactory resuscitation if extremely careful monitoring is done. All investigators working in this area agree that the hyperosmolality produced by hypertonic saline can be quite dangerous and even result in brain damage. Consequently, the widespread use of these hypertonic solutions, whether in burn patients or in postoperative patients, is probably not at the present time of any significant benefit. In fact, the potential hazards outweigh the benefits, in my opinion.—G.T. Shires, M.D.

Reference

1. Monafo WW, et al: *Surgery* 95:129, 1984.

Exercise-Mediated Peripheral Tissue and Whole-Body Amino Acid Metabolism During Intravenous Feeding in Normal Man

Albert JD, Matthews DE, Legaspi A, Tracey KJ, Jeevanandam M, Brennan MF, Lowry SF (New York Hosp–Cornell Med Ctr; Mem Sloan-Kettering Cancer Ctr, New York)
Clin Sci 77:113–120, July 1989   2–5

Preserving or restoring a patient's nutritional status during hospitalization after injury or surgery is crucial. The effect of a daily submaximal exercise regimen on whole-body and peripheral tissue amino acid metabolism during weight-stable intravenous feeding (IVF) was examined in 11 healthy volunteers. Five performed 1 hour of daily bicycle exercise at 75 W during IVF; the other 6 did not exercise during IVF and served as controls. Body nitrogen balance, leg and forearm plasma amino acid flux, and whole-body kinetics were determined before and 10 days after IFV.

At the end of IVF the exercising group had leg uptake of total amino acids significantly different from that in the control group. In the nonexercised forearm of the exercising volunteers, the total amino acid flux was significantly lower than in that of controls on the tenth day of IVF. Efflux of 3-methylhistidine was significantly lower in legs of the exercising group than in the legs of nonexercisers. Intravenous feeding increased whole-body leucine turnover in both groups, but only the exercising group had a significant rise in leucine oxidation, which was proportionate to a rise in muscle uptake of leucine. Whole-body protein breakdown also was significantly reduced in the exercising volunteers compared with nonexercising volunteers during IVF.

Daily submaximal exercise appears to function as a relative anticatabolic stimulus both locally and systemically. The local effects of this exercise during IVF were shown by the significantly increased uptake of total amino acids and reduced 3-methylhistidine efflux from the leg in the exercising group. The systemic effect of exercise was reflected in increased essential amino acid uptake and decreased alanine and glutamine efflux from the forearm, increased whole-body nitrogen retention, and decreased rates of whole-body protein breakdown.

▶ This interesting study attempted to answer the question of whether enhancing a patient's nutritional status during hospitalization after injury or surgery is possible. The study specifically examined the effect of a daily submaximal exercise regimen on whole-body and peripheral tissue amino acid metabolism during weight-stable intravenous feeding. The data demonstrate clearly that a daily submaximal exercise period produced systemic as well as limb-specific enhancement of amino acid balance in muscle providing an anticatabolic response under conditions of partial immobility induced by hospitalization. One can probably easily translate this into beneficial effects of submaximal exercise on patients who are immobilized by hospitalization.— G.T. Shires, M.D.

Addition of Glutamine to Total Parenteral Nutrition After Elective Abdominal Surgery Spares Free Glutamine in Muscle, Counteracts the Fall in Muscle Protein Synthesis, and Improves Nitrogen Balance
Hammarqvist F, Wernerman J, Ali R, von der Decken A, Vinnars E (St Göran's Hosp; Huddinge Univ Hosp; Wenner-Gren Inst for Experimental Biology; Univ of Stockholm)
Ann Surg 209:455–461, April 1989   2–6

Commercially available amino acid solutions for intravenous nutrition do not contain glutamine because it is not an essential amino acid. However, glutamine is central to the metabolism of free amino acids. In patients who have had elective abdominal surgery the protein synthesis in skeletal muscle is reduced, whether or not postoperative total parenteral nutrition (TPN) is given. Glutamine-supplemented TPN was given to patients after elective abdominal surgery to determine whether it would be beneficial.

Twenty-two patients were given either TPN with a conventional amino

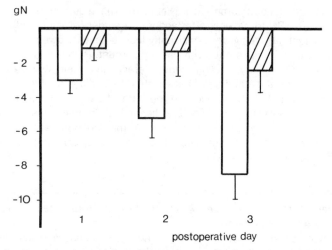

Fig 2–2.—Cumulative nitrogen balance during 3 days immediately after elective abdominal surgery. After the operation the patients received conventional TPN (n = 13, *open bars*) or TPN supplemented with glutamine (n = 9, *hatched bars*). On each day the cumulative nitrogen balance was negative in the control group ($P < .01$), whereas it was not significantly different from zero on any day in the glutamine-supplemented group. On the third postoperative day the cumulative nitrogen balance was significantly improved in the glutamine-supplemented group as compared with the control group ($P < .01$). Values are given as means ± SEM. (Courtesy of Hammarqvist F, Wernerman J, Ali R, et al: *Ann Surg* 209:455–461, April 1989.)

acid solution supplemented with glutamine or with a conventional amino acid solution without supplementation. Muscle biopsy specimens were obtained before surgery and 3 days afterward. The postoperative reduction in the intracellular concentration of free glutamine was less pronounced in the glutamine-treated group than in the controls. The concentration and size distribution of ribosomes indicated the protein synthesis. There were no significant differences in these parameters after surgery in the patients given the glutamine supplement. However, in the control group the total concentration of ribosomes dropped by 27.2% and the relative proportion of polyribosomes dropped by 10.6%. Although these changes in the control group were significant, the differences in these parameters between the control group and the experimental group were not. The cumulative nitrogen loss was significantly less in patients given the glutamine supplement than in those not given the supplement (Fig 2–2).

This glutamine-supplemented amino acid solution incorporated into TPN after elective surgery was beneficial. The intracellular free glutamine concentration in skeletal muscle improved significantly. Patients given the supplement had a less pronounced decrease in muscle protein synthesis. The administration of glutamine to catabolic patients is recommended.

▶ This is an interesting approach to augmentation of intravenous nutrition with glutamine. As the authors point out, glutamine, which is a primary nitrogen donor in muscle synthesis of protein, is not an essential amino acid and, consequently, is not added to commercial TPN fluids. These authors gave glutamine-supplemented TPN to patients after abdominal surgery. They found that accumulative nitrogen losses were significantly less in patients given the glutamine supplement than in those not given the supplement. In these patients sustaining relatively minor injury, no significant difference in protein synthesis was observed. However, the authors still believe that the addition of glutamine to TPN after surgery was beneficial, because the intracellular free glutamine concentration in skeletal muscle improved significantly. There was a less pronounced decrease in muscle protein synthesis even in this group of patients. This may well become a necessary standard for parenteral replacement of nutritional components.—G.T. Shires, M.D.

Total Parenteral Nutrition and Alternate Energy Substrates in Treatment of Severe Acute Pancreatitis
Sitzmann JV, Steinborn PA, Zinner MJ, Cameron JL (Johns Hopkins Med Insts)
Surg Gynecol Obstet 168:311–317, April 1989   2–7

Of 327 adults treated for acute pancreatitis in a 2-year period, 73 were given total parenteral nutrition (TPN). These patients were unable to take oral nutrition for at least 2 weeks, had lost weight, and had a total lymphocyte count of less than 1,500 and an albumin level of less than 3.5 mg/dL. Forty-four patients primarily received glucose and were given biweekly Intralipid infusions. Twenty patients with severe glucose intolerance received fat as their major calorie source. Nine patients received no lipid emulsion because of preexisting hyperlipidemia.

Total parenteral nutrition was initiated an average of 6 days after admission. Improvement was comparable in all groups, although more glucose recipients had improved nutritional indices. The average time of TPN was 29 days. Patients received an average of 2,487 kcal daily. Pancreatitis did not become worse in patients receiving Intralipid. No patient experienced hyperosmolar metabolic coma. The overall mortality rate was 11%; mortality was higher in patients who could not receive fat and in those with negative nitrogen balance.

Patients with severe acute pancreatitis generally are malnourished, and TPN effectively reverses the malnutrition. Lipid is well tolerated by glucose-intolerant patients and is the only calorie substrate available to meet energy needs.

▶ This interesting study of a large series of patients with acute pancreatitis examined the question of nitrogen balance and caloric intake source in such patients. It is clear from the results that TEN improved nutritional indices in the majority of patients in whom it was used. Further arms of the study showed that either lipid- or glucose-based TPN is a safe and effective therapy to reverse the malnutrition associated with acute pancreatitis. Furthermore, the results showed the striking finding of a tenfold increase in mortality in patients who did not achieve a positive nitrogen balance. This study tends to resolve the previous suggestions that TPN is not cost effective in the treatment of acute pancreatitis.—G.T. Shires, M.D.

Gallbladder Response to Enteral Lipids in Injured Patients
Merrell RC, Miller-Crotchett P, Lowry P (Univ of Texas, Houston)
Arch Surg 124:301–302, March 1989   2–8

Severe injury can be complicated by gallbladder stasis ranging from sludge formation and cystic duct occlusion by inspissation to acalculous cholecystitis. The effect of enteral lipids on the ability of the gallbladder to clear itself was studied in a double-blind, randomized trial.

Twelve injured patients aged 20–65 years were randomly assigned to receive either 40 mL of safflower oil or water. Gallbladders were assessed by ultrasonography for acute contractions, sludge, and dilation on the first, third, and seventh days after injury. There were no significant differences between the 2 groups. Both had modest enlargement of the gallbladder and contraction failure. The mean total bilirubin level was increased by day 7 in all patients.

In this population at risk for biliary complications, safflower oil appeared to have no impact on biliary dimensions. It is possible that, as a consequence of bowel edema and motility changes, there is no stimulation or cholecystokinin released by the enteral lipid. In severe injury the gallbladder may not be particularly responsive to circulating cholecystokinin. In either case, enteral lipid is ineffective for reflexive evacuation of the gallbladder in this patient population.

▶ This interesting study attempted to evaluate gallbladder stasis developing after trauma. All trauma surgeons recognize that acute acalculous cholecystitis is a significant problem following significant injury. The authors looked at the effect of enteric lipid on the ability of the gallbladder to clear itself and thereby reverse the stasis leading to acalculous cholecystitis. The fact that the gallbladders in these patients did not contract or respond to safflower oil confirms the previous suggestion by others that there is no stimulation by cholecystokinin released in response to the enteral lipid. It would appear that in severe injury the gallbladder may not be particularly responsive to circulating cholecystokinin, but, in any event, enteral lipid was ineffective for reflex evacuation of the gallbladder in this patient population.—G.T. Shires, M.D.

Total Parenteral Nutrition and Bowel Rest Modify the Metabolic Response to Endotoxin in Humans
Fong Y, Marano MA, Barber A, He W, Moldawer LL, Bushman ED, Coyle SM, Shires GT, Lowry SF (New York Hosp–Cornell Med Ctr, New York)
Ann Surg 210:449–457, October 1989   2–9

Intestinal mucosal atrophy secondary to total parenteral nutrition (TPN) or prolonged bowel rest might enhance the translocation of bowel endotoxin and alter host responses to infection. Twelve healthy persons received either enteral feedings or 1 week of TPN without oral intake. Metabolic tests were carried out during dextrose infusion starting 12 hours after the last feeding and continuing for 6 hours after an intravenous challenge with *Escherichia coli* lipopolysaccharide, 20 units per kg.

Body weight was maintained with the TPN. The pyrogenic response to endotoxin challenge was greater with TPN, as was the heart rate response. The mean blood pressure did not change significantly with either TPN or enteral feedings. Peak epinephrine and glucagon responses were significantly greater with TPN, and circulating levels of cachectin/tumor necrosis factor were higher than in the enterally fed participants. Peripheral lactate production was significantly increased in persons receiving TPN. Hypoaminoacidemia was noted in both groups. Levels of C-reactive protein were higher in persons receiving TPN than in those fed enterally.

It appears that bowel rest leads to changes in host resistance to injury independent of malnutrition. It seems clear that the route of feeding does affect injury and disease. Total parenteral nutrition can lead to an exaggerated counterregulatory hormone response and an enhanced systemic and splanchnic production of cytokines.

▶ This study examined the enhancement of bowel endotoxin translocation after TPN or enteral nutrition in healthy volunteers maintained for 1 week on weight-stable parenteral or enteric feedings. After administration of safe, national reference standard *E. coli* lipopolysaccharide, striking elevations of cachectin occurred in hepatic vein samples as well as in peripheral arterial samples. The peak responses were significantly higher in the group given TPN, as were C-reactive protein levels and the counterregulatory hormone levels. In the TPN group, then, after endotoxin challenge, a magnified acute-phase response, peripheral amino acid mobilization, and peripheral lactate production were noted. It may well be, therefore, that with prolonged bowel rest endotoxin translocation may alter host responses to infection.—G.T. Shires, M.D.

TEN Versus TPN Following Major Abdominal Trauma: Reduced Septic Morbidity
Moore FA, Moore EE, Jones TN, McCroskey BL, Peterson VM (Denver Gen Hosp; Univ of Colorado)
J Trauma 29:916–923, July 1989   2–10

Nutritional support of seriously injured patients is an important part of critical care. Recent research with animals suggests that total enteral feeding (TEN) is better than total parenteral nutrition (TPN) at improving resistance to infection. The effects of early TEN and TPN were compared in critically injured patients.

Seventy-five patients with abdominal trauma indices between 15 and 40 were randomly assigned at initial laparotomy to either a TEN or a TPN group. All feedings contained 2.5% fat, 33% branched chain amino

---

Nutritional Data From TEN vs. TPN Study Groups After Major
Abdominal Trauma

	TEN (n = 29)	TPN (n = 30)	p value
Caloric intake*			
Day 1	150 ± 15	180 ± 25	NS
Day 5	1,847 ± 123	2,261 ± 60	0.01
Nitrogen intake (gm)*			
Day 1	1.1 ± 0.1	1.2 ± 0.2	NS
Day 5	12.4 ± 0.8	15.4 ± 0.4	0.01
Nitrogen balance (gm)*			
Day 1	−11.5 ± 0.8	−12.2 ± 0.9	NS
Day 5	−0.3 ± 1.0	0.1 ± 0.8	NS

*Mean ± SEM; NS, not significant; caloric intake = nonprotein calories.
(Courtesy of Moore FA, Moore EE, Jones TN, et al: *J Trauma* 29:916–923, July 1989.)

---

acids, and a calorie-to-nitrogen ratio of 150:1. Total enteral nutrition was given through a needle catheter jejunostomy. Feedings were begun within 12 hours of surgery in both groups and were infused at a rate that achieved positive nitrogen balances. Eighty-six percent of the patients in the TEN group tolerated the jejunal feedings unconditionally. The nitrogen balance remained comparable throughout the study (table). The traditional markers of nutritional protein—albumin, transferrin, and retinol binding protein—were better restored in patients given TEN feedings. Infections developed in 17% of the TEN group and in 37% of the TPN group. Major septic morbidity occurred in 3% of the TEN group and in 20% of the TPN group.

Total enteral nutrition is significantly better than TPN feedings in reducing major septic complications in critically injured patients. It was also well tolerated in this population.

▶ This interesting clinical study revealed that TEN was far preferable to TPN in terms of the prevention of subsequent infection in sepsis. Both types of nutrition were given by needle catheter jejunostomy or via a central venous catheter, and nitrogen balance was maintained in both groups. The traditional markers of protein-bound albumin transparent in retinol-binding protein were better restored in patients given TEN. This study indicates that TEN was superior to TPN in reducing major septic complications in critically ill patients. Furthermore, TEN was well tolerated when given as feeding by jejunostomy needle catheterization.—G.T. Shires, M.D.

3 Shock

Platelet-Activating Factor: An Endogenous Mediator of Mesenteric Isch-emia-Reperfusion-Induced Shock
Mózes T, Braquet P, Filep J (Semmelweis Univ Med School, Budapest; Inst Henri Beaufour, Le Plessis Robinson, France)
Am J Physiol 257:R872–R877, October 1989   3–1

Current understanding of the role of platelet-activating factor (PAF), a novel mediator of inflammation and tissue injury in shock states, is based on studies showing that systemic administration of exogenous PAF to animals produced severe hypotension, shock, and death. Local concentrations of PAF at critical sites in shock are still unknown.

To determine whether PAF is released from the ischemic intestine during superior mesenteric artery occlusion (SMAO)-induced shock, and whether exogenous PAF mimics SMAO-shock, PAF levels in the superior mesenteric vein were measured in anesthetized dogs during reperfusion after 2-hour occlusion of the superior mesenteric artery. The effects of BN 52021, a specific PAF receptor antagonist, and the circulatory effects of exogenous PAF injected into the superior mesenteric vein also were assessed.

Removing the superior mesenteric artery occlusion produced an immediate dramatic reduction in mean arterial blood pressure with concomitant increases in mean portal venous pressure and hematocrit values. The PAF concentration in the superior mesenteric vein rose from 0.2 mg/mL to 2.8 ng/mL in the first 5 minutes of reperfusion. Injecting PAF, 0.1 µg/kg, into the superior mesenteric vein caused similar hemodynamic effects.

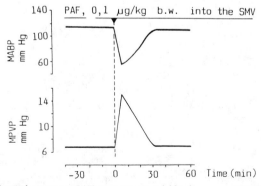

Fig 3–1.—Effects of exogenous PAF on mean arterial blood pressure (MABP) and mean portal venous pressure (MPVP). Platelet-activating factor (0.1 µg/kg) was injected over 1 minute into the superior mesenteric vein (SMV). Traces are representative for 4 experiments. (Courtesy of Mózes T, Braquet P, Filep J: *Am J Physiol* 257:R872–R877, October 1989.)

Pretreating the dogs with BN 52021, 4 mg/kg, prevented circulatory collapse (Fig 3–1).

There is evidence to support a role for PAF in the early phase of mesenteric ischemia-reperfusion-induced circulatory collapse. Platelet-activating factor concentrations were increased in the superior mesenteric vein during reperfusion. Also, BN 52021 treatment prevented almost all of the changes in the hemodynamic parameters and laboratory values that occurred after clamp removal. Exogenous PAF administration into the superior mesenteric vein mimicked most of the hemodynamic changes noted in SMAO-induced shock.

▶ This is another in the increasing number of articles indicating that PAF is a potent endogenous mediator of shock. In this particular experiment shock was induced by mesenteric ischemia and reperfusion. The study is interesting in that the bioactivity of a (PAF-like substance was actually measured using chromatography. This bioactivity was markedly increased after release of a superior mesenteric artery clamp. To obtain further proof, the authors administered PAF systemically. They showed that the animals experienced severe hypotension, shock, and death from PAF injection. In addition, a PAF antagonist, BN 52021, was given to prevent the circulatory effects of exogenous PAF injected into the superior mesenteric vein. Pretreatment with BN 52021 prevented the hemodynamic effects of PAF.

It is becoming increasingly clear that PAF is also a very proximal mediator in many forms of shock. Whether it is the proximal mediator or whether it is turned on endogenously primarily by cachectin as the prime mediator is yet to be determined.—G.T. Shires, M.D.

Promotion and Subsequent Inhibition of Plasminogen Activation After Administration of Intravenous Endotoxin to Normal Subjects
Suffredini AF, Harpel PC, Parrillo JE (Clinical Ctr, NIH, Bethesda, Md; New York Hosp-Cornell Med Ctr)
N Engl J Med 320:1165–1172, May 4, 1989   3–2

Sepsis with severe progressive failure of multiple organ systems is a common cause of death among patients in intensive care units. There is controversy over the role of endotoxin in the initiation of septic shock and subsequent multiple organ failure. Previous studies have suggested that, in seriously ill patients, endotoxin interferes with the fibrinolytic system. The effect of endotoxin on the fibrinolytic system was studied in healthy volunteers.

Escherichia coli endotoxin was administered intravenously to 13 men and 6 women aged 23–38 years. As part of another trial, 10 subjects also underwent pulmonary artery catheterization and 9 had bronchoscopy with bronchoalveolar lavage. Fibrinolytic proteins, protease inhibitors, neutrophil elastase, and von Willebrand factor were measured in serial blood samples collected during a 24-hour study period. All subjects were admitted to the intensive care unit.

One hour after endotoxin administration the tissue plasminogen activator (t-PA) antigen concentration increased from 10 ng/mL to 23 ng/mL, peaking at 52 ng/mL after 3 hours. The level of α-2-plasmin inhibitor-plasmin complexes increased by sevenfold, peaking at 3 hours. The plasminogen activator inhibitor-1 concentration increased more slowly, from 7 units per mL at baseline to a maximum of 49 units per mL at 5 hours. Neutrophil elastase and von Willebrand antigen levels were unchanged at 1 hour, increased by about threefold by 3 hours, and remained elevated at 24 hours. In a control group of 5 subjects given saline solution instead of endotoxin intravenously, no changes were observed in the base levels of the measured parameters. The functional activity of t-PA, measured in 4 subjects, increased rapidly from 1.2 ng/mL at baseline to 8.3 ng/mL at 1 hour to 13.9 ng/mL at 2 hours. At 3 hours, t-PA levels began to fall, reaching baseline values again at 24 hours.

In healthy subjects endotoxin activates the fibrinolytic system, starting with the release of t-PA in the blood within 1 hour and accompanied by plasmin generation. Early activation of the fibrinolytic system during endotoxemia may serve to prevent the initiation of microvascular thrombosis. The increased fibrinolysis is subsequently offset by the compensatory release of plasminogen activator inhibitory factors.

▶ This is another of the articles exploring the mediators and their tissue activation mechanisms in producing changes in response to endotoxin. In this study the specific target was plasminogen activation after administration of intravenous endotoxin to normal subjects. One hour after E. coli endotoxin administration, the t-PA antigen concentration more than doubled, peaking after 3 hours of administration. Subsequently, the plasminogen activator inhibitor complexes increased by sevenfold. It appears therefore, that endotoxin activates the fibrinolytic system, starting with the release of t-PA in the blood within 1 hour, accompanied by plasmin generation. Early activation of the fibrinolytic system during endotoxemia may serve to prevent the initiation of microvascular thrombosis. Although not discussed by these authors, it would appear that this sequence of events may well be initiated by mediators that are proximal but are turned on by the administration of endotoxin.—G.T. Shires, M.D.

Significance of Lipid Mediators in Shock States
Lefer AM (Thomas Jefferson Univ)
Circ Shock 27:3–12, 1989   3–3

Derivatives of fatty acids and phospholipids seem to be important mediators of a significant part of the pathophysiology of circulatory shock. The significance of lipid mediators in shock states was reviewed.

Evidence suggests that a variety of lipid mediators have an important role in the pathogenesis of different types of circulatory shock, including hemorrhagic, endotoxic, bowel ischemic, and traumatic. Thromboxane A_2, several leukotrienes, and platelet-activating factor (PAF) are mediators of shock. These substances produce significant pathophysiologic effects that mimic facets of the shock state, occur in biologic fluids of animals in shock states, and can be blocked by appropriate synthesis inhibitors or receptor antagonists that ameliorate shock. All of these lipid mediators also have a common chemical reaction to arachidonic acid. They can interact with one another and with other nonlipid shock mediators. Tumor necrosis factor is an important activator of lipid mediators, and PAF is an important focal distributor of eicosanoids. There appears to be a network of mediators interrelated in many complex ways.

Lipid mediators are potent substances having a variety of important biologic effects that contribute to cellular injury. Preventing the formation of these lipids by synthesis inhibitors, or blocking their action through specific receptor antagonism, improves shock states. Using sensitive chemical and immunologic detection techniques, researchers have identified greater amounts of these lipid mediators in body fluids during shock. Several lipid mediators are linked to the activation of other lipid and nonlipid mediators in a way that amplifies the actions of lipid mediators.

▶ This is a review article on shock research and discusses the significance of lipid mediators in shock states. The authors point out that derivatives of fatty acids and phospholipids are important mediators of a significant part, if not all, of the pathophysiology of various forms of shock. The types of shock studied were circulatory shock, including hemorrhagic, endotoxic, bowel ischemic, and post traumatic. Thromboxane A_2, several leukotrienes, and PAF are mediators of shock, as shown by a number of investigators. All of these substances produce significant pathophysiologic effects that mimic the shock state, occur in biologic fluids of animals, and, in some instances, man in shock states; they can be blocked by appropriate synthesis inhibitors or receptor antagonists. Furthermore, there is increasing evidence that these mediators can interact with one another as well as with other nonlipid shock mediators. Tumor necrosis factor (cachectin) is an important activator of lipid mediators, and it appears that PAF is an important focal distributor of eicosanoids.—G.T. Shires, M.D.

Effect of Morphine on the Hemodynamic and Neuroendocrine Responses to Hemorrhage in Conscious Rats
Feuerstein G, Sirén A-L, Goldstein DS, Johnson AK, Zerbe RL (Uniformed Services Univ of the Health Sciences; Natl Heart, Lung, and Blood Inst, Bethesda, Md; Univ of Iowa; Lilly Research Lab, Indianapolis)
Circ Shock 27:219–235, 1989   3–4

Activation of the endogenous opioid system is commonly believed to play a detrimental role in cardiorespiratory recovery after bleeding. If opioid-mediated cardiovascular depression is an important detrimental mechanism, administration of opiates to patients in cardiovascular shock would further compromise vital functions, aggravate the shock, and result in higher mortality. Analgesic doses of morphine accelerate the mortality of rats exposed to bleeding. The mechanisms involved in this phenomenon were studied.

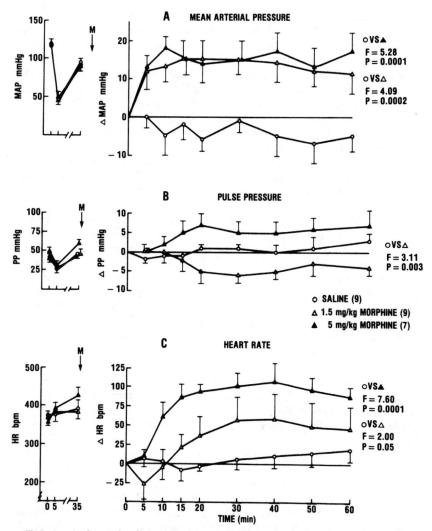

Fig 3–2.—Cardiovascular effects of morphine injected 30 minutes after hemorrhage (8.5 mL/300 g/5 min) in the conscious rat: mean arterial pressure (**A**), pulse pressure (**B**), and heart rate (**C**). The effect of bleeding is indicated in the lefthand panels. Bleeding was started at T_0 and completed at T_5. Time of intra-arterial morphine injection is given as ↓ M. *Vertical bars* indicate SEM. Number of rats in each group is given in parentheses. The statistical difference between morphine-treated and control groups was evaluated by analysis of variance with repeated measures, and F and P values for the variables are given in the figure. (Courtesy of Feuerstein G, Sirén A-L, Goldstein DS, et al: *Circ Shock* 27:219–235, 1989.)

Rats, chronically implanted with catheters in the femoral vessels, were given morphine, 1.5 mg/kg or 5 mg/kg, 30 minutes or 24 hours after hemorrhage. Arterial blood pressure and heart rate were monitored continuously. Rats chronically equipped with a minithermistor for cardiac output monitoring also were given morphine, 5 mg/kg.

Morphine given 30 minutes after bleeding produced a pressor response and tachycardia, in marked contrast to its depressor effect in intact rats. Morphine increased plasma renin activity and epinephrine but not vasopressin. Blood pH and gases showed no consistent change. Morphine administered after bleeding led to enhanced cardiac depression in response to a second hemorrhage of 2 mL/3000 g (Fig 3–2).

These findings confirm and extend previous findings showing depressor and bradycardic responses to morphine in rats. This study also found a still undocumented effect of morphine—a strong pressor response produced by an otherwise depressor dose of morphine in rats exposed to hypovolemic hypotension. Activation of pressor mechanisms by morphine during hypovolemic hypotension may enhance vasoconstriction in essential organs, depress cardiac function, and decrease effective tissue perfusion.

▶ These authors reported previously that analgesic doses of morphine accelerate the mortality of rats exposed to hemorrhage. The current study investigated the potential mechanisms involved in this phenomenon. Many variables were measured, including cardiac output, plasma catecholamines, and renin and vasopressin activity, as well as pH and blood gases. Interestingly, morphine administration produced a pressor response and tachycardia that were in marked contrast to its depressor effect in intact rats. These data suggest that activation of pressor mechanisms by morphine during hypovolemic hypotension might enhance vasoconstriction in essential organs, depress cardiac output, and therefore markedly reduce effective tissue perfusion.—G.T. Shires, M.D.

Prospective, Controlled, Randomized Trial of Naloxone Infusion in Early Hyperdynamic Septic Shock
Safani M, Blair J, Ross D, Waki R, Li C, Libby G (Mem Med Ctr of Long Beach, Calif)
Crit Care Med 17:1004–1009, October 1989   3–5

Naloxone reverses the hypotension of endotoxic shock in rats in a time- and dose-dependent fashion, but a beneficial effect in humans with late septic shock has not been found. To determine whether naloxone infusion is effective in patients with severe hyperdynamic septic shock, 22 patients were randomly assigned to receive naloxone or placebo. Treatment was begun at a mean of 12 hours after onset of shock. The mean arterial pressure was 63 mm Hg. All 22 patients had clinical evidence of an infectious process and were given dopamine.

Five of the 11 patients (46%) in the naloxone-treated group and 1 of the 11 patients (9%) in the placebo group had clinical responses. The mean arterial pressure in the responders rose from 62 mm Hg to 89 mm Hg within 20 minutes of naloxone treatment and was sustained throughout the clinical course. The mean arterial pressure did not significantly change in patients with no response to naloxone or in patients given placebo. Although the survival rate among treatment responders was 100%, overall survival in all groups was essentially the same. Naloxone produced no adverse effects except for mild agitation in some cases.

Naloxone infusion is clinically effective in some patients with severe early hyperdynamic septic shock. Almost half of the patients treated in this study had improved hemodynamic profiles. However, naloxone treatment does not appear to increase the overall survival rate.

▶ This is another of the many studies attempting to sort out the effects of naloxone as an antiendorphin in the setting of hyperdynamic septic shock. In this clinical study evaluating the use of naloxone in patients in septic shock, almost half of those treated had an arterial pressure response to treatment that was sustained throughout the course. The overall survival rate in these patients was not increased. No adverse effects were noted, but treatment with naloxone appeared to be ineffectual in improving survival in human septic shock. However, variations in time of administration and dose of naloxone should be studied continually because there is some evidence of at least a pharmacologic response to the drug in the septic shock patient.—G.T. Shires, M.D.

Triiodothyronine (T_3) Antagonizes Adverse Effects of High Circulating Reverse-T_3 (rT_3) During Hemorrhagic Shock
Yuan X-Q, Shatney CH, Dewitt DS, Prough DS, Smith RA (Wake Forest Univ; Stanford Univ; Mem Med Ctr, Jacksonville, Fla)
Am Surg 54:720–725, December 1988   3–6

Critical illness, including shock, is often accompanied by the euthyroid sick, or "low T_3," syndrome. Levels of reverse triiodothyronine (rT_3) rise and appear to affect outcome adversely after major blood loss. By contrast, T_3 improves hemodynamic variables and survival.

To determine whether T_3 can counteract the lethal effect of exogenous rT_3 in hemorrhagic shock, 21 anesthetized, heparinized dogs were given rT_3, 15 μg/kg intravenously. Thirty minutes later the dogs were rapidly bled. A mean arterial pressure of 40 mm Hg was achieved and maintained. After 60 minutes at this pressure to simulate compensated shock, the reservoir line was clamped for 30 minutes to simulate uncompensated shock. Blood was reinfused for 30 minutes. The dogs were monitored for another 60 minutes. At the beginning of uncompensated shock, 11 dogs were given 11 μg/kg or more of T_3 intravenously and 10 dogs were given saline. In the untreated group 80% of the dogs died during uncompensated shock. In the treated group, only 27% died. Long-term survival of the treatment group was 45%, significantly greater than the 10% survival of the control group.

A significantly greater number of dogs given T_3 at the beginning of uncompensated shock survived than those given saline. This and previous findings suggest that the therapeutic effect of T_3 in canine hemorrhagic shock might be related to the antagonism of the adverse effects of endogenous rT_3.

▶ This continuing study attempts to investigate the role of rT_3 in patients with critical illness, particularly including shock. In this study, the use of T_3 improved hemodynamic variables and survival. It does appear that a greater number of experimental animals will survive shock at the beginning of the uncompensated phase if treated with T_3.— G.T. Shires, M.D.

Quantitative Measurement of Bleeding Following Hypertonic Saline Therapy in "Uncontrolled" Hemorrhagic Shock

Gross D, Landau EH, Klin B, Krausz MM (Hadassah Univ Hosp, Jerusalem)
J Trauma 29:79–83, January 1989   3–7

How effective is small-volume hypertonic saline in "uncontrolled" hemorrhage? Rats had the terminal 10% of their tails resected to induce uncontrolled hemorrhagic shock. Treated animals received 0.9% or 7.5% saline, 5 mL/kg intravenously after 5 minutes.

Bleeding at 1 hour was somewhat less in animals given physiologic saline than in untreated animals, but the difference was not significant. The mean arterial pressure was significantly higher in the treated rats (Fig 3–3). Infusing hypertonic saline significantly increased bleeding at 1 hour and was associated with a fall in arterial pressure. Survival time was significantly shortened in the rats receiving hypertonic saline.

These findings suggest that hypertonic saline might be dangerous in patients in hemorrhagic shock after multiple trauma when injured vessels may continue to bleed. Hypertonic saline should be used cautiously in patients in shock after abdominal trauma before bleeding is controlled. "Controlled" bleeding does respond well to hypertonic saline.

▶ The authors point out that previous studies by others have used infusion of small volumes of hypertonic sodium chloride solutions for more rapid initial re-

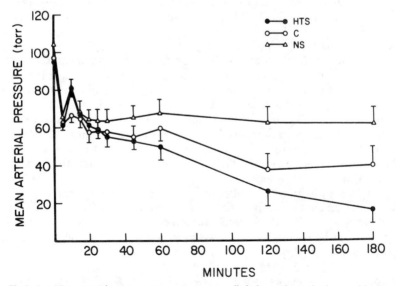

Fig 3–3.—Mean arterial pressure response in "uncontrolled" hemorrhagic shock treated by hypertonic saline (HTS) or normal saline (NS). C indicates untreated animals. (Courtesy of Gross D, Landau EH, Klin B, et al: *J Trauma* 29:79–83, January 1989.)

suscitation from hemorrhagic shock in dogs, sheep, pigs, and rats. There was a more rapid rise in cardiac output followed by peripheral vasodilation with an increase in the renal, mesenteric, splanchnic, and coronary flow. This study, however, tested the applicability of such resuscitation in hemorrhagic shock in a rat model in which injury to blood vessels was the source of continuous intra-abdominal bleeding. In this uncontrolled bleeding experiment, bleeding at 1 hour was somewhat less in animals given physiologic saline than in untreated animals, but the difference was not significant. However, after the infusion of hypertonic saline, significantly increased bleeding at 1 hour was associated with a fall in arterial pressure, and survival time was significantly shortened. These findings led the authors on to additional studies but suggested that hypertonic saline might be dangerous in patients in hemorrhagic shock after multiple trauma in whom injured vessels could continue to bleed.—G.T. Shires, M.D.

Crystalloid Versus Colloid Fluid Resuscitation: A Meta-Analysis of Mortality
Velanovich V (Letterman Army Med Ctr, Presidio of San Francisco)
Surgery 105:65–71, January 1989   3–8

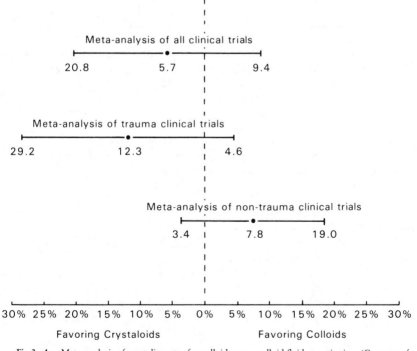

Fig 3–4.—Meta-analysis of mortality rates for colloid vs. crystalloid fluid resuscitation. (Courtesy of Velanovich V: *Surgery* 105:65–71, January 1989.)

The best fluid to use for resuscitation remains questionable, and there continues to be disagreement on the physiologic measures that determine the effectiveness of fluid resuscitation. Meta-analysis was employed to determine whether mortality rates differ with colloid and crystalloid fluid resuscitation. Mortality data from 8 randomized clinical trials were pooled. Four studies concerned trauma patients and 1 included both trauma and nontrauma patients.

When the data from all trials were pooled, the overall treatment effect was a 5.7% relative difference favoring the use of crystalloid solution (Fig 3–4). In trauma trials a 12.3% mortality difference favored crystalloid, whereas in nontrauma trials a 7.8% difference favored the use of colloid.

Patients with trauma may be resuscitated with the use of crystalloid solution. Colloid therapy may be more effective in resuscitating nontrauma patients. Colloid may not benefit patients with trauma who have sepsis and in whom capillary leakage leads to adult respiratory distress syndrome. In contrast, patients without sepsis and elective surgical patients have an intact basement membrane, and in this setting colloids are effective.

▶ This article uses a new technique, namely, meta-analysis, to approximate the effectiveness of fluid resuscitation primarily in the traumatized patient. This mathematical approach enables comparison of the relative efficacies of therapy between colloid and crystalloid fluid resuscitation.

Although one can argue the use of retrospective reported series because mortality rates and causes were not always reported, nevertheless, this approach does indicate the efficacy of crystalloid solutions in the trauma patient. Certainly, in the trauma patient with sepsis better survival and better resuscitation are achieved with crystalloid. Patients without sepsis and during elective surgical procedures can be equally resuscitated with colloid solutions. However, in view of the cost and potential side effects of colloid solutions, the advantages of crystalloid, even in the nontrauma, nonseptic setting, become obvious.—G.T. Shires, M.D.

Lung and Muscle Water After Crystalloid and Colloid Infusion in Septic Rats: Effect on Oxygen Delivery and Metabolism

Rackow EC, Astiz ME, Schumer W, Weil MH (Univ of Health Sciences/Chicago Med School, North Chicago)
J Lab Clin Med 113:184–189, February 1989   3–9

Compared with colloid infusion, saline infusion lowers plasma colloid osmotic pressure and promotes accumulation of lung water after plasmapheresis in animals without lung injury. When microvascular permeability is increased, the influence of plasma colloid osmotic pressure on fluid flux may be limited. The effects of physiologic saline and 10% low molecular-weight hydroxyethyl starch (hetastarch) were studied in rats with sepsis induced by cecal ligation and perforation. Rectus femoris and lung biopsies were performed at 6 hours.

Cardiac output was substantially higher after hetastarch infusion than after saline infusion at 6 hours. Colloid osmotic pressure was 16.1 mm Hg in controls, 21.6 mm Hg after hetastarch infusion, and 9.3 mm Hg after saline infusion. Differences in lung wet-dry to dry weight ratios were not significant, and alveolar-arterial oxygen gradients were comparable in all groups. Muscle wet-dry to dry weight ratios also were similar in the various groups. Skeletal muscle energy production was reduced in both treatment groups but did not differ in the hetastarch and saline groups.

Lung extravascular water was not increased by crystalloid compared with colloid infusion immediately after fluid administration, despite a fall in plasma colloid osmotic pressure. Crystalloid infusion did not appear to produce skeletal muscle edema or impede tissue energy metabolism compared with colloid in the initial stage of fluid repletion.

▶ This interesting experimental article compared the effects of physiologic saline as opposed to 10% low-molecular-weight hydroxyethyl starch in rats with sepsis induced by cecal ligation and perforation. As expected, the colloid osmotic pressure was 16 mm Hg in control animals. 21.6 mm Hg after starch infusion, and 9.3 mm Hg after saline infusion. However, differences in lung wet to dry weight ratios were nonsignificant, and alveolar-arterial oxygen gradients were comparable in all groups. Similarly, muscle wet to dry and wet-dry to dry ratios also were comparable. Skeletal muscle energy production was reduced in both treatment groups and did not differ between the starch and saline groups.

It is interesting that lung extravascular water was not increased by crystalloid compared with colloid infusion after fluid administration despite a fall in plasma colloid oncotic pressure associated with the crystalloid administration. Crystalloid infusion did not appear to produce skeletal muscle edema or impede tissue energy metabolism compared with colloid.

This type of study tends to confirm data from others that the anticipated reduction in plasma colloid oncotic pressure seen with crystalloids is not of sufficient magnitude to influence the development of edema. It would appear that a fall in tissue oncotic pressure to less than 20% of normal is necessary for this edema-forming tendency to develop, and this degree of fall in plasma oncotic pressure simply does not occur with crystalloid administration.—G.T. Shires, M.D.

Free Water Clearance After Supplemental Albumin Resuscitation for Shock
Moon MR, Lucas CE, Ledgerwood AM, Kosinski JP (Wayne State Univ, Detroit)
Circ Shock 28:1–8, 1989   3–10

Albumin supplementation appears to impede sodium and water excretion and increase renal insufficiency in patients with hypovolemic shock. The effects of albumin supplementation on free water clearance (CH_2O),

Free Water Clearance		
	Albumin (%)	Nonalbumin (%)
Group A		
$CH_2 < -0.25$ ml/min	22 (48)	35 (73)
Renal insufficiency	2 (9)	1 (3)
Group B		
$CH_2 = +/-0.25$ ml/min	5 (11)	4 (8)
Renal insufficiency	3 (60)	0 (0)
Group C		
$CH_2O > +0.25$ ml/min	19 (41)	9 (19)
Renal insufficiency	8 (42)	0 (0)

(Courtesy of Moon MR, Lucas CE, Ledgerwood AM, et al: *Circ Shock* 28:1–8, 1989.)

a sensitive indicator of renal tubular function, were examined in 94 patients receiving an average of 14.5 transfusions for shock. Forty-six patients received 31 g of albumin during operation and as much as 150 g daily postoperatively, whereas 48 received only electrolyte solution.

Sodium clearance was reduced significantly in the albumin-treated patients, but they were more likely to have abnormally increased CH_2O than a normal negative clearance (table). The filtered sodium load correlated positively with both sodium clearance and sodium excretion, and correlated inversely with CH_2O. Serum osmolarity did not change significantly after albumin administration. The increase in plasma volume correlated with the rise in sodium excretion but not with changes in CH_2O.

The combination of decreased sodium clearance and increased CH_2O after albumin reflects increased peritubular oncotic pressure, promoting sodium and water reabsorption. The increased plasma volume reduces reabsorption of both sodium and water. The changes are mediated by sodium-potassium exchange in the distal nephron.

▶ These authors and others have shown previously that in resuscitation from hypovolemic shock during which patients receive blood, albumin supplementation impedes sodium and water excretion and increases renal insufficiency. In the current study the authors examined the effects of albumin supplementation on free water clearance, a sensitive indicator of renal tubular function. These studies were conducted on 94 patients who were given an average of 14½ transfusions for shock. Half of the patients received additional albumin and half received only electrolyte solution.

Sodium clearance was reduced significantly in the albumin-treated patients; furthermore, there was abnormally increased free water clearance in the albumin-treated group. Interestingly, serum osmolarity did not change significantly after albumin administration. Thus the combination of decreased sodium clearance and increased free water clearance after albumin reflects increased peritubular oncotic pressure promoting sodium and water reabsorption. The adds one more nail to the coffin of extra albumin in the resuscitation of the patient in shock.—G.T. Shires, M.D.

Base Deficit as a Guide to Volume Resuscitation
Davis JW, Shackford SR, Mackersie RC, Hoyt DB (Univ of California, San Diego)
J Trauma 28:1464–1467, October 1988   3–11

Because the serum lactate level is nearly stoichiometric to base deficit (BD), an increased calculated BD may serve as a useful metabolic indicator of shock and volume deficit. The usefulness of BD in estimating blood volume deficits and titrating fluid therapy was examined in 209 trauma patients undergoing serial arterial blood gas measurements.

The initial BD was mild (2 to −5) in 70 patients, moderate (−6 to −14) in 110, and severe (less than −15) in 29. The mean arterial pressure declined with an increasingly severe BD, and the fluid volume required for resuscitation increased. When the BD became more negative as resuscitation progressed, continued bleeding was noted in two thirds of the patients. The BD increased in only 17 of 113 patients without ongoing hemorrhage after resuscitation began.

Base deficit is a helpful guide to volume replacement in trauma patients. Arterial blood gases should be measured whenever a victim of major trauma is admitted. If a moderate or severe BD is noted, measurement of blood gases should be repeated in 1 or 2 hours.

▶ This is a unique and interesting approach to the usefulness of BD in estimating continued bleeding in blood volume deficits. As the authors point out, excess in serum lactic acid occurs almost inevitably in the shock or low-flow state. Because determining the serum lactic acid level is time consuming, these authors used the BD as an estimate of lactic acidosis. As they correctly point out, the presence of a BD is a helpful guide to volume replacement in traumatized patients, particularly when unsuspected continuing blood loss or underreplacement of blood loss is present. Arterial blood gases should be measured in victims of major trauma, and if a BD develops, these blood gas measurements should be repeated. The authors suggest that the use of a cookbook fluid formula derived from the BD is not appropriate. However, the BD is a useful and powerful tool for guiding fluid management during resuscitation, particularly in the presence of untreated or continuing blood loss.— G.T. Shires, M.D.

Infusion of Small Volume of 7.5 Per Cent Sodium Chloride in 6.0 Per Cent Dextran 70 for the Treatment of Uncontrolled Hemorrhagic Shock
Rabinovici R, Gross D, Krausz MM (Hadassah Univ Hosp, Jerusalem)
Surg Gynecol Obstet 169:137–142, August 1989   3–12

Small volumes of hypertonic saline now are used to treat hemorrhagic shock. Dextran 70 has been used widely to expand blood volume but may produce bleeding abnormalities and aggravate blood loss in uncontrolled hemorrhagic shock. Rats having partial resection of the tail received 7.5% saline in 6% dextran 70, 5mL/kg. Controls received either physiologic saline, hypertonic saline, or dextran 70 alone.

Infusion of dextran 70 alone worsened blood loss, and hypertonic saline alone had a similar effect. Blood loss in the first 4 hours was greatest in animals given 7.5% saline in 6% dextran 70. Survival times for rats receiving hypertonic saline and hypertonic saline-dextran were shorter than those of untreated animals.

The potential danger of administering hypertonic saline in dextran 70 should be taken into account before its trial in either urban or military settings.

▶ This fascinating experimental study set out to evaluate the use of hypertonic saline with and without dextran as compared to other forms of fluid therapy, including normal saline, in hemorrhagic shock. As the authors point out, a favorable effect of 7.5% saline in dextran 70 in controlled hemorrhagic shock in animal studies has led to the suggestion by several groups that this combination should be useful clincally, both in hospitals as well as in the prehospital treatment of hemorrhagic shock. The current study, however, used uncontrolled hemorrhagic shock in that 10% of the tail of the rat was resected and various treatment regimes were evaluated. Infusion of 7.5% saline in dextran 70 resulted in increased bleeding following a decline in mean arterial pressure and early mortality. The suggestion is quite strong that if a vessel is opened in an injured patient, the powerful vasodilating effect of hypertonic solutions may increase blood loss, deplete blood volume, reduce blood pressure, and produce a much higher initial mortality. These authors warn that the use of hypertonic saline in dextran for resuscitation should be carefully considered because of its potential dangers.— G.T. Shires, M.D.

Early Versus Late Fluid Resuscitation: Lack of Effect in Porcine Hemorrhagic Shock

Chudnofsky CR, Dronen SC, Syverud SA, Hedges JR, Zink BJ (Univ of Cincinnati)
Ann Emerg Med 18:122–126, February 1989   3–13

The use of advanced life support (ALS) interventions, particularly the intravenous infusion of fluids, in the prehospital management of trauma is controversial. Some physicians believe that the delays associated with placing intravenous lines outweigh the benefits of early fluid resuscitation; others believe that paramedics can perform various ALS measures, including intravenous cannulation, expeditiously. An animal model was used to assess the utility of prehospital fluid resuscitation after trauma.

A reproducible, lightly anesthetized model of porcine continuous hemorrhage was used. Time delays associated with request and dispatch of ambulances, assessment and treatment of patients, and transport to the hospital were incorporated. Twenty-eight young swine were bled at the rate of 1.25 mL/kg/min. The 14 animals in the prehospital group were given fluid resuscitation at 1 mL/kg/min, beginning 20 minutes after bleeding was induced. The 14 animals in the inhospital group were given fluid at 3 mL/kg/min beginning 35 minutes after bleeding was induced. All animals were given blood and saline, 3 mL/kg/min, 45 minutes after hemorrhage began. In all animals hemorrhage was controlled within

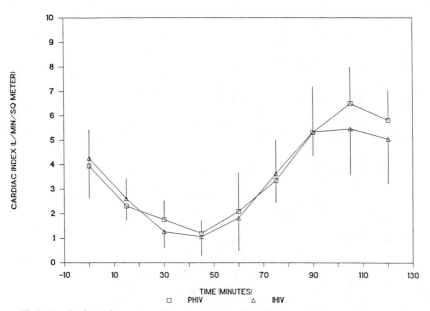

Fig 3–5.—Cardiac index vs. time (Courtesy of Chudnofsky CR, Dronen SC, Syverud SA, et al: *Ann Emerg Med* 18:122–126, February 1989.)

25 minutes after simulated hospital arrival. Fifty-seven percent of the animals in both groups survived. There were no significant differences in measured hemodynamic or biochemical parameters between groups (Fig 3–5).

These findings support the previous contention that intravenous fluid therapy is beneficial only in selected cases. Early intravenous therapy appeared to have no effect in this animal model. Higher rates of infusion or administration of hypertonic saline may justify placement of an intravenous line, but this has yet to be established.

▶ This experimental animal model attempted to evaluate the efficacy of the prehospital intravenous infusion of fluids. However, the experimental conditions that were set up probably mimic more closely the human trauma victim who has a relatively short transport time from injury site to hospital. In this setting, clinical studies have shown previously that the intravenous infusion of less than a liter during the average transport time of 5 or 10 minutes probably is of little benefit except in selected patients with severe volume deficit. It is not surprising, therefore, that this particular porcine model simply showed no significant advantage in the short time following bleeding.—G.T. Shires, M.D.

Traumatic Shock and Head Injury: Effects of Fluid Resuscitation on the Brain
Wisner D, Busche F, Sturm J, Gaab M, Meyer H (Univ of California, Davis, Sacramento; Hannover Med School, Hannover, West Germany)
J Surg Res 46:49–59, January 1989   3–14

Vigorous intravenous fluid resuscitation is a cornerstone of the initial therapy of multiple trauma victims. Large volumes of crystalloid solutions are administered, which can lead to a marked decrease in colloid osmotic pressure. An experimental study was conducted to determine the effects of fluid resuscitation on the traumatized brain. The effects of traumatic-hemorrhagic shock and resuscitation were assessed in 13 sheep without brain injury and 12 sheep with brain injury. The animals were resuscitated with either lactated Ringer's solution or 4% human albumin. Hemodynamics, intracranial pressure, electroencephalographic changes, and colloid osmotic pressure were monitored.

Traumatic-hemorrhagic shock alone resulted in no major change in intracranial pressure during the shock period. There was an increase in intracranial pressure with resuscitation in all groups, regardless of the resuscitation regimen used. Compared with control animals, those without brain injury had no increased brain water, as determined by the wet-to-dry weight data. Brain injury, however, significantly increased brain water content in the cortex of the injured hemisphere compared with both control animals and animals with traumatic-hemorrhagic shock and no brain injury.

These findings suggest that maintaining colloid osmotic pressure during initial resuscitation does not minimize cerebral edema in the presence or absence of brain injury. Both crystalloid and colloid solutions have similar effects on the brain. It appears that focal brain injury causes edema, but does not cause large increases in intracranial pressure with initial resuscitation.

▶ This interesting study evaluated intravenous fluid resuscitation in the experimental animal, the sheep, in the face of associated brain injury. The resuscitation solutions evaluated were lactated Ringer's solution and 4% human albumin. Traumatic and hemorrhagic shock alone resulted in no major change in intracranial pressure during the shock period, but there was an increase in intracranial pressure with resuscitation in all groups regardless of the regimen used. Brain injury, however, significantly increased brain water content in the cortex of the injured hemisphere compared both with control animals and animals with traumatic or hemorrhagic shock and no brain injury. These findings indicate that maintaining colloid osmotic pressure during initial resuscitation with the use of human albumin does not minimize cerebral edema in the presence or absence of brain injury. Both crystalloid and colloid solutions had similar effects on the brain. It appeared that the focal brain injury causes the edema but does not cause large increases in intracranial pressure with initial resuscitation, even with crystalloid alone or with colloid solution.—G.T. Shires, M.D.

The Percutaneous Common Femoral Vein Catheter for Volume Replacement in Critically Injured Patients
Mangiante EC, Hoots AV, Fabian TC (Univ of Tennessee, Memphis)
J Trauma 28:1644–1649, December 1988   3–15

Traditionally, large-bore catheters are placed in the upper extremity to restore intravascular volume in patients who sustain multiple trauma; however, circumstances may prevent placement of venous catheters in the arms or neck. A percutaneously placed 8.5-French common femoral vein catheter (CFVC) was inserted in 366 critically injured hypotensive patients in whom upper extremity veins were unavailable or inadequate for volume resuscitation. The CFVCs were removed on admission to the trauma intensive care unit or after completion of initial surgical procedures. Flow rates were further maximized by replacing standard intravenous tubing with genitourinary irrigating tubing; direct digital pressure was applied at the catheter site for 5 minutes after removal of the CFVC.

Trauma scores ranged from 1 to 16 (mean, 9.3); patients with blunt trauma had a mean injury severity score of 32.1. There were 139 deaths, 82% of which occurred within the first 24 hours. The CFVC was not related to death in any patient.

The fluid administration set-up used could transfuse 1 L of warm Ringer's lactate in 37 seconds. The mean volume infused in penetrating trauma victims was 4,451 mL, and 4,611 mL in blunt trauma victims. There was no evidence of major hematoma, iliofemoral thrombosis, local infection, or sepsis related to the catheter in the survivors. Use of the catheter resulted in 2 arterial injuries, both occurring when the catheter was placed in the absence of a femoral pulse. Venous access can be achieved safely and rapidly in patients with a potential need for massive volume infusion by use of the CFVC in conjunction with genitourinary irrigating tubing. The system is effective in trauma patients in whom upper extremity veins are either inaccessible or inadequate for volume resuscitation.

▶ This study is another in a series of attempts to increase the rapidity of resuscitation and the use of large-volume resuscitative fluids in the severely injured patients. As the authors point out, in the presence of hypovolemic shock, access to standard venous catheters in the arms or neck may be difficult and, similarly, in peripheral veins in the legs. These authors used a common femoral vein catheter in 366 critically injured hypotensive patients, and standard intravenous tubing was replaced with the larger genitourinary irrigating tubing. This system allowed the infusion of 1 L of warmed Ringer's lactate every 37 seconds. The authors concluded that the common femoral vein is a method of easy access in the hypotensive patient and affords massive volume infusion with the infusion system described.—G.T. Shires, M.D.

Evaluation of Blood-Warming Devices With the Apparent Thermal Clearance

Flancbaum L, Trooskin SZ, Pedersen H (Univ of Medicine and Dentistry of New Jersey, New Brunswick; Rutgers, The State Univ of New Jersey, New Brunswick)
Ann Emerg Med 18:355–359, April 1989   3–16

Hypothermia caused by massive transfusions is a life-threatening problem in seriously injured and critically ill patients. Maintenance of normal body temperature mandates the use of an efficient blood-warming device. The unit should have a low priming volume, a large heat transfer area, and a low pressure drop, and it should be able to warm blood from 4°C to 32°C or more without adverse effects.

The single-coil immersion heater, the single-channel dry wall electric heater, the multichannel countercurrent heat exchanger, and the single-channel countercurrent heat exchanger were compared. Thermal clearance values were estimated using saline and packed red blood cells.

Only the single-channel countercurrent unit met the requirements for an efficient blood warmer. The multiple parallel-channel countercurrent unit was adequate for saline but not for packed red blood cells, probably because of its large priming volume. Neither the single-coil immersion unit nor the single-channel dry wall heater achieved adequate flow rates with either saline or packed red blood cells. Apparent thermal clearance is a useful means of comparing and assessing blood-warming devices.

▶ Previous studies have shown the clear relationship between systemic hypothermia and a decrease in platelet function promoting clotting defect bleeding in patients who have had resuscitation with cold blood products and other fluids. As these authors point out, this hypothermia is a life-threatening problem in the seriously injured patient. Consequently, there have been a number of presumably efficient blood-warming and fluid-warming devices appearing on the market recently. These units should have a low priming volume, a large heat transfer area, and a low pressure drop, and also be able to warm blood efficiently from 4°C to 40°C without adverse effects on red blood cells. The present study compared single-coil immersion and a warm water bath with a single-channel dry wall electric heater; these 2 devices were then compared against a single- or multichannel countercurrent heat exchanger. Thermal clearances were calculated using saline and packed red blood cells as the infused fluid. The authors believe that the single-channel, countercurrent unit was preferable in terms of effective heat exchange and warming efficiency.—G.T. Shires, M.D.

An Improved Technique for Rapid Infusion of Warmed Fluid Using a Level 1 Fluid Warmer

Smith JS Jr, Snider MT (Milton S Hershey Med Ctr, Hershey, Pa)
Surg Gynecol Obstet 168:273–274, March 1989   3–17

In resuscitating trauma patients by rapidly administering warmed fluid, 3 devices are currently available. One of these, the Rapid Infusion System is expensive, and another, the Bard Infuser 37, is much less costly, but the temperature falls as the infusion rate increases. The Level 1 Fluid Warmer also delivers warmed fluid at body temperature but has been hampered by small-diameter tubing that precludes rapid flow rates.

Much less volume is needed to prime the circuit than with the Bard 37, and the unit is easily started and set up.

A system was designed incorporating 2 Alton Dean Pressure Infusion Boxes connected to an E-size oxygen cylinder and flow regulator mounted on the intravenous pole of the Level 1 Fluid Warmer. Peak flow rates as high as 425 mL/min are achievable. The temperature remains at about 37°C. Larger-bore tubing now is available, permitting flow rates of 735 mL/min under continuous pressurization at a temperature of 35°C.

This system has been used in 30 patients without hemolysis occurring. The modified Level 1 Fluid Warmer is a simple, cost-effective means of rapidly infusing normothermic fluids into critically ill patients.

▶ This is another of the flurry of articles appearing in the past year evaluating blood and fluid warmers for use during rapid and massive infusions of fluid and red blood cells in the severely injured patient. This particular study involved the clinical evaluation of a multiple-channel countercurrent warming device. The authors conclude that, with the Alton Dean Pressure Infusion Boxes and the multichannel countercurrent heat exchanger, extremely high peak flow rates are achievable with efficient temperature exchange and no adverse effects on the blood cells used in the experiment.—G.T. Shires, M.D.

4 Trauma

Comparison of Trauma Assessment Scores and Their Use in Prediction of Infection and Death

Cheadle WG, Wilson M, Hershman MJ, Bergamini D, Richardson JD, Polk HC Jr (Univ of Louisville)

Ann Surg 209:541–546, May 1989   4–1

The development of infection is the most common cause of late morbidity and mortality in the resuscitated trauma patient. However, none of the existing trauma scoring systems include assessment of immune competence as a predictor of subsequent infection or late death from sepsis. The ability of serum to support phagocytosis by normal neutrophils and of peripheral blood monocytes to express HLA-DR correlates independently with outcome. The Outcome Predictive Score (OPS) combines the Injury Severity Score (ISS) corrected for age, monocyte HLA-DR antigen expression, and degree of bacterial contamination at the time of hospital admission. To compare the OPS with other standard scales for predicting clinical outcome after trauma, 61 seriously ill trauma patients admitted with ISSs of 20 or more were evaluated.

The patients were divided into 3 clinical outcome groups: 18 had an uneventful recovery, 27 contracted major infections but survived, and 16 died, 13 of major infections with multiple organ failure. The OPS, the ISS, the ISS corrected for age, the Revised Trauma Score, and the Combined Trauma Score-ISS were calculated for each patient. The probability of mortality using the Anatomical Index was calculated for 22 patients.

Significant differences were noted between the mean ISS and the ISS corrected for age that distinguished survivors from those who died, but neither scoring system could distinguish between patients with a good outcome and those who would contract a major infection. The Combined Trauma Score-ISS also revealed significant differences between those who had a good outcome and the others, but because of the range of individual values within each of the 3 clinical outcome categories, the Combined Trauma Score-ISS could not distinguish survivors from those who died of major infection (Fig 4–1). The Revised Trauma Score also could not distinguish survivors from nonsurvivors. Only the OPS consistently distinguished between all outcome groups. As infection is a common complication after any type of trauma, a scoring system that early identifies patients who are at high risk of contracting infection would be useful.

▶ This interesting paper makes several points with regard to severity scoring in the injured patient. The data show that the mean ISS and $\%LD_{50}$ scores did distinguish between survivors and those who died, but the scoring systems

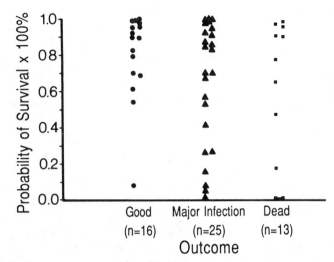

Fig 4–1.—Frequency scattergram of combined Injury Severity Score and Revised Trauma Score (TRISS). There was little predictive value of major infection or death in these patients from the individual TRISS value. (Courtesy of Cheadle WG, Wilson M, Hershman MJ, et al: *Ann Surg* 209:541–546, May 1989.)

could not distinguish between patients with a good outcome and those who contracted a major infection. Similarly, the Combined Trauma Score-ISS (TRISS) scores also showed significant differences between those who had a good outcome and the rest of the patients, but because of the range of TRISS values, they could not distinguish survivors from those who died of a major infection.

Only the OPS, which combined the ISS corrected for age with monocyte HLA-DR antigen expression and degree of bacterial contamination at the time of hospital admission, could consistently distinguish between a good outcome and death caused by major infection.

Because the development of infection is the most common cause of late morbidity and mortality in the resuscitated trauma patient, it is clear that the authors' conclusion that a scoring system that early identifies patients who are at high risk for acquiring infection is a necessary addition to the trauma scoring systems.—G.T. Shires, M.D.

Prospective Study of the Effect of Safety Belts on Morbidity and Health Care Costs in Motor-Vehicle Accidents

Orsay EM, Turnbull TL, Dunne M, Barrett JA, Langenberg P, Orsay CP (Univ of Illinois, Chicago)

JAMA 260:3598–3603, Dec 23–30, 1988   4–2

The effect of seat-belt use on the extent of injuries sustained during motor vehicle accidents was studied prospectively, and the economic impact of seat-belt use was evaluated. Data were collected on 1,364 patients seen at 4 Chicago-area hospitals after motor vehicle accidents. Physicians

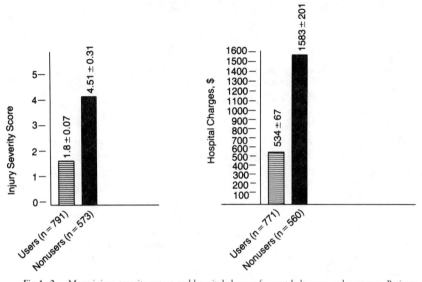

Fig 4–2.—Mean injury severity scores and hospital charges for seat belt users and nonusers. Patients who had worn seat belts had significantly lower injury severity scores (*P* < .01) and hospital charges (*P* < .001). (Courtesy of Orsay EM, Turnbull TL, Dunne M, et al: *JAMA* 260:3598–3603, Dec 23–30, 1988.)

ascertained seat-belt usage, patient's position in the automobile, mechanism of injury, posted speed limit at location of the accident, mode of transfer to the hospital, and final disposition. Evidence of alcohol use was also noted. Medical records of all patients were subsequently reviewed.

Seat belts had been worn by 58% of accident victims. The mean injury severity score for seat-belt wearers was 1.8 compared with 4.51 for unbelted passengers (Fig 4–2). Only 6.8% of belted passengers required hospital admission compared with 19.2% of unbelted passengers. Restrained occupants incurred charges of $534 compared with $1,583 in unrestrained occupants. Restrained passengers had a 60.1% reduction in severity of injury, a 64.6% reduction in hospital admissions, and a 66.3% decrease in hospital charges. These findings demonstrate that morbidity and costs of medical care could be reduced significantly if all automobile occupants wore safety seat belts.

► This is one of the few medical articles reporting a prospective study comparing injuries sustained in the presence or absence of seat-belt wearing. As expected, the mean injury severity score for seat-belt wearers was 1.8 compared to 4.5 in unbelted passengers. Also, 6.8% of belted passengers required hospitalization compared with 19.2% of unbelted passengers, and the restrained occupants incurred charges of $534.00 compared with $1,583.00 for unrestrained occupants. These findings suggest that the severity of injuries, hospital admission, and cost of care could be reduced significantly if automobile occupants would consistently wear seat belts.— G.T. Shires, M.D.

Impact of Helicopters on Trauma Care and Clinical Results
Moylan JA (Duke Univ)
Ann Surg 208:673–678, December 1988   4–3

Helicopter evacuation was first used in Korea, and experience in Vietnam confirmed the value of aeromedical evacuation. In civilian life the helicopter provides rapid transport to an appropriate trauma care facility. In addition, trained personnel are brought to the scene to begin early resuscitation and stabilization. Helicopters also are used to transport medical experts from a tertiary trauma center to outlying hospitals. Widely varying cost figures are cited for helicopter ambulance programs. Increased survival may relate more to a shorter interval between injury and institution of resuscitative measures than to more rapid arrival at the trauma center.

Helicopter service has improved survival most markedly in patients with low trauma scores. Continued efforts to improve triage at the scene are necessary. Key aspects of a civilian helicopter program include specially trained and experienced personnel, sophisticated equipment, and medical control. Proper education of the public agency involved in scene response will minimize the risks faced by ground health care providers as well as bystanders.

▶ This nice review of helicopter transport and its effect on trauma care needs to be more publicized. The article points out that the helicopter, in addition to providing rapid transport to an appropriate trauma facility, also has the trained personnel and medical helicopter life-saving capabilities that are simply not available with ground transport. Although some increased survival relates more to a shorter interval between injury and the start of resuscitative measures, as well as faster transport to the trauma center, it is clear that the immediate availability of a life-saving intensive care unit with its trained team is the critical factor in improving survival most markedly in patients with significant trauma scores. This article needs additional exposure, because the public agencies involved in scene response, as well as those involved in funding in helicopter transport, are simply not educated as to the striking benefits, quite apart from the decrease in transport time.—G.T. Shires, M.D.

Zero-Time Prehospital IV
O'Gorman M, Trabulsy P, Pilcher DB (Univ of Vermont, Burlington)
J Trauma 29:84–86, January 1989   4–4

The necessity of Advanced Trauma Life Support before transport to the hospital is still debated. Many authors advocate little or no paramedic prehospital involvement, whereas others think that on-scene airway control and fluid replacement can be life-saving. Resolving this question is especially important in rural areas, where transport times to the hospital may be longer. The efficacy of attempting to start an intravenous infusion at the scene was compared with that of attempting intravenous access only after patients were en route to the hospital.

From 1985 to 1986, intravenous access attempts were made in 350 consecutive patients. Seventy intravenous lines were begun at the scene and 213 were begun en route to the hospital. Of 90 attempts to start intravenous lines at the scene, 77% were successful; of the 260 attempts to start them during transport, 81% were successful. Among patients whose blood pressure never dropped below 100 mm Hg at the scene or during transport, intravenous placement was successful 80% and 85% of the time, respectively. In patients with blood pressures of less than 100 mm Hg the success rate was 66% on the scene and 72% en route, not a significant difference. The average times required to start intravenous lines were 3.8 minutes at the scene and 4.1 minutes en route.

The success rate of intravenous placement en route to the hospital is equal to that of intravenous placement at the scene. Therefore, in patients who are not trapped, intravenous access should be initiated only during transport. It is not possible to justify any delay at the scene, even if that delay is minimal.

▶ This article examines a controversial aspect of prehospital treatment. As is pointed out, many authors advocate little or no prehospital paramedic involvement, whereas others believe that on-the-scene airway control and fluid replacement can be life-saving. This study looks specifically at the efficacy of starting intravenous infusion at the scene compared with that of attempting access only after patients were enroute to the hospital. It is interesting that the success rate for intravenous access was just as good during transport as it was at the scene. As expected, the success rate was higher if the patient was not in shock; even if the patient were in shock, however, the success rate still was 72%. The authors conclude that the success rate of intravenous placement en route to the hospital is equal to that attempted at the scene; therefore, access in patients who are not trapped should be initiated during transport rather incur any delay at the scene.

Most authors would now agree that airway control at the scene is highly desirable, but that intravenous access can probably be done equally well en route to the hospital.—G.T. Shires, M.D.

Prospective MAST Study in 911 Patients

Mattox KL, Bickell W, Pepe PE, Burch J, Feliciano D (Baylor College of Medicine, Houston; Ben Taub Gen Hosp, Houston)
J Trauma 29:1104–1112, August 1989 4–5

The use of military anti-shock trousers (MAST) in the prehospital care of hypotensive trauma patients has received unqualified support from providers of emergency medical service, emergency physicians, and surgeons. However, no prospective, controlled trials have demonstrated the effectiveness of MAST in prehospital management of injury. In 1986 the first prospectively randomized study of prehospital MAST showed no benefit or advantage of MAST use, and no other controlled trials have since been published. The final results of a continuation study that was done under the same protocol as the 1986 study were assessed.

During a 3.5-year period, 911 injured patients with systolic blood pressures of 90 mm Hg or less were randomly assigned to treatment with MAST or without MAST on an alternate-day protocol. Trauma patients randomized to receive MAST were given the same treatment as the no-MAST trauma patients, except that MAST garments were applied before intravenous placement of catheters. All patients were taken to the same level I trauma center.

Of 784 evaluable patients, 345 received treatment with and 439 received treatment without MAST. The population cohorts were statistically identical. The principal sites of injury were the thorax in 41%, abdomen in 32%, extremity in 16%, head in 7%, and neck in 4%. Among 185 patients whose initial systolic blood pressure was between 51 mm Hg and 70 mm Hg, survival in the no-MAST group was 11.4% greater than in the MAST group. The mortality rates among 320 patients with thoracic injuries were 31.7% in the no-Mast group and 41.8% in the MAST group. Prehospital mortality rates among patients with thoracic injuries were 5.2% in the no-MAST group and 16.4% in the MAST group. Among 484 patients who had total prehospital times of 30 minutes or more, MAST application did not increase the length of survival. In all, 222 of the 784 trauma patients died. The overall mortality rates were 31% in the MAST group and 25% in the no-MAST group. The difference was statistically significant.

Because survival among hypotensive trauma patients not treated with MAST was significantly better, the pneumatic antishock garment is no longer used in ambulances of the Houston fire department, and all inventory has been removed from the emergency department at the hospital studied.

▶ This article is another of the very few prospective, randomized, controlled trials to evaluate the MAST garment in the prehospital care of hypotensive trauma patients. As pointed out by the authors, these trousers have received unqualified support from many sources, including emergency medical services providers, emergency physicians, and the like. In this 3.5-year study of 911 injured patients with systolic blood pressure below 90 mm Hg, patients were randomly assigned to MAST or no-MAST on an alternate-day protocol. All of the treatment was kept constant, and the results were quite clear. Survival in hypotensive trauma patients not treated with MAST was significantly better. As a consequence, the Houston Fire Department, the site of the study, has now removed the pneumatic antishock garment from its ambulances and the related hospital has pulled the MAST garments from its inventory.

Although the controversy continues, the results of the only prospective, controlled, randomized studies in an urban setting, even those reporting transport times of frequently less but occasionally more than 30 minutes, are definitive. It seems that it is very difficult to get rid of a practice that was initiated based largely on animal studies, even though it has now been shown to be detrimental clinically.— G.T. Shires, M.D.

Venous Air Embolism From Head and Neck Wounds
Adams VI, Hirsch CS (Office of Chief Med Examiner, New York City; State Univ of New York, Stony Brook)
Arch Pathol Lab Med 113:498–502, May 1989   4–6

Air embolism is common in persons with fatal penetrating head injuries and may also occur in victims of blunt trauma. Venous, or pulmonary, air emboli originate from breaches of systemic veins and progress centrally through negative intrathoracic pressure on inspiration. There must be a pressure gradient between the breached vein and the right side of the heart, but this can be as low as 5 cm of water. Stiff-walled veins (e.g., sinuses in cancellous bone and the dural sinuses) form the most effective communication with atmospheric air. Small air emboli lodge in pulmonary arterial branches and large ones in the pulmonary artery and right ventricular outflow tract.

Air emboli in the right heart and pulmonary artery were found in 16 autopsies of persons with shotgun and gunshot wounds of the head and traffic fatalities. One neck incision was included. The shotgun wounds were incurred at contact range and involved explosive comminution of the vault and base of the skull. In traffic fatalities skull fracture crossing a dural sinus was a consistent finding.

Air emboli may be present in most contact shotgun wounds of the head and in many gunshot wounds of the head. The dura must be examined in situ. Roentgenography of the chest and the head/neck is very helpful in evaluating trauma victims if skull fracture or a breach of neck veins is suspected.

▶ These authors make the point that air embolism is quite common in persons with fatal penetrating head injuries as well as in patients with neck wounds. In a series of autopsy studies air emboli were found to be present in most contact shotgun wounds of the head and in many gunshot wounds of the head. When a skull fracture or breach of neck veins is suspected, x-ray examination of the chest, head, and neck would be very helpful in evaluation. The authors' point that this is frequently overlooked in the early management of head and neck trauma victims, is probably a very important one.— G.T. Shires, M.D.

Penetrating Injury to the Carotid Artery: A Reappraisal of Management
Timberlake GA, Rice JC, Kerstein MD, Rush DS, McSwain NE Jr (US Naval Hosp, San Diego; Tulane Univ)
Am Surg 55:154–157, March 1989   4–7

The proper management of penetrating carotid artery injuries remains uncertain. Twenty-four patients with penetrating cervical carotid artery injuries were evaluated between 1981 and 1986. The average age was 34 years, and the mean trauma score at admission was 10.6. There were 15 gunshot wounds, 5 stab wounds, and 4 shotgun wounds. Thirteen patients had neurologic deficits related to the ipsilateral hemisphere. Fourteen of the 24 patients survived.

Three patients had carotid injuries in zone I of the neck, and 8 had zone III injuries. Two patients in each of these groups were taken directly to surgery because of clinical instability. Four patients with zone III injuries required ligation of the vessel at the skull base. Among 13 patients with zone II injuries, all 3 with external carotid injuries had ligation without neurologic sequelae. Indwelling shunts were used during carotid artery repair in 4 patients. The average postoperative hospital stay was 8½ days.

These findings support the repair of all common and internal carotid artery injuries in neurologically intact patients, when feasible. Neither repair nor vessel ligation has altered the outcome in patients with preoperative neurologic deficit.

▶ This is another in a series of articles appearing in the past few years supporting the change in approach to common and internal carotid injuries. These articles now support repair of internal carotid artery injuries in all neurologically intact patients, which is generally accepted. However, the current study indicates that an attempt should be made to repair carotid injuries in a patient with neurologic deficits unless the patient is comatose with profound and probably irreversible neurologic damage, in which case there is no difference in outcome between ligation of the major carotid artery and repair. This approach seems to be becoming more and more standardized as new articles appear.—G.T. Shires, M.D.

The Role of Abdominal CT in the Evaluation of Stab Wounds to the Back
Meyer DM, Thal ER, Weigelt JA, Redman HC (Univ of Texas, Dallas)
J Trauma 29:1226–1230, September 1989   4–8

Retroperitoneal injuries from stab wounds to the back often are difficult to evaluate. To determine whether CT is useful in the evaluation of stab wounds to the back, during a 2.5-year period, 205 patients aged 9–68 years were evaluated by CT scanning with both oral and intravenous contrast material used. Patients with a positive CT scan or clinical suspicion of injury, or both, underwent operation. Patients whose scans, whether negative or positive, suggested only minor insignificant injury were admitted to the hospital for observation.

Thirteen patients with a positive CT scan who were treated nonoperatively and 3 with an equivocal scan were excluded from statistical analysis. Of the remaining 189 patients, 169 had a negative scan, but 30 of these were operated on because of clinical concern. Injuries were found in only 2 of these 30 patients: One had a diaphragmatic injury, and the other had a liver injury. None of the 139 patients not operated on had any adverse sequelae.

Of the 20 patients operated on because of a positive scan, 16 had positive findings confirmed at operation; 4 had falsely positive scans. Seven of the 16 with true positive CT scans had additional significant injuries that were not detected on CT, including 4 diaphragmatic injuries, 2 hepatic injuries, and 1 injury each to the spleen, stomach, pancreas, and gallbladder. The 4 false positive CT scans had suggested a retroperitoneal hematoma, a small bowel injury, and 2 splenic injuries, none of which was found at operation. Only 2 of 8 confirmed diaphragmatic injuries were identified on CT scans.

Statistical analysis revealed that CT scanning of stab wounds to the back had a sensitivity of 89%, a specificity of 98%, and an accuracy of 97%. Thus CT is reasonably reliable in evaluation of patients with stab wounds to the back.

▶ This is another comparative study concerning the use of CT, but in this instance in evaluation of penetrating wounds to the back. All surgeons dealing with traumatized patients agree that evaluation of the significance of a penetrating back wound is difficult at best. In this study the sensitivity of the CT scan was 89%; the specificity, 98%; and accuracy, 97%. Thus, in this series, CT was reasonably reliable in evaluation of patients with stab wounds to the back. This may become a very important modality in determining the significance of back injuries in patients who have no clinical signs of significant injury or clinical suspicion of injury who probably all should be operated on. The only other alternative, i.e., local exploration of the back wound, may still be used, but it is probably not nearly as sensitive or specific as a combination of clinical findings and CT.—G.T. Shires, M.D.

Sonography Versus Peritoneal Lavage in Blunt Abdominal Trauma
Grüessner R, Mentges B, Düber Ch, Rückert K, Rothmund M (Univ of Mainz, West Germany)
J Trauma 29:242–244, February 1989   4–9

The usefulness of sonography and diagnostic peritoneal lavage (DPL) in determining the need for immediate exploration was examined in a prospective series of 71 patients with blunt abdominal trauma. Those who had definite indications for emergency laparotomy were excluded. Twenty patients were in shock when admitted, and 45 had a depressed sensorium. Forty-four patients had multiple injuries.

Thirty-five patients underwent laparotomy. Three others died shortly after admission. Peritoneal lavage was 100% sensitive and 99% accurate, and had a predictive value of 97%. In comparison, sonography was 84% sensitive and 86% accurate, and had a predictive value of 89%. These differences were statistically significant. Peritoneal lavage was considered positive if a bright red return was obtained, if the amylase concentration exceeded 175 units per dL, or if frank gastrointestinal contents were identified.

Peritoneal lavage is an invasive procedure but is highly reliable in determining the need to explore a victim of blunt abdominal trauma. Sonography is a useful screening measure; DPL may be done if the clinical or sonographic findings are equivocal. The procedures are considered to complement one another.

▶ This is another of the few articles appearing in the past 2 years relating sonography to DPL in determining the need for immediate exploration in patients with blunt abdominal trauma. In this study DPL was 100% sensitive and 99% accurate, and had a predictive value of 97%. In comparison, sonography was 84% sensitive and 86% accurate, and had a predictive value of 89%. The authors conclude correctly that sonography is probably a useful, complementary screening procedure. Diagnostic peritoneal lavage is an invasive procedure, but it is highly reliable in determining the need to explore a victim of blunt abdominal trauma and certainly should be done if clinical or sonographic findings are equivocal. It would appear that these 2 approaches to evaluation are beginning to emerge as useful complementary procedures, with sonography preceding DPL, with the realization that sonography is not nearly as definitive as lavage.— G.T. Shires, M.D.

Evaluation of Computed Tomography and Diagnostic Peritoneal Lavage in Blunt Abdominal Trauma
Meyer DM, Thal ER, Weigelt JA, Redman HC (Univ of Texas, Dallas)
J Trauma 29:1168–1172, August 1989   4–10

In a 2.5-year study, the accuracy of CT was compared with that of diagnostic peritoneal lavage (DPL) in the assessment of blunt abdominal trauma. The series included 301 hemodynamically stable patients aged 1 month to 76 years (mean, 26 years) all of whom had sustained blunt abdominal injuries. They were evaluated by CT, using both oral and intravenous contrast medium, and by DPL. Patients with a positive CT scan, positive findings on DPL, or both, underwent celiotomy. Those with both a negative CT scan and a negative findings on DPL were hospitalized for observation. The diagnostic results were compared with the intraoperative findings.

Of 271 evaluable patients, 194 had both negative CT and negative DPL results and were considered true negatives. Fifty-one patients had both positive CT and positive DPL results, and all had injuries identified at operation. Seven of these patients had significant injuries at operation that had not been identified on the CT scan. Nineteen patients had negative CT and positive DPL results, all of whom had significant injury confirmed at operation. Five patients had positive CT and negative DPL results, 3 of whom had false negative DPL results. Two patients with negative CT scans and false positive DPL results experienced complications of DPL requiring operation. Diagnostic peritoneal lavage was more sensitive than CT. The tests were equally specific. The accuracy of DPL was 98%, and of Ct, 93%.

Both CT and DPL had an acceptable accuracy. Both tests have a place in the assessment of blunt abdominal trauma, and the selection of 1 test over the other should be based on individual circumstances.

▶ This article is one of the huge number of articles appearing in the past several years concerning the use of CT with or without DPL in the assessment of blunt abdominal trauma. The reports in the literature have been variable, some considering CT superior to DPL and others the reverse. The current study was a large one examining 301 hemodynamically stable patients with blunt abdominal injuries. Diagnostic peritoneal lavage had a sensitivity of 96%, compared with 74% for CT. Both modalities had a specificity of 99%. Further, DPL had an accuracy of 98.2% and CT an accuracy of 92.6%.

These authors suggest, has have many others, that CT is a useful adjunct in the hemodynamically stable patient with blunt abdominal trauma. However, sensitivity is higher with DPL, as is accuracy. Consequently, it would appear that, even in the stable group, care should be exercised in deciding which patient might benefit more from CT. However, DPL remains the gold standard in the diagnosis of blunt abdominal trauma.—G.T. Shires, M.D.

Computed Tomography Versus Diagnostic Peritoneal Lavage: Usefulness in Immediate Diagnosis of Blunt Abdominal Trauma

Frame SB, Browder IW, Lang EK, McSwain NE Jr (Naval Hosp, San Diego; Tulane Univ; Louisiana State Univ)

*Ann Emerg Med*18:513–516, May 1989   4–11

The use of CT in place of diagnostic peritoneal lavage (DPL) in the assessment of patients with blunt abdominal trauma is controversial. The accuracy of the 2 techniques in the early diagnosis of blunt abdominal trauma was compared prospectively in 54 patients with acute injuries to the abdomen.

Patients brought to the emergency room with unstable vital signs, peritoneal signs on abdominal examination, or overt evisceration were excluded from the trial and taken to the operating room for immediate surgical exploration. The remaining patients had diagnostic abdominal CT and DPL. They underwent surgical exploration if either technique indicated intra-abdominal injury. The CT scans were read immediately, and clinical decisions on patient care were made on the basis of these interpretations.

Eighteen patients underwent abdominal exploration, 15 of whom actually required surgical intervention. The criteria for surgical exploration were positive DPL findings in 12 patients, positive DPL findings plus positive CT scans in 3 patients, and false positive DPL results in 3 patients with negative CT findings. In the latter 3 patients, DPL had been unsuccessful because of previous abdominal operations. Computed tomography missed splenic injuries in 6 patients and liver lacerations in 3, but all 9 definitely required surgical repair.

Diagnostic peritoneal lavage is the gold standard against which new diagnostic modalities must be measured. This prospective trial confirmed that DPL is more accurate than CT and thus remains for now the diagnostic test of choice in assessment of patients with acute blunt abdominal trauma.

▶ This is another comparison of the use of CT as opposed to DPL in assessment of patients with blunt abdominal trauma. Once again, the authors carefully point out that only injured patients who were hemodynamically stable and without signs of peritoneal injury were included. Once again, DPL emerged as more specific, more sensitive, and more accurate than CT.

This study confirms others in the past 2 years indicating that selection of a patient with abdominal injury for CT diagnosis, even though vital signs are stable, should be done very carefully. The need for immediate operation is far more accurately determined with DPL.— G.T. Shires, M.D.

Microscopic Hematuria After Blunt Trauma: Is Pyelography Necessary?
Thomason RB, Julian JS, Mostellar HC, Pennell TC, Meredith JW (Bowman Gray School of Medicine, Winston-Salem, NC)
Am Surg 55:145–150, March 1989   4–12

Hematuria is frequent in patients with multiple blunt abdominal injuries, but it is not clear whether routine intravenous pyelography (IVP) is necessary. In a 17-month period, 102 consecutive patients underwent IVP after blunt abdominal trauma. Twenty-six patients had gross and 76 had microscopic hematuria.

Abnormal IVPs were found in 27% of the patients with gross hematuria; 2 of these patients required urologic surgery. Of the 76 patients with microscopic hematuria only 1 (1.3%) had an abnormal IVP and did not require urologic surgery. If pyelography had been done only for gross hematuria, all surgically significant urinary tract lesions would have been found and 75% of the patients would have been spared the procedure.

Microscopic hematuria alone is not an indication for emergency IVP. Intravenous pyelography should be done if any other indication of urologic injury is present and in stable patients with gross hematuria. Renal pedicle injuries are best diagnosed by contrast CT or angiography.

▶ This paper was written to challenge the concept that IVP is necessary for patients with microscopic hematuria following blunt trauma. The authors believe it should be reserved for those patients who have gross hematuria or clinical evidence of renal injury. This is a very small series of patients, however, and most authors would agree that the presence of microscopic hematuria is an adequate indication for pyelography following blunt trauma.— G.T. Shires, M.D.

Complications of Negative Laparotomy for Trauma
Weigelt JA, Kingman RA (Univ of Texas, Dallas)
Am J Surg 156:544–547, December 1988   4–13

Morbidity of Negative Laparotomy

Reference	Mechanism of Injury	Patients	Complications	
			n	%
Petersen & Sheldon [18]	Stab, gunshot, & blunt	109	19	17
Bagwell & Ferguson [7]	Blunt	4	0	0
Moore et al [9]	Gunshot	13	0	0
Thompson et al [10]	Stab	26	2	8
Peck & Berne [11]	Stab	30	4	13
Demtriades & Rabinowitz [8]	Stab	11	2	18
Lee et al [2]	Stab	14	2	7
Total	...	207	28	14

(Courtesy of Weigelt JA, Kingman RA: *Am J Surg* 156:544–547, December 1988.)

Routine abdominal exploration in patients with blunt and penetrating trauma yields a high negative rate of findings, but conservative management may result in missed injuries. A key issue is complications, especially small bowel obstruction. The records of patients with negative laparotomies were reviewed retrospectively to assess early and late morbidity.

The charts of 185 patients with penetrating injuries and 63 with blunt injuries who had negative laparotomy findings were examined; 125 patients were asymptomatic; 29 had shock. Results of abdominal examination were normal in 98 patients; 117 patients had localized abdominal tenderness; 18 patients had wound tenderness. There were no associated injuries in 52% of patients. Pneumothorax, long-bone fracture, and brain injury were the most common associated injuries. Acute perioperative morbidity occurred in 53% of patients with associated injuries and in 22% of patients without associated injuries.

On long-term follow-up, 5 had small bowel obstruction. The incidence of small bowel obstruction was related to the type of operative dissection, with greatest incidence in patients requiring peritoneal and retroperitoneal dissection.

Early morbidity after negative laparotomy is more common in patients with associated injuries (table). The risk of postoperative small bowel obstruction is small, especially when extensive dissection is not required. Abdominal exploration is a viable diagnostic and therapeutic procedure in patients with equivocal findings.

▶ This paper is one of the few in recent times to examine the concept of laparotomy being an acceptable form of management of patients with blunt and penetrating trauma when it may be likely that operative findings will be negative. The authors attempted to define these complications and found that the perioperative morbidity that occurred after laparotomy in trauma victims was significant only in those with positive intra-abdominal findings. Early morbidity after a negative laparotomy was quite low and mortality was zero. The authors conclude correctly that abdominal exploration certainly should not be discarded as a viable diagnostic and therapeutic procedure in patients with equivocal physical findings or equivocal CT or diagnostic peritoneal lavage assessments, either one.—G.T. Shires, M.D.

Safety and Efficacy of Mezlocillin: A Single-Drug Therapy for Penetrating Abdominal Trauma

Lou MA, Thadépalli H, Mandal AK (Charles R Drew Postgrad School of Medicine; Univ of California, Los Angeles; Martin Luther King Jr Gen Hosp, Los Angeles)

J Trauma 28:1541–1547, November 1988   4–14

Polyantimicrobial therapy increases the risk of superinfection and produces more toxicity, expecially potential nephrotoxicity from aminoglycosides. Mezlocillin was evaluated as a single-drug treatment for patients with penetrating abdominal trauma. In all, 173 such patients were entered into an open, randomized trial comparing mezlocillin in an intravenous dose of 4 g every 6 hours with combined clindamycin-gentamicin therapy. The latter drugs also were given intravenously, clindamycin in a dose of 600 mg every 6 hours and gentamicin in a dose of 80 mg every 8 hours, adjusted to body weight and renal function.

Of 73 evaluable patients given combined drug therapy, 18 had infectious complications. Five of them failed to respond promptly, but only 1 required a change in treatment. Seventeen of 74 patients given mezlocillin had infectious complications. Infection was not eliminated in 4 patients, and 2 patients required a change in antibiotic treatment. No failure in either group resulted from *Enterococcus* or *Pseudomonas* infection and there were no deaths. More than 90% of patients in each group had a good to excellent therapeutic response. One in each group had azotemia.

Single-agent treatment with mezlocillin was as effective as combined clindamycin-gentamicin therapy in these patients with penetrating abdominal injuries. The routine use of aminoglycosides in this setting is not necessary.

▶ This paper is representative of a number of recent efforts assessing the efficacy of presumptive antibiotics in patients with abdominal trauma. The present study used a safe, single-drug, broad-spectrum antibiotic, mezlocillin, and compared it with combined clindamycin and gentamicin. There were no deaths in either group, and more than 90% of the patients in each group had a good to excellent therapeutic response.

This study fits with several other recent papers indicating that the use of a broad-spectrum, safe, single antibiotic in a presumptive mode given immediately after arrival in the hospital to patients with penetrating abdominal trauma is probably the preferred approach. Furthermore, other recent studies indicate that the use of such therapy can be terminated after a very short period of time, frequently within 24 hours.—G.T. Shires, M.D.

Presumptive Antibiotics for Penetrating Abdominal Wounds
Moore FA, Moore EE, Ammons LA, McCroskey BL (Denver Gen Hosp; Univ of Colorado)
Surg Gynecol Obstet 169:99–103, August 1989   4–15

An optimal antimicrobial spectrum remains the most controversial aspect of presumptive antibiotic therapy in the management of penetrating abdominal wounds. Previous trials suggested that extended-spectrum penicillins are as effective as combination regimens in this setting. A new extended-spectrum penicillin, mezlocillin, was compared with a proven combination antimicrobial regimen that has been given presumptively for acute penetrating abdominal wounds.

During a 3-year period, 317 patients undergoing celiotomy for penetrating abdominal wounds were assigned randomly and prospectively to receive either mezlocillin, 4 g every 6 hours, or the combination regimen of gentamicin, loading dose of 2 mg/kg and then 1.5 mg/kg every 8 hours, and clindamycin, 600 mg every 6 hours. Antibiotic therapy was started in the emergency room. The duration of coverage was determined by the types of injury observed at laparotomy: 5 days for injury to the colon or distal part of the ileum, 2 days for other hollow visceral perforations, and 1 day for all other injuries. Sixteen patients died within 48 hours after injury, and 23 patients were excluded because of breach of protocol. Of the remaining patients, 136 received mezlocillin and 142 received the combined drugs.

No significant difference was noted in any of the measured parameters between the 2 groups. Septic morbidity occurred in 21 of the 136 mezlocillin-treated patients (15%) and in 19 of the double-antibiotic-treated patients (13%). The incidence of major infections, including lobar pneumonia and intra-abdominal abscess, was 13% in both groups. The incidence of multiple organ failure was 1% in the mezlocillin-treated group and 2% in the gentamicin/clindamycin-treated group. Both groups had a 1% septic mortality rate. Analysis of bacterial culture indicated that gram-negative *Escherichia coli* and *Klebsiella* species, as well as gram-positive *Enterococcus* and anaerobic *Bacteroides* species, were the most commonly isolated pathogens.

The results achieved with mezlocillin were similar to those obtained with the combined drugs. Because the latter treatment is more expensive and potentially toxic, mezlocillin is an optimal antibiotic for patients with acute penetrating abdominal wounds.

▶ This is another study comparable to that described in Abstract 4–14 using an extended-spectrum penicillin as a single-drug, presumptive agent in the treatment of penetrating abdominal injuries. This large study included 317 patients undergoing laparotomy for penetrating abdominal wounds and randomly assigned to receive either an extended-spectrum penicillin (mezlocillin) or the combination of a gram-negative bactericidal drug (gentamicin) and an anaerobic drug (clindamycin). The important key here is that antibiotic therapy was started in the emergency room. Results in the 2 groups were comparable. There was a 1% septic mortality rate in both groups, and the instance of multiple organ failure was 2% or less in both groups. Consequently, the use of single-drug, presumptive antibiotic therapy for penetrating abdominal injuries appears to be the preferable approach at the present time. The abdominal infections that did occur were caused by *E. coli, Klebsiella,* and *Enterococcus,* as well as by the anaerobic *Bacteroides.* However, the development of such abscesses after presumptive antibiotic therapy was the same, both with single-drug therapy and the combined drugs as presumptive antibiotics.—G.T. Shires, M.D.

The Role of Intra-Aortic Balloon Occlusion in Penetrating Abdominal Trauma
Gupta RK, Khaneja SC, Flores L, Eastlick L, Longmore W, Shaftan GW (State Univ of New York, Brooklyn)
J Trauma 29:861–865, June 1989   4–16

Control of bleeding is the primary goal in abdominal trauma victims, particularly those near death because of penetrating injury to the torso. Intra-aortic balloon occlusion was attempted in 21 consecutive patients who had missile injuries of the abdomen and were hemodynamically unstable (Fig 4–3). Five patients had no recordable blood pressure, 6 others had refractory hypotension of 80 torr systolic or below, and 10 patients deteriorated to this point while being prepared for or undergoing celiotomy.

Intra-aortic balloon occlusion was effective in 20 patients, whose blood pressure increased. One patient required thoracotomy for clamping of the aorta. Operative control of bleeding was achieved in 11 patients, 7 of whom survived and were discharged in a functional state. Three patients in refractory hypotension and 4 who deteriorated also survived.

Intra-aortic balloon occlusion offers a relatively easy and versatile means of controlling bleeding in patients with penetrating abdominal injury. Thoracotomy has had variable success in these patients. There is a risk of spinal cord damage from any means of thoracic aortic occlusion.

▶ This article reports a technique that is being used increasingly in patients with severe intra-abdominal bleeding after trauma. An intra-aortic balloon introduced through the superficial femoral artery was used to control bleeding in 21 consecutive patients who had missile injuries to the abdomen and were hemodynamically unstable. Effective bleeding control was accomplished in 20 patients, even though operative control was achieved subsequently in only 11.

As the authors state, intra-aortic balloon occlusion offers a relatively easy, quick, and versatile means of controlling bleeding in patients with penetrating

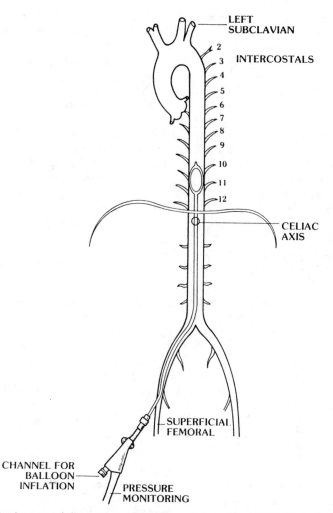

LEFT
SUBCLAVIAN

2
3 INTERCOSTALS
4
5
6
7
8
9
10
11
12

CELIAC
AXIS

SUPERFICIAL
FEMORAL

CHANNEL FOR
BALLOON
INFLATION

PRESSURE
MONITORING

Fig 4–3.—Intra-aortic balloon catheter has been inserted via the right superficial femoral artery; the balloon occludes the descending thoracic aorta just cephalad to the celiac axis. (Courtesy of Gupta RK, Khaneja SC, Flores L, et al: *J Trauma* 29:861–865, June 1989.)

abdominal injury, particularly with massive bleeding and hemodynamic instability. There is, of course, the risk of spinal cord damage, but this will be true with any method used to control the thoracic aorta.—G.T. Shires, M.D.

The Effect of Viable Omentum on Early Bile Leakage and Healing of Liver Lacerations

Trooskin SZ, Pierce RA, Deak SB, Flancbaum L, Mackenzie JW, Greco RS, Boyd CD (Univ of Medicine and Dentistry of New Jersey, New Brunswick)
J Trauma 29:47–50, January 1989   4–17

Viable omentum effectively controls bleeding and abscess formation in patients with severe liver injuries. The added blood and lymphatic supply may reduce sepsis and promote wound healing. The effects of suturing viable omentum into liver lacerations were studied using a rabbit model of a complex laceration with ligation of hepatic lobar blood vessels. After creating the laceration and achieving hemostasis by vessel ligation and electrocoagulation, the wound either was left open or omentum was sutured to its base.

Dye extravasation, simulating bile leakage, did not occur when omentum was present in the wound. Studies of procollagen mRNA, a measure of wound healing, indicated similar healing in both groups. Scar hydroxyproline content was similar in both groups of animals, and the DNA content of wound-edge tissue also was similar.

These findings do not rule out a role for omentum in treating major liver lacerations. It may well promote hemostasis through gentle tamponade and also supply factors that promote coagulation. However, bile leakage and collagen synthesis are not affected. Omentum may decrease the risk of liver wound infection.

▶ This interesting experimental study sought to evaluate the purported benefits of using viable omentum to cover major liver lacerations. Interestingly, studies of procollagen mRNA, a measure of wound healing, indicated similar healing with and without omental patch. Scar hydroxyproline content also was similar, as was the DNA content of wound-edge tissue. The conclusions that bile leakage and collagen synthesis were not affected led the authors to conclude that if there is any role for omentum in the treatment of liver lacerations, it may be as a gentle tamponade. Most investigators in this area have concluded that omentum is probably not of benefit in the management of liver lacerations.—G.T. Shires, M.D.

Hypotension and Bleeding With Various Anatomic Patterns of Blunt Splenic Injury in Adults

Buckman RF JR, Dunham CM, Kerr TM, Militello PR (Univ of Maryland; Temple Univ Hosp, Philadelphia)
Surg Gynecol Obstet 169:206–212, September 1989   4–18

The rethinking of the belief that the spleen is a useless organ, and the development of new surgical techniques for its repair, have led to unprecedented efforts to preserve the injured spleen. Selective nonoperative management of spleen injuries in children is the latest and most radical concept to evolve in this area. However, the applicability of this approach in adults with blunt ruptures of the spleen is controversial. To predict more accurately which patients would be amenable to selective nonoperative management of spleen injuries, the records of 112 adults with blunt splenic lacerations were analyzed retrospectively to determine whether a relationship exists between anatomical extent of splenic injury and splenic bleeding.

All patients had operative anatomical grading of their splenic injuries according to a prospective protocol. Patients with subcapsular hematoma were excluded. Overall, 55% of the patients were hypotensive before operation and 77% were bleeding from the spleen at operation.

No correlation was noted between preoperative hypotension and the incidence of bleeding at operation; many patients who were not hypotensive before operation were bleeding from the spleen at operation. Although patients with severe anatomical grades were more likely to be hypotensive, no significant difference was noted between severe and mild lacerations with respect to the incidence of bleeding from the spleen at operation.

Neither the absence of hypotension nor the presence of a superficial splenic laceration can predict whether or not a patient is bleeding from the spleen. Therefore, before nonoperative management of blunt splenic injury in adults is adopted widely, further investigation is required.

▶ This investigation attempts to answer the question of whether it is safe to undertake the nonoperative management of splenic injuries. This evolves from the radical approach in children with splenic injuries, which are generally low-velocity, confined, handle bar injuries. The present studies were done in adults, and all patients had operative anatomical grading of their splenic injuries. There was no correlation between preoperative hypotension and the incidence of bleeding at operation, as many patients who were not hypotensive before operation were found to be bleeding from the spleen at operation. Furthermore, there was no significant difference between severe and mild lacerations with respect to the incidence of bleeding from the spleen at operation. These authors correctly conclude that neither the absence of hypotension nor the presence of a superficial splenic laceration can predict whether a patient is at risk from severe bleeding from the spleen.—G.T. Shires, M.D.

A Simplified Approach to Techniques of Splenic Salvage
Trooskin SZ, Flancbaum L, Boyarsky AH, Greco RS (Univ of Medicine and Dentistry of New Jersey, New Brunswick)
Surg Gynecol Obstet 168:547–548, June 1989   4–19

In an effort to prevent overwhelming postsplenectomy sepsis, splenic conservation techniques after iatrogenic splenic injury and blunt and penetrating splenic injuries have become common practice. Partial splenectomy recently was recommended as the procedure of choice in the treatment of benign cystic lesions of the spleen. Numerous techniques to control bleeding from the splenic parenchyma after traumatic splenic laceration or during partial splenectomy have been developed.

Technique.—Sharp dissection is used to completely mobilize the spleen from its attachments to the diaphragm, colon, and left kidney so that the spleen is teth-

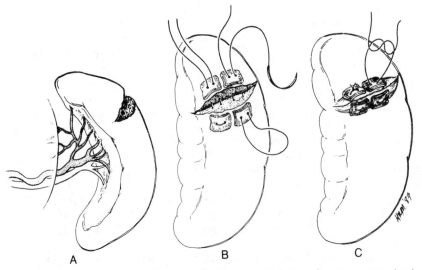

Fig 4–4.—**A,** injuries to the lateral surface of the upper pole. **B,** horizontal mattress sutures placed through pledgets of folded oxidized cellulose. **C,** sutures tied snugly. (Courtesy of Trooskin SZ, Flancbaum L, Boyarsky AH, et al: *Surg Gynecol Obstet* 168:547–548, June 1989.)

ered only by its blood supply. The spleen is suspended by the splenic hilar and short gastric vessels to allow easy visual inspection of all surfaces. Appropriate hilar and short gastric vessels supplying the area to be resected are ligated individually with silk ligatures. Bleeding is minimized by placing a noncrushing clamp at the junction of viable and nonviable splenic tissue. Devitalized splenic tissue then is débrided. Bleeding from lacerations deep into the splenic parenchyma is controlled by compressing raw or oozing splenic tissue between bolsters of folded sheets of oxidized cellulose placed parallel to the laceration. Horizontal mattress sutures are placed through the cellulose bolsters and tied snugly (Fig 4–4). The spleen is then replaced in the left upper quadrant. Drains are not used routinely.

This procedure was successful in 14 patients, 11 of whom required extensive repairs of splenic injuries and 3 of whom had partial splenectomies. None of the patients experienced postoperative bleeding.

▶ Various techniques have been reported in the past few years to increase the rate of splenic salvage after injury from both blunt and penetrating trauma. The technique described by these authors recommends vascular isolation of the splenic vessels and removal of the devitalized splenic tissue with suture control by the compression of splenic tissue between bolsters of folded sheets of absorbable oxidized cellulose placed parallel to the laceration. Horizontal mattress sutures are placed through the cellulose bolsters and tied snugly.

We have performed a technique similar to this and find the use of bolsters in splenic tissue to be advantageous. Another recent technique involves use of the stapler to amputate the vitalized spleen.—G.T. Shires, M.D.

Posttraumatic Autotransplantation of Spleen Tissue

Mizrahi S, Bickel A, Haj M, Lunski I, Shtamler B (Regional Hosp of Western Galilee, Nahariya, Israel)
Arch Surg 124:863–865, July 1989 4–20

The spleen has an important role in host defense, and splenectomy may expose children and adults to the danger of overwhelming pneumococcal infection. Consequently, splenic injury now is managed by salvage procedures whenever possible. When the spleen is damaged beyond repair and splenectomy is unavoidable, autotransplantation of spleen tissue into omental pouches within the peritoneal cavity provides some splenic function.

During a 3-year period 16 patients sustained blunt abdominal trauma that shattered their spleen and required splenectomy for hemostasis after all salvage attempts had failed. Follow-up data were available for 10 patients aged 8–34 years who underwent autotransplantation of approximately 50 g of the removed spleen tissue into the peritoneal cavity. Patients were followed up 4, 8, and 12 weeks after splenectomy to monitor serum IgM levels and to examine blood smears for Howell-Jolly bodies. Splenic scans were performed 10 weeks after tissue implantation. All patients received prophylactic antipneumococcal vaccine and antibiotics after operation.

At 4 weeks after operation IgM levels were still significantly reduced, but they had increased to normal range by 8 weeks after operation. Radioisotope scanning of the spleen performed 10 weeks after operation revealed that the implanted splenic tissue was functioning in all 10 patients. Peripheral blood smear examinations 4 weeks after operation confirmed the disappearance of Howell-Jolly bodies. None of the patients experienced severe infection during a follow-up period of 12–36 months.

Reimplantation of splenic tissue into omental pouches is a safe procedure that provides some splenic function. However, whether this procedure will be functionally efficient and sufficient has not been confirmed, and splenic autotransplantation remains an unproven measure.

▶ This abstract describes another of the many attempts in recent years to preserve splenic tissue after injury. This technique of autotransplantation of splenic tissue has been advocated by a number of surgeons. It is still unknown whether the antipneumococcal or anti-gram-positive organism effects of salvaged spleen when autotransplanted will be effective. However, interesting data are presented concerning the patients followed by the authors. These patients were followed to monitor serum IgM levels and to examine blood smears for Howell-Jolly bodies. In addition, splenic scans were performed 10 weeks after tissue implantation. The authors showed that, by 2 months after operation, IgM levels had returned to normal, and radioisotope scanning of the spleen performed 10 weeks after operation revealed implanted splenic tissue functioning in all patients. Peripheral blood smear examinations 4 weeks after operation confirmed the disappearance of Howell-Jolly bodies. The authors probably conclude correctly that reimplantation of splenic tissue into omental pouches is a safe procedure that provides some splenic function. However, whether this procedure will be functionally efficient and sufficient in the long term is not known.—G.T. Shires, M.D.

Colostomy and Drainage for Civilian Rectal Injuries: Is That All?
Burch JM, Feliciano DV, Mattox KL (Baylor College of Medicine, Houston; Ben Taub Gen Hosp, Houston)
Ann Surg 209:600–611, May 1989   4–21

The routine use of colostomy, presacral drainage, antibiotics, and blood transfusions have dramatically decreased the mortality of traumatic rectal injuries (table). However, the more destructive MK-47 rifle used in the Viet Nam War caused more severe rectal trauma, which required additional measures such as diverting colostomy, débridement and repair of rectal perforations, and irrigation of the distal rectum. There is no agreement among civilian centers about the value of some of these additional therapeutic options. A study was conducted to determine to what extent additional therapeutic options such as those used in Viet Nam are applicable to the treatment of traumatic rectal injuries in civilian urban trauma centers.

During a 10-year period, 88 men and 12 women (average age, 28 years) were treated at an urban trauma center for extraperitoneal rectal injuries. Mechanisms of injury included firearms in 82 patients, stab wounds in 3, other penetrating injuries in 10, and blunt trauma in 5. Rectal examinations were performed in 99 patients, and proctoscopy was performed in 67. Treatment of the rectal injury was determined by the operating surgeon's bias, the patient's condition, and the magnitude of the rectal injury.

Diversion of the fecal stream was achieved by proximal loop colostomies in 44 patients, diverting colostomies in 51, a Harmann's procedure in 4, and abdominoperineal resection in 1. Extraperitoneal rectal perforations were closed in 21 patients; 46 patients underwent rectal irrigation. Transperineal presacral drainage was used in 93 patients. Infectious complications occurred in 11 patients that were directly attributabed to rectal wound management. Four patients died of their injuries.

Mortality and Morbidity From Collected Series of Civilian Rectal Injuries Published During This Decade

Author	Date	Number of Patients	Mortality (%)	Pelvic or Abdominal Abscess (%)	Rectal Fistula (%)
Vitale et al.	1982	32	6	6	0
Grasberger and Hirsch	1983	20	10	25	5
Tuggle and Hubber	1984	47	0	2	6
Mangiante et al.	1985	43	0	9	0
Shannon et al.	1987	26	4	27	15
Present series	1988	100	4	4	3

(Courtesy of Burch JM, Feliciano DV, Mattox KL: *Ann Surg* 209:600–611, May 1989.)

Statistical analysis revealed that only the failure to drain the presacral space increased the likelihood of infectious complications. It could not be determined with certainty that any of the other therapeutic options correlated with outcome. Therefore, a totally diverting colostomy and presacral drainage remain for now the hallmark of treating traumatic rectal injuries.

▶ This study evaluated the treatment of civilian rectal injuries. Standard treatment has evolved using colostomy, presacral drainage, presumptive antibiotics, and blood and fluid requirements as necessary; there is no question that the mortality associated with traumatic rectal injuries has decreased. I reported on this same combination of therapeutic modes in 1973. The current study simply adds to the conclusions. The one thing that is reemphasized dramatically in this series is that presacral drainage is an important and necessary part of the initial treatment of rectal injuries. Similarly, we would agree that most often the diverting double-barrel colostomy is far more effective in diversion than is a simple loop colostomy.—G.T. Shires, M.D.

Percutaneous Drainage of Intra-Abdominal Abscesses Following Abdominal Trauma
Stylianos S, Martin EC, Starker PM, Laffey KJ, Bixon R, Forde KA (Columbia Univ College of Physicians and Surgeons; Presbyterian Hosp, New York)
J Trauma 29:584–588, May 1989   4–22

Intra-abdominal abscess as a complication of emergency celiotomy in the management of abdominal penetrating injuries remains an important cause of morbidity and mortality. Intra-abdominal abscesses traditionally have been treated by reoperation and drainage, but percutaneous catheter drainage (PCD) has become a feasible alternative in the management of abdominal abscesses.

During a 42-month period, 408 patients underwent emergency celiotomy after sustaining abdominal injuries. Twenty-five of the 380 patients who survived for at least 7 days after operation had postoperative intra-abdominal fluid collections that required treatment. Nine patients had biliary, urinary, or enteric fistulas associated with the abscesses.

Twenty-one patients with intra-abdominal fluid collections were managed successfully by PCD, 3 patients underwent reoperation, and 1 had transrectal drainage of pelvic abscess. Cultures were positive in 86% of the abscesses. The median interval from injury to PCD was 13 days. The duration of catheter drainage was less than 4 weeks in 62% of the patients. None of the patients required subsequent operative procedures because of an inadequately drained fluid collection. In 1 patient with a complex subphrenic collection after splenectomy, a small, self-limited pneumothorax developed from the unintended transpleural path of the catheter. No other complications occurred. In retrospect, even the 4 patients who underwent reoperation could have been treated safely with PCD.

Percutaneous catheter drainage is recommended for all postoperative trauma patients with accessible abdominal abscesses. Reoperation should be reserved for patients in whom safe acccess to the abscess is not available, or in whom PCD has failed to control the sepsis.

▶ This is a large series of patients with intra-abdominal abscesses after emergency abdominal procedures for trauma. Intra-abdominal fluid collections that required treatment developed in 6.6% of the patients who survived for 1 week after operation. This is about what is reported on most trauma services. In this series, all of the patients in whom intra-abdominal fluid collection management was done with PCD had a successful outcome. In 21 instances 3 patients underwent reoperation, and 1 patient had transrectal drainage of a pelvic abscess. Certainly, with data from a series as large as this, it should be clear that postoperative trauma patients with accessible abdominal abscesses can be treated safely, in competent hands, by PCD. Reoperation should be reserved as the authors point out, for patients in whom safe access to the abscess is not available or in whom PCD has failed to control the sepsis.— G.T. Shires, M.D.

Pediatric Trauma: Need for Surgical Management

Kaufmann CR, Rivara FP, Maier RV (Univ of Washington)
J Trauma 29:1120–1126, August 1989   4–23

Trauma surgeons now are initially responsible for the resuscitation, triage, and follow-up care of injured children. However, some pediatricians propose that *they* be made primarily responsible for resuscitation and triage, with surgical care being initiated only through consultation with the surgeon. This concept is advocated via the Advanced Pediatric Life Support course. If a significant number of injured children would require emergent or urgent surgical intervention, however, primary care by pediatricians would be inappropriate, as adding this echelon of responsibility would cause a delay in definitive operative management.

To determine the frequency of operative intervention in pediatric trauma victims, a retrospective study was made of 376 injured children aged less than 15 years (mean, 7.9 years) who were admitted during a 30-month period to 1 trauma center. Sixty-two children were severely injured. The mean emergency room Revised Trauma Scores were 10.2 in the entire patient population and 4.7 in the severely injured subgroup. The mean Injury Severity Scores were 16 in the entire group and 42 in the severely injured subgroup. Operations were classified as emergent, urgent, and elective.

Of the 376 children, 52% required at least 1 operation, with 194 children undergoing a total of 254 operations during their hospital stay. There were 27 deaths, yielding an overall mortality of 7.2%. Twenty-two children with severe injuries arrived in the hospital with persistent hemodynamic instability; 76% underwent emergent operation. However, only 6 of these 22 children survived. Furthermore, 42% of the 90 moderately injured children and 14% of the 224 children with only minimal injuries also required emergent operation.

Surgery was necessary for more than half of the injured children brought to this trauma center. The addition of triage by pediatricians as another echelon of care in an already complex trauma system would delay definitive care and create the potential for catastrophic outcomes.

▶ These courageous authors took a significant problem head-on, namely, the recent proposal by pediatricians that they be made primarily responsible for the resuscitation and triage of injured children. They examine the question of whether a significant number of injured children would require urgent surgical intervention, in which case primary care by pediatricians would be inappropriate as an additional echelon of responsibility. This added responsibility might well cause a delay in definitive operative management. Of the 376 injured children studied, more than half brought to a trauma center required operation. The authors conclude that the addition of triage by pediatricians as another echleon of care in an already complex trauma system would delay definitive care and create the potential for catastrophic outcomes. This article should stimulate a lot of discussion in trauma centers around the nation.—G.T. Shires, M.D.

5 Wound Healing

Enhancement of Wound Healing by Topical Treatment With Epidermal Growth Factor
Brown GL, Nanney LB, Griffen J, Cramer AB, Yancey JM, Curtsinger LJ III, Holtzin L, Schultz GS, Jurkiewicz MJ, Lynch JB (Emory Univ; Vanderbilt Univ; Univ of Louisville)
N Engl J Med 321:76–79, July 13, 1989   5–1

Topically applied epidermal growth factor accelerates epidermal regeneration of skin-graft donor sites and partial-thickness burns in animals. In a prospective, randomized, double-blind study to test its effect on humans, 12 patients requiring skin grafting for reconstructive surgery or burns had paired donor sites prepared. One site from each patient was treated with silver sulfadiazine cream alone and the other with cream containing epidermal growth factor (10 μg/mL). Healing was assessed by planimetric analysis of daily photographs.

Compared with unaugmented silver sulfadiazine, treatment with epidermal growth factor significantly lessened the average time to 25% and 50% healing by about 1 day and to 75% and 100% healing by approximately 1.5 days. Punch-biopsy sections taken from donor sites 3 days after healing began supported these results. Follow-up a maximum of 1 year later showed no complications or evidence of neoplasia.

The ability to accelerate regeneration could be valuable for patients with large burns but limited donor areas. The full clinical implications of these observations require further exploration.

▶ The treatment of a skin donor site is about the only conceivable indication for increasing epidermal migration kinetics. The data in this paper are important in the study of epidermal growth factor; clinical usefulness is not obvious at this time.—E.E. Peacock, Jr., M.D.

Reconstitution of Structure and Cell Function in Human Skin Grafts Derived From Cryopreserved Allogeneic Dermis and Autologous Cultured Keratinocytes
Langdon RC, Cuono CB, Birchall N, Madri JA, Kuklinska E, McGuire J, Moellmann GE (Yale Univ)
J Invest Dermatol 91:478–485, November 1988   5–2

Skin grafts consisting of allogeneic dermis and stratified keratinocyte cultures derived from autologous epidermis were used to provide skin replacement in 6 severely burned patients.

Technique.—Cryopreserved split-thickness cadaveric skin was grafted onto débrided wounds. Autologous keratinocytes were cultured from uninjured donor areas. Allograft epidermis was abraded and replaced with keratinocyte cultures several weeks later. The final grafts were therefore composites of autologous cultured epidermis and allogeneic dermis.

Patient, followed for 28 months, underwent immunohistochemical and ultrastructural studies of the graft. Just before grafting, thawed cryopreserved skin reacted with antibodies against laminin and type IV collagen in normal patterns. On day 29 after grafting, the dermal-epidermal basement membrane zone (BMZ 1) reacted weakly with both antibodies, and anticollagen type IV reactivity was absent from the microvascular basement membrane zone (BMZ 2). Antilaminin reactivity of BMZ 2 was moderately intense. The allograft epidermis was replaced with autologous keratinocyte cultures 29 days after grafting. Twenty-five days after this, staining of both BMZs was intense with both antibodies. Forty-seven days after culture placement BMZ 1 revealed only small hemidesmosomes, a few incipient anchoring fibrils, and a discontinuous lamina densa. The BMZ 2 was fully reconstituted. By day 124 both BMZs were normal. On day 76 the presence of lymphocytes, organellar debris, and hyperactive collagen fibrillogenesis, which indicated dermal remodeling, was noted in the dermis. The microvasculature was well differentiated. No elastic fibers or nerves were found, however. In the epidermis, melanocytes and evidence of melanosome transfer were noted 5, 47, and 95 days after culture placement.

The immunohistochemical and ultrastructural findings indicated normal cell function in the composite skin graft used to treat this severely burned patient. The composite procedure reconstitutes skin with excellent textural and histologic qualities.

▶ The use of allogeneic dermis may provide the best answer so far to the problem of epidermal adherence. The frontier in this research is reconstitution of basement membrane adherence.—E.E. Peacock, Jr., M.D.

In Vitro Toxicity of Topical Antimicrobial Agents to Human Fibroblasts
McCauley RL, Linares HA, Pelligrini V, Herndon DN, Robson MC, Heggers JP
(Univ of Texas, Galveston; Shriners' Burns Inst, Galveston)
J Surg Res 46:267–274, March 1989   5–3

Burn wound closure ultimately is dependent on the cellular effects of topical antimicrobial agents. The in vitro responses of human diploid fibroblasts and dermal fibroblasts to both silver sulfadiazine and mafenide acetate were examined.

Both types of fibroblasts were much less numerous within 48 hours of exposure to silver sulfadiazine. A concentration of 0.01% markedly reduced cell counts, and matrix protein content was decreased in parallel. Filtered silver sulfadiazine exhibited dose-related destructive cellular effects. Cell counts also were much reduced by exposure to mafenide acetate. Progressive cell destruction was evident with this antimicrobial agent as well.

The toxic effects of commonly used topical antimicrobial agents on fibroblasts may help to explain observations of delayed wound healing.

▶ There is no doubt that topical antimicrobial agents inhibit clinical wound healing in burned patients. The results reported in this paper indicate a possible mechanism and point out the need to prevent overuse of sulfadiazine and mafenide as well as to find some way to counteract the deleterious effects of antimicrobials on fibroblast activity.—E.E. Peacock, Jr., M.D.

Reversal of Adriamycin-Impaired Wound Healing by Transforming Growth Factor-Beta
Curtsinger LJ, Pietsch JD, Brown GL, von Fraunhofer A, Ackerman D, Polk HC Jr, Schultz GS (Univ of Louisville; Univ of Texas, San Antonio; Univ of Florida)
Surg Gynecol Obstet 168:517–522, June 1989   5–4

Recent data suggest that locally produced peptide growth factors may mediate normal healing. Impaired wound healing, caused by doxorubicin (Adriamycin), may be reversible with early exposure of regenerating tissue cells to growth factors. Rats pretreated with doxorubicin, 8 mg/kg, received locally applied biosynthetic transforming growth factor-β or epidermal growth factor (EGF) to standardized incisions. The tensile strength of the incisions was measured.

Compared with normal rats, pretreated rats had significantly decreased wound tear strength and wound tear energy at 7 days and 10 days. Wound healing impairment was reversed by a single, 2-μg dose of transforming growth factor-β in a collagen vehicle. Wound tear strength and energy became nearly normal. Tensile strength was not increased by 1 50-μg dose of EGF in hyaluronic acid, perhaps because of failure to formulate EGF in a release-prolonging vehicle.

The findings suggest that growth factors may promote incision healing. More studies of various growth factors, alone and in combination, as well as in other vehicles, are needed.

▶ So much attention is being placed on macrophage-derived growth factors now that it seems appropriate to review this article in the YEAR BOOK. It seems to me, however, that if any of these factors are to be useful clinically, they will most likely be helpful in overcoming the lag phase of wound healing in normal individuals rather than stimulating wound healing in abnormal individuals.—E.E. Peacock, Jr., M.D.

The Stretched Scar: The Benefit of Prolonged Dermal Support
Elliot D, Mahaffey PJ (St Andrew's Hosp, Essex, England)
Br J Plast Surg 42:74–78, January 1989   5–5

The rate of scar stretching after surgery is maximal during the first 6 months. To determine the effect of dermal support with a nonabsorbable suture during this period, 86 skin wounds (divided into 3 study groups) of the arm and forearm resulting from elliptical excisions of tattoos were compared after 1 year.

In 31 wounds there was a highly significant and numerically considerable reduction (37.5%) of scar stretching with the subcuticular polypropylene (Prolene) suture remaining in situ for 6 months compared with the conventional percutaneous nylon suture. In 26 wounds a significant reduction in scar width (15.7%) was noted when the subcuticular polypropylene suture remained in situ for 6 months compared with 3 weeks. In 29 wounds subcuticular polyglycolic acid (Dexon) suture achieved no reduction in scar width compared with the conventional interrupted suture.

Scar stretching after surgery is no longer an uncontrollable factor. A comparison study of polypropylene and polyglyconate (Maxon), the newer generation of absorbable suture with complete absorption at 180 days, is needed.

▶ Permanent suture material that is either white or clear is more difficult to obtain because white silk is no longer available. The need for a permanent subcuticular suture to prevent stretch of a scar has been confused in the past but seems clearly justified in view of this paper and several others substantiating the usefulness of permanent dermal approximation.—E.E. Peacock, Jr., M.D.

Topical Silicone Gel: A New Treatment for Hypertrophic Scars

Ahn ST, Monafo WW, Mustoe TA (Washington Univ; Catholic Univ, Seoul, South Korea)
Surgery 106:781–787, October 1989   5–6

Hypertrophic scars, particularly those developing after deep burn injury, are difficult to treat. Available evidence on the efficacy of elastic compression is anecdotal. Because reports from the United Kingdom suggested that sheets of silicone gel can soften hypertrophic burn scars, that approach was evaluated prospectively in 10 adults who had 14 hypertrophic scars. All but 2 had scars resulting from burn injury that were 2 months to 4 years old. Silicone gel sheets 3.5-mm thick were applied for 8 consecutive weeks.

Eleven scars were treated for at least 12 hours a day, and all of them were improved at the end of treatment. The 3 scars treated less intensively did not improve clinically. The outcome was not related to the age of the patient or the scar, or to the site of the scar. Complications included superficial maceration of the scar and a rash. Elastometry confirmed increased elasticity of the treated scars. Evaluation of biopsy specimens gave no evidence of inflammation or foreign body reaction and showed no change in vascularity.

Measurable clinical improvement occurs in 8 weeks of treatment of hypertrophic scars with Silastic gel. There appears to be no leakage of silicone into the scars; side effects were minor and transient.

▶ If I had seen this myself I would not believe it, but the quality of the work and the report are such that the observations cannot be overlooked. There must be something here, although it is difficult to see now what the explanation is.—E.E. Peacock, Jr., M.D.

Polypropylene Mesh Closure of Infected Abdominal Wounds
Jones JW, Jurkovich GJ (Univ of South Alabama, Mobile)
Am Surg 55:73–76, January 1989   5–7

Closing large infected abdominal wall defects after traumatic tissue loss or necrotizing fasciitis is a difficult surgical problem. Polypropylene mesh, which has proved safe and effective in the closure of clean, elective hernias, has been advocated for this purpose. Polypropylene mesh was used in closure of infected or dehisced midline abdominal incisions in 5 patients seen during a 3-year period. An average of 200 cm^2 of the mesh was placed. It was secured with 0-prolene in a horizontal mattress fashion in all cases. All wounds were packed open with saline-soaked gauze.

Complications related directly to the use of polypropylene mesh occurred in 80% of the patients: a small bowel fistula developed in 4 and wound dehiscence in 1. One of these patients died. All 4 patients with complications subsequently required removal of the mesh. Two patients had significant weight loss that allowed mesh removal and primary fascial closure after a bowel fistula was surgically repaired. In a third patient with a bowel fistula and wound dehiscence, fistula repair, removal of the mesh, and wound closure with rectus rotational flaps were performed. The fourth had mesh removal and fistula repair but died subsequently of multisystem organ failure. Complications occurred from 14 to 487 days after placement of polypropylene mesh.

In this small series the overall complication rate was 80%. The incidence of serious complications may be reduced by covering the mesh with full-thickness skin or muscle flaps in the early postoperative period, or removing the mesh at the earliest time conducive to fascial closure. It is often impossible, however, to predict in which patients early removal of the mesh will be possible, and full-thickness coverage of a persistently infected wound usually fails. The use of polypropylene mesh in the emergency setting is associated with an unacceptably high complication rate, and alternative ways of caring for such patients should be explored.

▶ In my view, there is no reason to put polypropylene mesh into an infected wound. Evisceration can be prevented by use of a proper dressing and binder until fibrin adhesions develop. Skin grafts can be applied directly to bowel after evisceration is no longer a danger. The long-term results of putting polypropylene mesh into an infected wound are so well known now that the practice should be abandoned, even though short-term results are acceptable.—E.E. Peacock, Jr., M.D.

Recent Trends in the Management of Incisional Herniation
Read RC, Yoder G (John L McClellan Mem VA Hosp, Little Rock; Univ of Arkansas for Med Sciences, Little Rock)
Arch Surg 124:485–488, April 1989   5–8

Incisional herniation remains a problem despite technical advances in wound closure materials. Data on an unselected consecutive series of 206 patients, operated on for incisional hernia, were analyzed retrospectively.

In 56.1% of the patients the incisional hernia had appeared more than 1 year after initial celiotomy. Sutures were used to repair 82%; 18% had a plastic prosthesis. After primary repair the recurrence rate was 24.8%, and after reoperation, 41.7%. The rate was similar in both groups because protrusion around the edges occurred with plastic prostheses. Most of the hernia sites were in the abdominal midline. The infection rate was slightly less than 20% after celiotomy.

Delayed herniation may have been caused by "buttonholing" of the rectus sheath by a gradual sawing motion of the continuous nonabsorbable suture. Use of synthetic, longer lasting sutures may reduce delayed herniation. Problems with polypropylene mesh (Marlex) may occur without sufficient external and internal overlap where it attaches to the edge of the defect (Fig 5–1). Subxiphoid epigastric hernias after sternotomy do not require plastic prostheses.

▶ Polypropylene mesh has solved many problems in abdominal wall reconstruction. The search for normal tissue, relief of tension, and simplification of

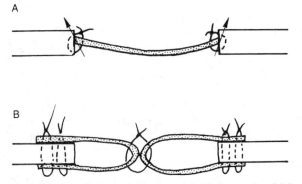

Fig 5–1.—A, limited fixation of knitted polypropylene mesh (Marlex) to edge of defect. **B,** sandwich repair giving good lateral fixation. (Courtesy of Read RC, Yoder G: *Arch Surg* 124:485–488, April 1989.)

operative technique argue strongly for the use of a patch rather than approximation of living tissue.—E.E. Peacock, Jr., M.D.

Modified Gluteus Maximus V-Y Advancement Flaps
Heywood AJ, Quaba AA (Bangour Gen Hosp, Broxburn, West Lothian, England)
Br J Plast Surg 42:263–265, May 1989   5–9

Closure of wide surgical defects is difficult with a simply advanced V-Y flap because of tension in the center. A modification of a gluteus

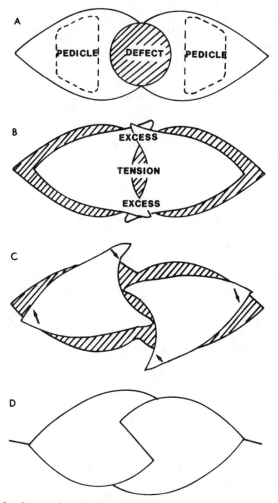

Fig 5–2.—**A,** flap design with attachment to pedicle retained in middle third. **B,** advancement alone fails to make optimum use of flap tissue. **C,** flaps advanced and rotated. *Arrows* indicate direction of transpositions. **D,** lines of final closure. (Courtesy of Heywood AJ, Quaba AA: *Br J Plast Surg* 42:263–265, May 1989.)

maximus V-Y advancement flap was designed to add rotation and transposition.

Technique.—The flap design provides extra tissue at the advancing edge corners in the shape of horns (Fig 5–2). The flap is undermined at the surface of the gluteus maximus muscle and elevated, leaving a pedicle in its middle third. The flap is rotated so that a horn of 1 flap and the advancing edge of the other meet at midpoint. The 2 other horns and flap apices fill the remaining defect sections by transposition. The suture forms a Z-shaped line across the defect's midsection.

This method was successful in 7 patients, 6 of whom had a pressure ulcer. In 1 a large skin tumor had been removed. A similar method has been used for head and neck defects and may also be used elsewhere. The extra tissue allows the flap to be sutured in position without tension, and obviates the need to use muscle detachments for blood supply.

▶ The development of gluteus maximus musculocutaneous flaps has made a real contribution to one of the hardest problems in the care of bedridden patients. Continued experience has shown that almost any defect can be closed by development of these relatively simple flaps. The rotation advancement technique reported in this paper increases the usefulness of local tissue repair of very large midline defects.—E.E. Peacock, Jr., M.D.

Local Fasciocutaneous Flaps for Cutaneous Coverage of Lower Extremity Wounds
Hallock GG (Allentown Hosp, Allentown, Pa)
J Trauma 29:1240–1244, September 1989   5–10

Some form of vascularized flap is often needed to repair a soft tissue deficit resulting from severe lower extremity trauma. Transposition of the neighboring soleus or gastrocnemius muscles is a lengthy procedure and is associated with a high rate of major complications. A new method was developed that involves inclusion of the deep crural fascia with local skin flaps.

The best results with local fasciocutaneous flaps are obtained in patients whose wounds are of moderate size and relatively uncontaminated. Ideally, the flap is oriented with a proximal base overlying the known direct cutaneous, musculocutaneous, or septocutaneous perforators. These perforators ramify within the suprafascial plexus and in turn nourish the overlying skin. The dominant longitudinal orientation of circulation throughout the lower leg should be taken advantage of by designing vertically oriented flaps.

In a 7-year period 41 local fasciocutaneous flaps were used to cover lower leg wounds in 38 patients (Fig 5–3). All but 2 were successful; flap necrosis required limb amputation in 1 of these patients. Successful flaps healed without need for further reconstruction. Some type of complica-

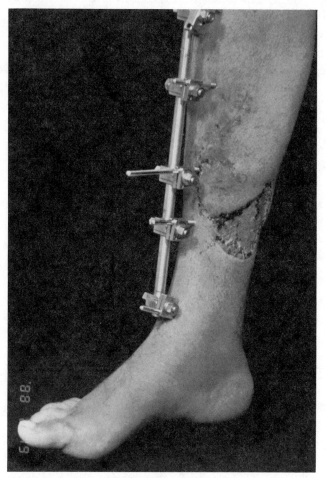

Fig 5–3.—Medial, superior-based fasciocutaneous flap at 10 weeks. (Courtesy of Hallock GG: *J Trauma* 29:1240–1244, September 1989.)

tion occurred in 8 flaps, most in the subset used for distal third lower leg wounds.

These patients might have otherwise required a complex microsurgical tissue transfer. Advantages of the fasciocutaneous flap include simplicity, diminished morbidity, and low risk of hematoma. Although larger or infected defects require local muscle or free tissue transfers, fasciocutaneous flaps are ideal for small and moderate-sized defects in the lower leg.

▶ More simple methods are still needed to replace soft tissue in the lower leg, ankle, and foot. This is a welcome addition to the almost encyclopedic stable of highly technical and often unreasonably expensive techniques.—E.E. Peacock, Jr., M.D.

6 Infections

Preincisional Intraparietal Augmentin in Abdominal Operations
Pollock AV, Evans M, Smith GMR (Scarborough Hosp, Scarborough, Yorkshire, England)
Ann R Coll Surg Engl 71:97–100, March 1989   6–1

Intravenous injection of antibiotic at induction of anesthesia was substituted for direct placement of an antibiotic solution in the wound before closing when studies showed no advantage to the latter method of wound prophylaxis. Now "preincisional intraincisional" injection has been proposed as a means of achieving both adequate serum levels of the antibiotic and high local concentrations. The incidence of wound infection was compared in 328 patients receiving Augmentin intravenously and in 296 patients given the antibiotic intraparietally.

The patients, who were randomly assigned to 1 of the 2 treatment methods, were scheduled for major abdominal surgery. They were evaluated according to a Preoperative Assessment of Fitness Score, with higher scores indicating a greater risk of major postoperative complications and death.

The mortality rate was similar in the 2 groups; 19 given intravenous and 21 given intraincisional prophylaxis died. Two patients in each group died of intraperitoneal sepsis, and 4 in each group died of pneumonia. Preoperative Assessment of Fitness Scores of 6 or more had been recorded for all but 6 of the 41 patients who died. The rates of complications were similar in the 2 groups, but infections occurred nearly twice as often in the patients treated intravenously. The difference in wound infection rate—15.9% vs. 8.4%—was highly significant. Measurements obtained at the incision site showed much higher concentrations of amoxycillin and clavulanic acid in the group given intraparietal prophylaxis. Thus preincisional intraparietal injection is more effective than intravenous injection of Augmentin in preventing surgical wound infection.

▶ It appeared first that systemic antibiotics were needed before surgery. Then it appeared that intravenous antibiotics would be just as effective during surgery. And now it appears that injection of antibiotics directly into tissue at the time of surgery is the most effective way to prevent soft tissue infection. One cannot help but wonder if we are not reaching a point of diminishing returns in searching for ways to administer antibiotics.—E.E. Peacock, Jr., M.D.

Local Antibiotic Infusion After Primary Closure of Heavily Contaminated Wounds
ReMine SG, Organ CH (Lahey Clinic Med Ctr, Burlington, Mass)
Infect Surg 7:55–59, February 1989   6–2

Contaminated (class 3 and class 4) operative wounds have usually been treated by delayed primary closure. An alternative method, primary closure followed by local antibiotic infusion, offered good results. Ninety-seven patients with a total of 100 heavily contaminated wounds underwent primary closure.

Procedure.—After the skin is scrubbed and sutured, a 3-mm soft Silastic Jackson-Pratt infusion catheter is placed in the subcutaneous tissue along the long axis of the wound. The subcutaneous space is irrigated with 500 mL of a triple antibiotic solution (neomycin, polymyxin, and gentamicin) before the wound is closed. After closure, 5–10 mL of the solution is administered every 8 hours for 3–4 days. Systemic antibiotic therapy is started before surgery and continued until the patient's discharge from the hospital.

Of the 100 wounds, 61 were judged class 4—dirty and infected wounds with pus encountered during surgery. The rate of postoperative complications was 16%, and the incidence of local wound fluid accumulation was 5%. Only 1 of the fluid collections was considered major. Wound infections were associated with younger age (less than 8 years), extensive intra-abdominal abscesses, and the use of stainless steel staples.

The exceptionally low rate of wound infection after primary closure in this study suggests that this method is safe and effective and may give a better cosmetic appearance after healing. In selected dirty traumatic wounds, delayed primary closure may be unnecessary.

▶ One cannot help but wonder why it is necessary to close 100 wounds that are heavily contaminated, but if it is necessary to do so, the technique outlined in this paper appears helpful.—E.E. Peacock, Jr., M.D.

Timing of Prophylactic Antibiotics in Abdominal Surgery: Trial of a Pre-Operative Versus an Intra-Operative First Dose
Bates T, Siller G, Crathern BC, Bradley SP, Zlotnik RD, Couch C, James RDG, Kaye CM (William Harvey Hosp, Willesborough, Kent, England)
Br J Surg 76:52–56, January 1989   6–3

When prophylactic antibiotics are used for abdominal surgery, the first dose is usually given before the operation. Infection rates were compared in a randomized, double-blind trial of antibiotics begun preoperatively and after initial abdominal exploration in patients undergoing emergency or at-risk abdominal surgery.

Data on 700 procedures were analyzed; 3 intravenous doses of 500 mg of metronidazole plus 1 g of cefazolin were administered. At the end of surgery, antibiotic plasma concentrations were significantly lower in the group in whom antibiotics were given preoperatively but were well within the therapeutic range. Wound infection rates, including minor and delayed infections, were 16.7% in the preoperative antibiotic group and 15.4% in the group receiving antibiotics after initial exploration; the difference was not statistically significant. In appendicitis the wound infection rates were 12.1% and 13.9% in the 2 groups, respectively. Nonfatal deep sepsis was more common in the group receiving preoperative antibiotics. Postoperative infection was twice as common in obese patients with body mass indexes of 26 or higher than in patients whose body mass indexes were lower than 24.

This study found no advantage in starting prophylactic antibiotics preoperatively in patients scheduled for abdominal surgery, even in patients with appendicitis, in which this could be considered a treatment rather than prophylaxis. Obesity was a risk factor for wound infection, with body mass index proving to be a sensitive discriminator.

▶ Previous studies indicating that "a load of antibiotics should be on board" before surgery apparently were not correct. Considerable experience has been accumulated to show that antibiotics can be started intravenously when the need for antibiotic therapy appears during surgery with just as good a result as if prophylactic antibiotics were started before surgery. Such data make it possible to reduce the use and expense of antibiotics in many patients.—E.E. Peacock, Jr., M.D.

Prevention and Treatment of Endotoxin and Sepsis Lethality With Recombinant Human Tumor Necrosis Factor
Sheppard BC, Fraker DL, Norton JA (Natl Cancer Inst, Bethesda, Md)
Surgery 106:156–162, August 1989   6–4

Tumor necrosis factor (TNF) released in response to endotoxin has been implicated in the toxic and lethal effects of bacterial sepsis and endotoxemia. Previous experimental studies in rats have shown that repetitive twice-daily intraperitoneal administration of sublethal doses of recombinant human TNF (rTNF) confers protection against a subsequent challenge with a lethal dose of rTNF or endotoxin. More recent studies have shown that the same treatment regimen reduces the morbidity and mortality in a rat model of cecal ligation and puncture. Whether a single low-dose intravenous injection of rTNF can rapidly induce tolerance and confer protection from a septic insult was investigated.

Pretreatment with a single low intravenous dose of rTNF protected rats from a lethal dose of rTNF or endotoxin administered 24 hours later, yielding a significant advantage when compared with vehicle-pretreated control rats. Pretreatment with intravenous administration of rTNF also protected against a lethal challenge with endotoxin given 24 hours later. In addition, intravenously administered rTNF protected against the lethal effects of cecal ligation and puncture. Protection did not occur when rTNF was given 24 hours after cecal ligation and puncture.

Pretreatment with a single dose of rTNF does confer protection against a subsequent lethal septic insult with rTNF or endotoxin. Protection appears to occur rapidly. Early administration of low-dose rTNF may have clinical application in the prevention and treatment of the lethality of sepsis.

▶ If we keep looking we are going to find a real use for various growth factors and similar chemical messengers. There are plenty of companies ready to produce these factors; all they need is some evidence that they can be injected into human beings with beneficial results.—E.E. Peacock, Jr., M.D.

Monitoring of Postoperative Intra-Abdominal Septic Complications Following Major Abdominal Surgery

Schöffel U, Kopp K-H, Lausen M, Ruf G, Farthmann E-H (Univ of Freiburg, West Germany)
Surg Res Comm 5:49–53, 1989   6–5

Every inflammatory response results in activation of cellular and plasmatic systems that can characterize a septic development. This response has been shown in early peritonitis. The use of parameters that represent the activation state of the single systems was assessed during the postoperative course after major abdominal surgery.

The time sequence pattern of the levels of the inflammatory parameters studied was determined in 21 patients considered to be at high risk for the development of intra-abdominal complications. In an earlier series the C3 split product C3a, the fibrinogen split product fibrinopeptide A (FPA), and the elastase-α_1 proteinase inhibitor-complex ($E\alpha_1PI$) were significantly different between survivors and nonsurvivors at the time of admission and during the postoperative period. In the current series the uncomplicated postoperative course was characterized by slight increases in FPA, C3a, $E\alpha_1PI$ in the first 3–4 postoperative days, followed by gradual renormalization. A persistent increase or later increase of fivefold to tenfold closely correlated with postoperative complications, necessitating relaparotomy in 7 patients. When the 3 parameters exceeding their cut-off levels were taken as a positive result, a sensitivity of 100% and a specificity of 100% was obtained on the third day after surgery.

▶ Fibrinogen split product, elastase α_1, appears significantly different in survivors than nonsurvivors with intra-abdominal sepsis. Other parameters measured such as plasma fibronectin have not been found to be significantly different. The question of whether abnormal levels can favorably influence treatment is not clear.—E.E. Peacock, Jr., M.D.

Management of Severe Intra-Abdominal Sepsis: Single Agent Antibiotic Therapy With Cefotetan Versus Combination Therapy With Ampicillin, Gentamicin and Metronidazole

Huizinga WKJ, Baker LW, Kadwa H, van den Ende J, Francis AJ, Francis GM (Natal Univ, Durban, South Africa)
Br J Surg 75:1134–1138, November 1988   6–6

Single-drug therapy with the new semisynthetic cephamycin, cefotetan, was compared with standard combined drug therapy in 100 adults who required surgery for intra-abdominal sepsis. Cefotetan was given intravenously in a dose of 2 g every 12 hours. The comparison patients received 1 g of ampicillin every 6 hours and 80 mg of gentamicin plus 500 mg of metronidazole every 8 hours, all intravenously.

Sites of infection were comparable in the 2 groups. Antibiotics were given for 5–6 days on average. Sixty-five of the 97 surviving patients had a satisfactory response to treatment. In 11 patients wound infections developed, and 10 had respiratory or urinary tract infections. Cefotetan-treated patients did better clinically but not to a significant degree. Abnormalities in laboratory values were more frequent in the cefotetan-treated group.

Treatment with a single broad-spectrum antimicrobial agent, cefotetan, was as effective as combined drug therapy in patients with severe intra-abdominal sepsis. Adverse effects were not frequent in this study. Antibiotic therapy is only an adjunct to appropriate surgery and supportive management of organ dysfunction in patients with intra-abdominal sepsis.

▶ These data are encouraging. There are many advantages to using a single agent, and it appears that cefotetan fulfills all of the objectives that a combination of other agents is prescribed for. Anything that will simplify antimicrobial therapy in the surgical patient is appreciated.—E.E. Peacock, Jr., M.D.

Small-Bowel Perforation Complicating the Open Treatment of Generalized Peritonitis
Mastboom WJB, Kuypers HHC, Schoots FJ, Wobbes T (St Radboud Hosp, Nijmegen, The Netherlands)
Arch Surg 124:689–692, June 1989   6–7

Nontraumatic small-bowel perforations rarely occur spontaneously, although their appearance has been noted during open abdominal treatment of patients with generalized peritonitis. Studies were made in patients with such perforations to learn the cause and optimal treatment.

In some cases of relaparotomy performed on patients who remain septic during the treatment of generalized peritonitis, the abdominal wall is left open to avoid extreme tension on the fascial sutures and a mesh is applied. In a 10-year period, 135 of 394 patients seen at 1 institution had the abdominal wall left open during this procedure; in 27 of them perforations of the jejunum or ileum developed. Data on 14 of these who had no predisposing pathophysiologic factors for perforations developing were reviewed.

The mean age was 51 years. All 14 had undergone from 4 to 20 laparotomies. Small-bowel perforations of unknown origin were diagnosed 43 times, from 1 to 13 times per patient. The mean time to occurrence was the eighth postoperative day after laparotomy. All 14 patients required treatment in the intensive care unit for intra-abdominal sepsis; the mean length of stay was 74 days. Most of the perforations were diagnosed when patients were fed parenterally. Microorganisms cultured from blood samples and abdominal foci showed no relation with occurrence of the lesions. Nine patients died of underlying diseases.

Although no common cause was found, the perforations were clearly related to open abdominal treatment. They may result from weak spots affected by traction forces that are prevalent in the granulating wound. The preferred treatment includes mobilization of the bowel with resection of the affected part and primary anastomosis.

▶ Reluctance to operate on small bowel perforations in an infected abdomen has always been dangerous, even though parenteral alimentation seemed for awhile to reduce the need to resect bowel in an infected field. There is still an important need for surgery when this potentially devastating complication occurs during open treatment of peritonitis; aggressive surgical removal of areas with multiple perforations should be performed in most patients.—E.E. Peacock, Jr., M.D.

Postoperative Necrotizing Fasciitis in Children

Farrell LD, Karl SR, Davis PK, Bellinger MF, Ballantine TVN (Univ Hosp; Milton S Hershey Med Ctr; Pennsylvania State Univ, Hershey)
Pediatrics 82:874–879, December 1988   6–8

Necrotizing fasciitis, a progressive soft tissue infection of the fascia, subcutaneous tissue, and skin, is a rare but life-threatening postoperative complication in children. It can result in systemic sepsis and death. The most important factors in survival are early diagnosis and aggressive surgical therapy. Four children with necrotizing fasciitis were treated at 1 center from 1978 to 1985.

Necrotizing fasciitis in these 4 children and 7 others reported in the literature developed after appendectomy for ruptured appendix, bilateral inguinal herniorrhaphy, and gastrostomy closure. There were 3 girls and 8 boys aged 6 days to 15 years. Five surgical procedures were clean, 5 were clean-contaminated, and 1 was contaminated. None of the children had evidence of malignancy or diabetes. Two had evidence of failure to thrive. One had an intra-abdominal abscess. In 10 cases the infection began in the abdominal wall, and in 1, it began in the chest wall. Of the 4 patients newly reported on, 3 had neutropenia and fever, all had tachycardia, and 2 had wound crepitation and radiographic evidence of subcutaneous gas.

Cultures of all 10 wounds were positive for bacteria, and in 6 more than 1 organism was grown. Blood culture results were positive in all 5 children who died and in only 2 of 5 patients who survived. All of the survivors underwent wide surgical débridement and were treated with broad-spectrum antibiotics. Overall, the death rate was 45%. In the 4 newly reported cases the only death occurred in a child with Down's syndrome and failure to thrive whose parents refused further treatment.

Necrotizing fasciitis can complicate clean surgical procedures in pediatric patients without risk factors. Septicemia is a late, ominous sign.

Early wide surgical débridement and broad-spectrum antibiotic treatment are needed for survival, and skin grafting is often required for late coverage of the defects.

▶ The key is systemic signs of sepsis greater than can be explained by local findings. Fascial biopsy is the only way to make the diagnosis early enough to prevent a high mortality. The need for wide excision and appropriate antibiotics is generally appreciated. The importance of making the diagnosis by fascial biopsy before gross findings are typical is still a neglected factor.—E.E. Peacock, Jr., M.D.

Pneumococcal Vaccine Improves Pulmonary Clearance of Live Pneumococci After Splenectomy
Hebert JC (Univ of Vermont, Burlington)
J Surg Res 47:283–287, October 1989   6–9

Overwhelming sepsis, particularly from *Streptococcus pneumoniae*, is a well-known complication after splenectomy. Although postsplenectomy vaccination with polyvalent pneumococcal capsular polysaccharide vaccines continues to be recommended, the efficacy of this practice remains controversial. The value of pneumococcal vaccination in animal models is also unclear. A study in splenectomized mice identified a defect in early pulmonary defenses against pneumococci. Whether pneumococcal polysaccharide vaccine would increase early pulmonary defenses against pneumococcal infection was studied in mice.

One week after splenectomy or sham operation in adult male mice, 0.1 mL of a 23-valent pneumococcal polysaccharide vaccine or 0.1 mL of saline solution was administered intraperitoneally. Two weeks later the mice were exposed to pneumococcal aerosol. Groups of mice were killed immediately and at 6 hours and 24 hours after aerosol exposure. The remaining exposed animals were observed for survival.

Splenectomy impaired clearance of pneumococci from mouse lungs and caused increased translocation of pneumococci to tracheobronchial lymph nodes in comparison with findings in sham-operated animals. Pneumococcal vaccine improved lung clearance in splenectomized and sham-operated mice in comparison with saline-treated controls. However, the number of live pneumococci recovered from the lungs of splenectomized mice was greater than that recovered from the lungs of sham-operated animals. Although vaccination improved survival in animals undergoing splenectomy, survival remained well below that of sham-operated controls that received saline. Thus pneumococcal vaccine given to mice after splenectomy improves pulmonary defenses against pneumococcal infection, but not to the same extent as it does in animals with intact spleens.

▶ These data clarify the possible use of pneumococcal vaccine after splenectomy. It is still not clear, however, whether the standard of care of patients requires pneumococcal vaccination after splenectomy.—E.E. Peacock, Jr., M.D.

Incidence of Septic and Thromboembolic-Related Deaths After Splenectomy in Adults

Pimpl W, Dapunt O, Kaindl H, Thalhamer J (Landeskrankenanstalten Salzburg, Austria)

Br J Surg 76:517–521, May 1989   6–10

The risks of splenectomy have led to controversy regarding optimal surgical management of the ruptured spleen. Some authors have recommended repair of the traumatically ruptured spleen or reimplantation of splenic tissue. Because these techniques may also result in complications, investigators sought to determine the risk of septic and thromboembolic-related deaths—both early postoperative and long term—after splenectomy.

In a retrospective review of 37,012 autopsies performed in Salzburg in the past 20 years, 202 adults were identified who had undergone splenectomy. Reasons for the procedure included trauma (30.2%), injury during abdominal surgery for nonmalignant diseases (31.2%), cancer surgery (27.7%), and hematologic disorders (10.9%). Patients were divided into 2 subgroups: those who died within 3 months of surgery and those who died more than 3 months afterward. In the control group were 403 patients who had undergone similar surgery without splenectomy.

Mortality at 3 months in the splenectomy group was 50.5%. Within the first 3 postoperative years another 28.2% of the patients died. Compared with controls, death in the splenectomized group was caused significantly more often by pneumonia, pulmonary embolism, and sepsis. Both lethal sepsis with multiple organ failure and purulent pyelonephritis were significantly more frequent among splenectomized patients (6.9% and 7.9%, respectively) than in the control group (1.5% and 2.2%).

Splenectomy was associated with considerable risk for infection and thromboembolism, even years after surgery. The greatest risk of complications (78.7%), however, is in the first 3 postoperative years. To prevent such complication, patients of all ages should receive perioperative antibiotic prophylaxis and preoperative pneumococcal vaccination. A broad spectrum penicillin and a low-dose aspirin regimen are advised for at least 3 years. The same precautions should be followed with patients undergoing spleen autotransplantation.

▶ For years it was impossible to show that splenectomy produced any significant hazard to health and longevity. There seem to be more data now than we can evaluate, and most of the findings support the importance of the spleen in preventing infection and thromboembolism. One can only hope that there is a corresponding reduction in splenectomy, particularly during nonrelated procedures such as vagotomy.—E.E. Peacock, Jr., M.D.

7 Burns

Smoke Inhalation Injury: Evaluation of Radiographic Manifestations and Pulmonary Dysfunction
Peitzman AB, Shires GT III, Teixidor HS, Curreri PW, Shires GT (New York Hosp–Cornell Med Ctr)
J Trauma 29:1232–1239, September 1989   7–1

Smoke inhalation injury is a frequent complication in burned patients. Upper airway injury is diagnosed reliably by endoscopy, but the early diagnosis of primary pulmonary parenchymal injury is less reliable. Various techniques for diagnosing pulmonary parenchymal injury have been recommended, including chest radiography and pulmonary function testing. However, the sensitivity of the chest radiograph (CXR) as an indicator of inhalation injury is controversial. To correlate the degree of change in CXR with measurements of pulmonary function during the first 5 days after inhalation injury, 29 patients with burn injuries were examined, 25 of whom were intubated on admission.

The average percentage of body burns was 59%. Pulmonary function was assessed daily, including measurement of the intrapulmonary shunt fraction, the extravascular lung water volume, static pulmonary compliance, and the plasma colloid osmotic pressure-pulmonary artery wedge pressure gradient. Daily CXRs were graded without knowledge of the patient's clinical condition (table). Patients were examined until death or for 5 days post burn.

Twenty of 29 patients died of their injuries. In all, 108 CXRs were obtained. Of the 25 patients who had serious inhalation injury requiring intubation, 84% had some abnormality on CXR within 48 hours after injury. When any abnormality was noted on CXR, 92% of the patients had some evidence of pulmonary dysfunction. Radiographic findings in inhalation injury correlated well with the degree of pulmonary dysfunction. When serious abnormalities were noted on CXR, patients also had evi-

---

Radiologic Criteria for Estimation of Pulmonary Parenchymal
Damage in Inhalation Injury

0:   Normal
1+: Peribronchial cuffing or perivascular edema (vessels are prominent and fuzzy but not obliterated)
2+: Edema, alveolar or interstitial, involving 1/3 of lung field
3+: Edema, involving 2/3 of lung field
4+: Edema, involving entire lung field

(Courtesy of Peitzman AB, Shires GT III, Teixidor HS, et al: *J Trauma* 29:1232–1239, September 1989.)

---

dence of marked pulmonary dysfunction. These findings suggest that the grading scale used in this trial may be useful in reports of CXR findings in inhalation injury.

▶ Smoke inhalation injuries are a frequent complication in burn patients. The current study examined the sensitivity of the CXR as an indicator of inhalation injury. The findings were interesting in that, when any abnormality was present on CXR after burn injury, 92% of the patients had some evidence of pulmonary dysfunction. Pulmonary dysfunction was assessed in these patients daily and included measurement of the intrapulmonary shunt fraction, the extravascular lung water, static pulmonary compliance, and plasma colloid osmotic pressure–pulmonary artery wedge pressure gradient. This is a unique study in that there were consistent physiologic data measurements made to correlate closely with blinded x-ray evaluations. Of the 25 patients who had serious inhalation injury, some abnormality on the CXR was seen in 84% within 48 hours. More importantly, the radiographic findings in inhalation injury correlated well with the degree of pulmonary dysfunction. It would appear that a grading scale, as used in this study, would have utility in reporting CXR findings in those patients with inhalation injury.—G.T. Shires, M.D.

Temporal Analysis of Murine Lymphocyte Subpopulations by Monoclonal Antibodies and Dual-Color Flow Cytometry After Burn and Nonburn Injury
Hansbrough JF, Gadd MA (Univ of California, San Diego)
Surgery 106:69–80, July 1989   7–2

Sepsis remains the chief cause of late morbidity and death after trauma, and it may relate to immune defects that follow severe injury. Many studies have shown depressed in vitro lymphocyte responses after burn injury. Monoclonal antibodies and dual-color flow cytometry were used to examine the expression of lymphocyte phenotypes in mice after hind limb amputation and controlled burn injury. Gradient procedures that can entail the selective loss of some lymphocyte groups were avoided.

Helper/inducer cells and suppressor/cytotoxic cells in the spleen of burned-injured mice were depressed. Proportions of non-B, non-T lymphocytes were increased. Changes in nodal cells were minimal. Subsets of Ia$^+$ cells, possibly activated or proliferating cells, were depressed in the peripheral blood, but levels of circulating suppressor/cytotoxic cells were increased late after burn injury. Burned animals but not those subjected to limb trauma had marked splenic hypertrophy. Eschar excision studies showed that both splenic hypertrophy and the splenocyte phenotypic changes were related to the presence of burned tissue.

Prolonged changes in lymphocyte subsets occur after burn injury and are accompanied by splenic hypertrophy. The presence of burn-injured tissue may help to mediate the immune changes that accompany severe thermal injury. Changes following limb trauma are less marked and last a shorter time, and splenic hypertrophy does not occur.

▶ Recent suggestions that the apparent advantages of early burn eschar excision may be attributable to the unintentional selection of patients who can tolerate anesthesia and surgery may not be correct. There are a number of potential and some theoretical dangers in leaving dead burned tissue on the body. Immunologic factors have not been considered major risks in the past; the reduction in infection after early excision may, however, be the result of preventing immunologic depression.—E.E. Peacock, Jr., M.D.

Improved Myocardial Oxygen Utilization Following Propranolol Infusion in Adolescents With Postburn Hypermetabolism
Minifee PK, Barrow RE, Abston S, Desai M, Herndon DN (Shriners Burns Inst, Galveston; Univ of Texas, Galveston)
J Pediatr Surg 24:806–811, August 1989   7–3

Major thermal injury is characterized by catecholine-mediated hypermetabolism, tachycardia, and hyperdynamic cardiac activity, which may lead to postburn cardiac dysfunction and death. Whether propranolol, administered intravenously to patients with burns at the height of the postburn hypermetabolic response, attenuates the catecholamine-induced cardiac effects was investigated.

Six severely burned patients aged 14–21 years (median age, 17 years) with burns over 82% of the total body surface area underwent complete early excision and débridement with patch grafting 2–8 days before propranolol therapy was initiated. Propranolol was administered a mean of 20 days postburn when patients were in a catecholamine-induced, hypermetabolic phase of response. All patients had continuous monitoring of hemodynamic parameters. The pressure-work index and the rate-pressure product, clinically derived indices of myocardial oxygen consumption, are used to estimate the energy expenditure of the working heart. These indices were calculated to determine whether propranolol could lower cardiac work during the hypermetabolic state.

All 6 patients survived and were discharged home with ongoing rehabilitation. None experienced side effects from propranolol administration. Both the mean pressure-work index and the mean rate-pressure product were significantly decreased after propranolol administration, indicating a reduction in cardiac workload. The mean heart rate and mean arterial blood pressure also were significantly decreased after propranolol administration. However, overall oxygen delivery and total body oxygen consumption remained elevated throughout drug treatment. Thus propranolol administered to burn patients during the hypermetabolic state effectively decreases myocardial oxygen requirements by lowering the patients' heart rate and blood pressure without adversely affecting essential oxygen delivery or total body oxygen consumption.

▶ Cardiac failure in burned children has always been a difficult problem; digitalization never produced the results that were anticipated. Propranolol appears to be of more specific value to cardiac function. If these data hold up, particularly in the treatment of younger children, propranolol will be a welcome addition to the methods of burn therapy available.—E.E. Peacock, Jr., M.D.

Effects of Fish Oil on Postburn Metabolism and Immunity
Trocki O, Heyd TJ, Waymack JP, Alexander JW (Shriners Burns Inst, Cincinnati)
J Parenter Enteral Nutr 11:521–528, November–December, 1987   7–4

An earlier study of burned guinea pigs found enteral formulas containing 5% to 15% of nonprotein calories as fat to be optimal in promoting protein synthesis and preserving muscle mass after burn injury. The effects of different levels of fish oil in the enteral formulas on metabolic and immune responses after burn injury were investigated in 37 burned guinea pigs with previously placed gastrostomy feeding tubes. They were given diets containing 5%, 15%, 30%, or 50% of nonprotein calories as fish oil. The diets were isonitrogenous, isocaloric, and contained identical amounts of vitamins and minerals.

After 14 days of feeding no significant differences were observed in resting metabolic expenditure or serum transferrin and albumin levels. Animals receiving 30% and 50% fish oil had significantly greater weight loss than those receiving 5% and 15% fish oil. Carcass weights and liver weights in the 2 groups receiving diets with higher lipid content also were significantly lower. The groups did not differ in cell-mediated immunity, macrophage bactericidal indices, or opsonic indices.

The findings confirm that diets containing lower levels of lipids are more effective for enteral nutritional support than those containing higher levels. Unlike linoleic acid-rich lipid sources, higher levels of fish oil did not have adverse effects on immunity, possibly because the fish oil contained high concentrations of $\omega 3$ fatty acids, which are not precursors of immunosuppressive prostaglandin E_2

▶ What we need now is to find a few Eskimos with coronary insufficiency. Fish oil appears to be very overrated as a therapeutic or prophylactic modality for almost everything it has been studied for.—E.E. Peacock, Jr., M.D.

Hemodynamic and Oxygen Transport Effects of Pentastarch in Burn Resuscitation
Waxman K, Holness R, Tominaga G, Chela P, Grimes J (Univ of California Irvine Med Ctr, Orange)
Ann Surg 209:341–345, March 1989   7–5

Albumin solutions, used in large volumes for fluid resuscitation of seriously burned patients, are effective but costly. In a search for alternatives, hydroxyethyl starch (HES) was developed as a colloid volume expander. An HES preparation, hetastarch, has many of the advantages of albumin solutions but a long tissue retention time. Pentastarch, a newer HES, is less highly hydroxyethylated and thus has less potential to cause reticuloendothelial impairment than hetastarch. Pentastarch was compared with albumin in 12 patients (mean age, 42 years) requiring acute burn resuscitation. The mean burn size was 39% of the total body surface.

In a randomized, crossover schedule, patients received 500 mL of 5% albumin and 500 mL of 10% pentastarch. Central venous pressure (CVP) and wedge pressure (WP) significantly increased with both colloid solutions. Pentastarch brought about more significant increases in cardiac index, stroke volume, and right and left ventricular stroke work than did albumin infusion. Colloid infusion had little effect on blood gases. Oxygen delivery increased significantly after pentastarch infusion; both solutions increased oxygen consumption over the supernormal baseline levels.

Pentastarch was an effective plasma expander during resuscitation within a mean of 23.6 hours after burn injury. The effects of the solution were equal to or better than those of albumin.

Although these patients had normal vital signs, urine output, and cardiac function at baseline, the effects of colloid fluid administration suggest that plasma volume increases are required to meet their increased metabolic needs.

▶ The need and the search for plasma substitutes continues. The public health and economic disadvantages to the use of human plasma and human plasma products are significant. Pentastarch may be an answer if it can be given safely in large volumes.—E.E. Peacock, Jr., M.D.

Precise Diagnosis of Infection in Burn Wound Biopsy Specimens: Combination of Histologic Technique, Acridine Orange Staining, and Culture
Mitchell V, Galizia J-P, Fournier L (C Huriez Hosp, Lille, France)
J Burn Care Rehabil 10:195–202, May–June 1989   7–6

Clinical bacteriologic monitoring of burned patients is important for the early diagnosis of infection. Because sepsis is the main cause of death in severely burned patients, a rapid method of detecting microorganisms was sought. A review was made of 86 biopsy specimens that were processed using a rapid manual histologic technique, acridine orange (AO) fluorescent staining, and quantitative culture.

Burn wound biopsy specimens were obtained several times weekly using conventional incision techniques; 1 of 2 adjacent specimens from each patient was sent to the microbiologic laboratory and the other to the histologic laboratory. Two segments of the latter specimen were processed by the rapid manual technique and the third by the traditional method. Within 4 hours sections processed by the rapid method can be evaluated by the histologist. The adjacent biopsy specimen was processed for detection of microorganisms with AO staining, also within 4 hours. Complete quantitative results require 48 hours.

Grading of the specimens using the rapid histologic method was based on both degree and depth of microbial penetration. Grading was on a scale of 0 (no microorganisms observed throughout the entire tissue) to IV (an important microbial invasion in burn wound eschar and hypodermis). Grades 0 and Ia show good infection control. Grades Ib and II indicate a need to change the topical agent. Grades III and IV signal that vigorous therapy is needed to prevent sepsis. Thus important information is available early for therapeutic choices. These 3 complementary techniques are recommended for routine monitoring of burned patients.

▶ Most burn units should be able to perform the techniques described in this paper. Although qualitative data have been available in most units, quantitative evaluation of sepsis is important in obtaining a healed wound; it is not always available when wound closure is contemplated.—E.E. Peacock, Jr., M.D.

Risk Factors Associated With Intravascular Catheter Infections in Burned Patients: A Prospective, Randomized Study
Franceschi D, Gerding RL, Phillips G, Fratianne RB (Cleveland Metropolitan Gen Hosp)
J Trauma 29:811–816, June 1989   7–7

Although strict guidelines exist for catheter insertion and maintenance, infectious complications remain a major problem. The rate of catheter infection is especially high among burned patients. The role of tubing manipulation and skin contamination in the etiology of catheter infection was examined in a prospective study of 89 adult burn patients.

The patients' average burn size was 37.8% of the total body surface. They were randomized to have tubing changed on new catheters every 24 or 48 hours. Skin cultures were obtained at the insertion site before the catheter was placed and at its removal 72 hours later.

Overall, 25.7% of catheters were infected: 35% of the arterial catheters, 27% of the central venous catheters, and 12% of the peripheral venous catheters. The most common isolates were *Pseudomonas* species (33%) and coagulase-negative *Staphylococcus aureus*. More frequent changing of the tubing did not lower infection rates. Burn size was not related to the incidence of catheter infection, but the day post burn correlated positively. The incidence of infection correlated inversely with the distance of the insertion site from the burn wound.

Frequent changes of intravenous tubing are of no benefit to burn patients. As much distance as possible should be kept between the burned area and the catheter insertion site. An important cause of catheter infection appears to be skin contamination with migration of bacteria along the catheter.

▶ The bottom line remains the same: There is no substitute for surface cleanliness. The term "no substitute" includes betadine.—E.E. Peacock, Jr., M.D.

Acute Septic Cholecystitis in Patients With Burn Injuries
Slater H, Goldfarb IW (Western Pennsylvania Hosp, Pittsburgh)
J Burn Care Rehabil 10:445–447, September–October 1989   7–8

Acute septic cholecystitis in patients with extensive burns may go undetected or be delayed because these patients often have fever and leukocytosis, abdominal distention, and abnormal liver enzymes as a result of the burn injury itself. Deeply burned abdominal skin may also obscure clues from physical examination.

During an 18-month period 5 patients with burn injuries aged 13–40 years had acute septic cholecystitis. The burn surface area ranged from 30% to 75%. Cholecystitis was suspected on the basis of unexplained sepsis, abdominal distention, and abnormal findings on gallbladder sonography and hepatobiliary scintigraphy.

Four patients underwent cholecystectomy and 1 patient had a cholecystostomy between 18 and 61 days after burn injury. Four patients had positive blood cultures before operation, and all 5 had positive bile cultures at operation. One patient died on day 61 after burn injury, 13 days after cholecystostomy. This patient had third-degree burns over 75% of his body, and he had already undergone bilateral below-knee amputations because of severe burns. The other 4 patients recovered and were discharged. All patients had received narcotics intravenously and total parenteral nutrition or nasojejunal tube feedings, which increase the susceptibility for cholecystitis. None had received oral feedings or orally administered drugs for at least 1 week before acute septic cholecystitis was diagnosed.

A missed or delayed diagnosis of acute cholecystitis may lead to increased mortality or morbidity. Serial sonography and hepatobiliary scanning should be performed in all patients with burns who have unexplained sepsis, ileus, abdominal pain, and elevated bilirubin or liver enzymes. The availability of portable ultrasound and radionuclide devices has facilitated such examinations in the burn unit.

▶ The usual cause of cholecystitis is treatment of pain with drugs such as Demerol or morphine, which increase smooth muscle tone. A parasympathetic block of T–9 and T–10 ganglia relieves spasm and can make emergency cholecystectomy unnecessary.—E.E. Peacock, Jr., M.D.

The "Sponge Deformity" After Tangential Excision and Grafting of Burns
Engrav LH, Gottlieb JR, Walkinshaw MD, Heimbach DM, Grube B (Univ of Washington)
Plast Reconstr Surg 83:468–470, March 1989   7–9

Excision and grafting of deep burns solves some problems and creates others. A "sponge deformity" can occur in areas of tangential excision and grafting where, in multiple small areas around the periphery, the bed underneath the graft heals with or without slough of the overlying graft. A pockmark forms if the graft sloughs; if it does not, an overlying bridge forms. This deformity is distressing to patients because it is difficult to wash, catches on objects, bleeds, and is unsightly. Findings in 16 patients with sponge deformity were reviewed (Fig 7–1).

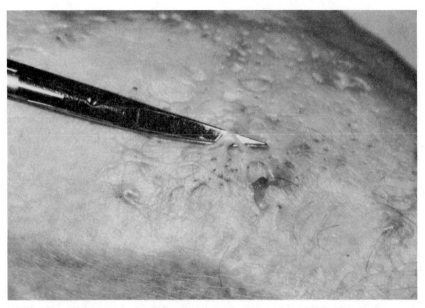

Fig 7–1.—Demonstration of a skin bridge. (Courtesy of Engrav LH, Gottlieb JR, Walkinshaw MD, et al: *Plast Reconstr Surg* 83:468–470, March 1989.)

The series included 2 females and 14 males aged 11–59 years. Fifteen were white, and 1 was black. Nine deformities were on the arm and 5 were on the hand. Graft thickness varied from 0.01 to 0.015 in. Nine were sheet grafts; 5 were meshed. Typically, the grafts appeared to take well initially, but about 2 weeks after grafting, small foci of inflammation developed in the periphery. The foci responded to local wound care and disappeared over several weeks, leaving pockmarks and bridges. The deformity was treated with simple excision of the edges and bridges in all cases. The wounds healed well in 14 patients, with the resultant surface smooth. In 2 patients the excision had to be repeated.

Sponge deformity usually occurs at the periphery of the excised area where the excision is shallower and when thicker grafts are used. The bed underneath the graft may epithelialize from residual epithelial elements before autograft vascularization occurs. If this is true, it may be possible to prevent this deformity by excising the wound deeper, applying thinner grafts, or applying allograft or xenograft.

▶ The deformity described here is the result of regeneration of surface elements from skin appendages that were not destroyed by thermal injury. If there is adequate skin, the problem is not a serious one. If sufficient skin is a major problem, however, questionably third-degree burns should be saved until the last to allow maximum opportunity for regeneration of deep appendages.— E.E. Peacock, Jr., M.D.

The Fate of Meshed Allograft Skin in Burned Patients Using Cyclosporin Immunosuppression

Frame JD, Sanders R, Goodacre TEE, Morgan BDG (Mount Vernon Hosp, Northwood, Middlesex, England)
Br J Plast Surg 42:27–34, January 1989   7–10

A team of researchers reported the use of azathioprine to prolong allograft survival in a small number of burned patients in 1974. However, they excised the allograft and replaced it with autograft before meaningful results of allograft survival could be obtained. They did not expect allograft survival. Whether the immunosuppressant cyclosporine could prolong allograft survival or allow a state of immunotolerance to allograft was investigated in 3 burned patients.

The patients were treated with cyclosporine after allograft skin was applied. They had burns over 25%, 35%, and 60% of their bodies. Allograft biopsies were taken at different intervals (Fig 7–2). Cyclosporine treatment was continued for 3 weeks in 2 patients and for 3 months in the third. None of the patients experienced any adverse treatment effects. The allografts survived during cyclosporine treatment but were rejected 12 days after cyclosporine was discontinued in 1 patient and after 5–7 days in another. In the third patient, in whom a meshed autograft-al-

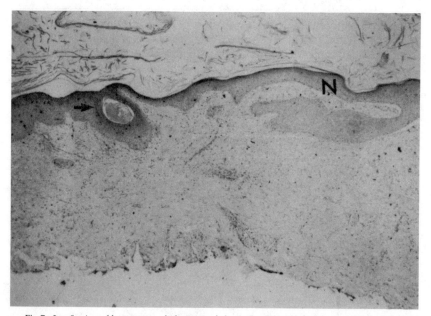

Fig 7–2.—Section of homogeneously keratinized skin at 3 weeks. Section is taken from a biopsy of the dorsum of the right foot and stained with S100. The original allograft mesh, which contains part of a hair follicle *(arrow)*, contains S100-positive Langerhans cells, but the newly keratinized region *(N)* does not. S100 stain; original magnification, ×28.80. Courtesy of Frame JD, Sanders R, Goodacre TEE, et al: *Br J Plast Surg* 42:27–34, January 1989.)

lograft sandwich technique was used, there was no evidence of rejection. The allograft in this case was probably replaced by a process of "creeping substitution" associated with the sandwich technique.

It appears that cyclosporine created a state of immunotolerance to the antigenic load while the patient was receiving the drug. After the treatment was stopped, rejection occurred in 2 of 3 cases. The absence of visible rejection of the more finely meshed allograft in the third patient suggests a process of "creeping subsitution." The Langerhans cells are probably not solely responsible for rejection of allograft.

▶ Using cyclosporine to inhibit the immune response in a burned patients is burning the candle at both ends. Success or failure is probably dependent upon how long the candle is.— E.E. Peacock, Jr., M.D.

The Use of Non-Viable Glycerol-Preserved Cadaver Skin Combined With Widely Expanded Autografts in the Treatment of Extensive Third-Degree Burns
Kreis RW, Vloemans AFPM, Hoekstra MJ, Mackie DP, Hermans RP (Dutch Burns Centre at Beverwijk, The Netherlands)
J Trauma 29:51–54, February 1989   7–11

Using expanded autologous split-skin grafts for reepithelialization of primarily excised deep burn wounds is an established procedure. Grafted wounds have been overlaid with split-skin donor allograft to protect the autograft when expansion ratios are greater than 1:4. However, rejection of the allogeneic donor skin is unpredictable. Preserving skin allografts with 98% glycerol simplifies the conservation of cadaver skin and attenuates the rejection reaction enough to enhance the uninterrupted outgrowth of widely expanded autograft. The use of nonviable glycerol-preserved cadaver skin combined with widely expanded autographs to treat extensive third-degree burns was investigated.

Fifty-eight sandwich grafting procedures were performed in 39 patients. Forty-five grafting procedures done within 10 days of the burn injury resulted in an epithelialization rate of at least 75% within 5 weeks. Thirty-three of the operations achieved complete wound closure. Of 13 procedures done after the 14th postburn day, 10 resulted in wound epithelialization of 75% or more. Epithelial quality and cosmetic results were judged to be good. The mean length of stay in the hospital was 56 days. One patient died of unrelated respiratory problems.

Allograft skin lyophilized in 98% glycerol was an effective overlay for widely expanded autografts. In this series the good results achieved may have been partly the result of apparent attenuation of allograft antigenicity conferred by the action of 98% glycerol. Cadaver skin preservation in 98% glycerol is a simple, inexpensive process.

▶ The technique appears reliable. Wound healing by epithelialization is only a temporary advantage, however. The concept that there is "uninterrupted outgrowth of widely expanded autografts" except by epithelialization is not justified. Actually, wound contraction in some areas is the major disadvantage of a widely expanded graft.—E.E. Peacock, Jr., M.D.

8 Transplantation

Experience With Anencephalic Infants as Prospective Organ Donors
Peabody JL, Emery JR, Ashwal S (Loma Linda Univ, Calif)
N Engl J Med 321:344–350, Aug 10, 1989   8–1

Although anencephalic infants are potential organ donors for other infants, under current law they cannot be used as such until brain stem activity ceases. With the usual care given, the solid organs commonly undergo irreversible hypoxic injury and, by the time of total brain death, are unsuitable for donation. A modification of the care of live-born anencephalic infants for 1 week to maintain organ viability was attempted.

Six anencephalic infants received intensive care from birth, and 6 others only when signs of imminent death were present. Only 2 infants met criteria for total brain death within 1 week, and no solid organs were procured. Intensive care from the time of birth maintained organ function, but brain stem activity ceased within the first week in only 1 instance. When intensive care was withheld until death was imminent, most organs were so damaged as to be unsuitable for transplantation.

With current restrictions it usually is not feasible to obtain solid organs for transplantation from anencephalic infants. Possible alternatives include xenotransplantation and a legal change to allow organ procurement from anencephalic infants as a separate category of donors to whom current standards for total brain death would not apply.

The Use of Anencephalic Infants as Organ Sources: A Critique
Shewmon DA, Capron AM, Peacock WJ, Schulman BL (Univ of California, Los Angeles; Univ of Southern California, Los Angeles)
JAMA 261:1773–1781, March 24–31, 1989   8–2

Obtaining infant cadavers with artificially supported vital functions to serve as organ donors is difficult. The use of organs from anencephalic infants has been proposed, and Loma Linda University began an active program for harvesting organs for transplant from such infants. This program has since been suspended, however.

Harvesting organs from anencephalic donors is inherently problematic, both ethically and practically. Various evidence suggests that surprisingly few organs from anencephalic donors would actually benefit other children. Attempts to revise the Uniform Anatomical Gift Act or the Uniform Determination of Death Act to permit removal of organs from spontaneously breathing anencephalic newborns elicit major ethical objections. Such radical revisions in the law would undermine the goal of promoting organ transplantation and result in moral confusion that may constitute a greater evil than the good done to the relatively few surviving organ recipients. Providing intensive care to anencephalic infants would tend to preserve the brain stem as effectively as the other organs, making the occurrence of brain death unlikely.

The proposal for using anencephalic infants as organ sources was well intended but shortsighted. The number of children who die each year of congenital kidney, heart, and liver disease would be reduced insignificantly, even if existing laws were changed to allow organ harvesting from live anencephalic infants. Important ethical issues include the consequences for the anencephalic newborn and expansion of the category of potential donors to infants with less serious defects. Thus anencephalic infants are not as attractive a source of organs as some had hoped.

▶ In an effort to treat terminal infants with fatal cardiac anomalies by heart transplantation, the team at Loma Linda University developed and implemented a protocol of maintaining life support for anencephalic donors hoping to maintain organ function until total brain stem activity ceased, at which time transplantation would be accomplished. This failed, however, because the intensive care used to maintain the donor also maintained brain stem function. The group suggests that anencephalic donors be deemed a separate category in order to facilitate organ procurement. Shewmon and colleagues (Abstract 8–2) argue against this proposal, feeling that public confidence in organ donation will be undermined by making an exception. This is a difficult issue and either viewpoint is debatable; however, a moratorium has been placed on organ procurement from anencephalic infants. Unfortunately, it will be difficult to find other donors for the few infants who might have benefited from this donor source. As others involved in transplantation of infants and small children have pointed out, events leading to brain death of infant donors are rare and small organs are difficult to come by.—O. Jonasson, M.D.

Decreased Immunogenicity of Fetal Kidneys: The Role of Passenger Leukocytes

Velasco AL, Hegre OD (Univ of Minnesota)
J Pediatr Surg 24:59–63, January 1989   8–3

Organ rejection is a complicated biologic process influenced by the immunologic status of the host and the immunogenicity of the donated organ. Traditionally, it was thought that antigen recognition was a sufficient requirement for recipient lymphocyte activation. Now, however, it appears that 2 signals are needed for lymphocyte activation: donor leukocytes traveling with the graft serve as antigen-presenting cells (APC), and APCs produce the second signal—interleukin-1—necessary for lymphocyte activation. The dendrite cell is probably the most potent stimulator of recipient lymphocytes. In rats, fetal kidneys early in gestation are less immunogenic than fetal kidneys in later stages and than early-gestation fetal hepatic tissue. This observation was tested in an allogeneic model.

Kidneys and livers were harvested from fetal rats at different gestational ages. Either 1 kidney or a 3-mm piece of liver was grafted under the kidney capsule of incompatible adult rats. By the tenth day after surgery all hepatic grafts were completely rejected. The degree of kidney rejection, however, was dependent on age. Kidneys from younger fetuses had a minimal or moderate rejection, and kidneys from older fetuses were completely rejected by the tenth day.

Early in gestation the fetal liver probably contains dendritic cells that act as APCs and provide the 2 signals needed for recipient lymphocyte activation, However, kidneys from fetuses aged 15 gestational days—the youngest fetuses used—lack dendritic cells in the parenchyma and thus fail to produce an allogeneic reaction. Later in gestation, fetal kidneys may become immunogenic as dendritic cells from bone marrow arrive in their parenchyma.

▶ These are nice experiments that demonstrate the critical role of the passenger APCs (dendritic cells?) in initiating allograft rejection. These investigators capitalized on differences in the population of various organs by dendritic cells during fetal development and showed that the organs with dendritic cells were rejected, whereas those without this population of cells were accepted.— O. Jonasson, M.D.

Transplantation Tolerance Correlates With High Levels of T- and B-Lymphocyte Activity

Bandeira A, Coutinho A, Carnaud C, Jacquemart F, Forni L (Inst Pasteur, Paris; Hôpital Necker, Paris; Basel Inst for Immunology, Basel, Switzerland)
Proc Natl Acad Sci USA 86:272–276, January 1989   8–4

It has been suggested that clonal deletion by elimination of specific cells or clonal anergy after downregulation of molecules needed for the functional performance of tolerant cells represents the prototype mechanism of natural self-tolerance. However, induced tolerance might follow different rules, especially because the processes of self-tolerance are thought to occur intrathymically, whereas neonatal transplantation tolerance is likely to be attained in the periphery. This latter kind of tolerance is critical for experimental systems aimed at intervening in organ transplantation.

Tolereance to transplantation antigens was induced neonatally in CBA/ Ca, CBA/J, and C57BL/6J mice. Tolerant adult mice contained very large numbers of activated lymphocytes in their spleens. Acceptance of allogeneic tissues by tolerant mice is associated with a high level of lymphoid activity, even higher than that needed for rejection in normal mice. Lymphocyte hyperactivity in tolerant mice involved B, CD4$^+$, and CD8$^+$ cells and both host and donor lymphocytes. Lymphocyte activity in tolerant mice also showed anamnestic recall after a second graft.

Adult mice made tolerant to transplantation antigens at birth maintain a high level of immune activity involving both host and donor lymphocytes. This observation is less compatible with theories of clonal anergy or suppression than with models considering a positive definition of self, in which tolerance shares many of the cellular characteristics associated with immunity.

▶ In these interesting experiments, tolerance induced in neonatal mice was found to be a very active immune phenomenon, not a clonal deletion or suppression. Tolerance, or the induction of specific "nonresponsiveness" to an allograft, may more resemble active immunity than a passive nonreactive state.— O. Jonasson, M.D.

Immunoregulation of Transfusion-Induced Immunosuppression With Inhibitors of the Arachidonic Acid Metabolism
Perez RV, Babcock GF, Alexander JW (Univ of Cincinnati)
Transplantation 48:85–87, July 1989   8–5

Blood transfusions have a beneficial effect on allograft survival. Several researchers report an increase in metabolism of arachidonic acid (AA) after transfusion and suggest that prostaglandin E compounds mediate transfusion-induced immunosuppression (TII). However, not all AA metabolites are immunosuppressive. Also, increased metabolism of AA after transfusion could lead to the production of the immunostimulatory compounds thromboxane and the leukotrienes. It is therefore possible that inhibiting that potentially deleterious pathways during transfusion could result in augmentation of TII.

To further define the role of AA metabolites in TII, AA metabolism was manipulated pharmacologically in a rodent model. Lewis rats were given donor-specific transfusions from Buffalo rats in conjunction with cyclo-oxygenase or lipoxygenase. Two weeks later they were given intra-abdominal Buffalo heart allografts or were used for mixed lymphocyte responses. Inhibition of cyclooxygenase partly abrogated TII; cardiac allograft survival was shortened. Lipoxygenase inhibition augmented TII; the mixed lymphocyte reaction was depressed, and allograft survival was prolonged. Thromboxane synthetase inhibition had no effect.

These findings support the hypothesis that AA metabolites are important mediators of TII. The prostaglandin E compounds are probably the main AA metabolites involved in mediation of TII.

▶ In these investigations of the "transfusion effect," wherein blood transfusion is immunosuppressive in allograft recipients and augments graft survival, prostaglandin E compounds are identified as important factors. New information on the immunosuppressive effect of prostaglandins has appeared in other studies, including a clinical renal transplantation series in which administration of a prostaglandin E analogue (misoprostol) appeared to prevent rejection events in most patients receiving conventional cyclosporine immunosuppression. These are potentially very important observations.— O. Jonasson, M.D.

Suppression of the Humoral Response to Anti-CD3 Monoclonal Antibody
Hirsch R, Chatenoud L, Gress RE, Sachs DH, Bach J-F, Bluestone JA (Natl Cancer Inst, Bethesda, Md; Hôp Necker, Paris; Univ of Chicago)
Transplantation 47:853–857, May 1989   8–6

Clinicians administer anti-CD3 monoclonal antibodies (mAbs) to treat organ allograft rejection. However, their use is limited by the humoral response of patients against mAbs, resulting in loss of therapeutic benefit. An animal model was used to examine the in vivo effects of anti-CD3 mAbs.

Mice were exposed to the antimurine CD3 mAb 145–2C11. Exposure resulted in suppression of graft rejection but also stimulated a strong humoral response, abrogating the efficacy of further treatment. An additional dose of anti-CD3 mAb did not prolong skin graft survival. In some instances it produced a lethal anaphylactic reaction. In an attempt to suppress this humoral response, anti-CD4 mAb was administered before anti-CD3 mAb treatment. Pretreatment almost completely suppressed the humoral response to anti-CD3 mAb and allowed the anti-CD3 mAb to be given again without a loss of efficacy.

The use of anti-CD4 mAb to suppress the humoral response against anti-CD3 mAb should be attempted clinically. It may allow repeated courses of anti-CD3 administration, significantly improving the efficacy of these drugs in the treatment of organ allograft rejection.

▶ A monoclonal antibody to the CD4 helper T cells in mice has essentially eliminated the humoral, presumably the anti-idiotypic, response that renders further OKT3 treatment ineffective. This is very exciting information and, although the data are in an experimental model system, there is an implication that tolerance was produced and that tolerance could possibly be achieved toward other antigens such as the transplant antigens. Administration of the CD4 antibody was accompanied by mortality in the mice as a result of infections, as severe depletion of the helper T cells occurred, an event similar to what occurs in AIDS.—O. Jonasson, M.D.

Immunosuppression by Anti-CD4 Treatment In Vivo: Cellular and Humoral Responses to Alloantigens
Weyand CM, Goronzy J, Swarztrauber K, Fathman CG (Heidelberg Univ, West Germany; Stanford Univ)
Transplantation 47:1039–1042, June 1989   8–7

Most therapeutic models allowing immune response suppression in transplant recipients make use of the antiproliferative effects of cytotoxic agents. Treatment with monoclonal antibodies to $CD4^+$ helper T cells has been used to induce long-term tolerance by foreign body administration during severe helper cell depletion. Generating primary cytolytic responses to viral antigens depends completely on the presence of $CD4^+$ cells. Treatment with anti-CD4 mcAb in vivo may not be sufficient to suppress humoral and cytolytic memory cell responses. Immunosuppression by anti-CD4 treatment in vivo was examined in mice.

The administration of anti-CD4 mcAb did not suppress allospecific CTL responses. However, the formation of alloantibodies initially was inhibited parallel to the deficiency in CD4$^+$ helper cells. After CD4$^+$ T-cell regeneration, the mice regained the capability of producing specific IgG alloantibodies.

The dichotomy of helper pathways in humoral and cellular alloreactive responses casts doubt on the concept of a single CD4$^+$ helper cell population. A better understanding of the functional heterogeneity of helper cells for primary, secondary, and allospecific responses may open new avenues for selective manipulation of helper subpopulations.

▶ In further experiments using a monoclonal antibody to the CD4$^+$ helper T cell marker, it was found that primary humoral immune responses were inhibited and tolerance achieved, but memory cell humoral responses in primed animals were not suppressed. There appeared to be different helper cell requirements for the generation of cytotoxic cellular responses than for humoral responses. The authors suggest that the elimination of CD4$^+$ cells will be ineffective in averting cellular allograft rejection and may increase vulnerability to viral infection.— O. Jonasson, M.D.

Successful Transplantation After Conversion of a Positive Crossmatch to Negative by Dissociation of IgM Antibody
Tellis VA, Matas AJ, Senitzer D, Louis P, Glicklich D, Soberman R, Veith FJ (Montefiore Med Ctr, New York)
Transplantation 47:127–129, January 1989   8–8

Performing transplantations in patients with a high percentage of panel-reactive antibody continues to be problematic. Because the number of such sensitized patients is increasing, the problem has become more pressing. Despite current positive crossmatches, successful transplantation was attained in a group of patients by eliminating the activity of IgM antibodies, thus converting the donor-specific crossmatch to negative.

The sera of 25 highly sensitized patients were analyzed for cytotoxicity against a selected panel of 40 cells. Patients whose monthly percentage of panel reactive antibody (%PRA) against a panel of 35–50 cells showed an increase of more than 30% were given dithiothreitol (DTT). Sera treated with DTT were tested on minipanels of 6 cells, against which the untreated sera showed cytotoxicity. The decrease or elimination of cytotoxicity after DTT suggested that IgM had been at least partly responsible for the high %PRA. The sera of patients with long-term cytotoxicity demonstrated no effect after DTT treatment when tested against a minipanel. Sera treated with DTT and from the highly sensitized patients did not change in cytotoxicity if the high %PRA was related temporally to transfusions or previous transplants. However, the sera of 2 patients in whom high %PRA developed without a clear cause had little reactivity after DTT treatment. Five patients with crossmatches currently positive by standard methods but negative after DTT treatment underwent renal transplant. All 5 kidneys were functioning 3–15 months after surgery.

Transplantation has been contraindicated for patients with a current positive donor-specific crossmatch. If the lymphocytotoxic antibodies are of the IgM class of immunoglobulins, successful transplantation is possible, despite a positive current donor-specific crossmatch.

▶ The highly sensitized patient is essentially nontransplantable under ordinary circumstances, because a compatible nonreactive donor is difficult to identify. The recognition that a positive crossmatch may be caused by extraneous IgM antibodies that are not cytotoxic or transplantation antigen directed has allowed successful transplantation to proceed even in the face of the strict contraindication of a positive crossmatch. Survey of sensitized patients on the waiting list by exposing their cytotoxic serum to simple, readily available reagents to dissociate the IgM antibody may make transplantation possible for a number of patients.—O. Jonasson, M.D.

Recipient Pool Sizes for Prioritized HLA Matching
Mickey MR, Cook DJ, Terasaki PI (Univ of California, Los Angeles)
Transplantation 47:401–403, February 1989   8–9

Renewed interest in objectivity-based organ sharing stresses the need for calculating the predictable consequences of various organ allocation protocols. Three priority protocols were assessed to determine what fractions of the transplants will have the various degrees of compatibility for a variety of sizes of recipient pools.

The protocols were specified to the extent of sequences of HLA matching categories. The protocols considered were (1) O-A,B,DR mismatch, O-B,DR mismatch, O-A,B mismatch, O-DR mismatch, other; (2) O-A,B,DR mismatch, 1-A or B, O-DR mismatch, O-A or B, 1-DR mismatch, other; and (3) 6-antigen match, HLA identical but with fewer than 6 antigens, O-A,B,DR mismatch, 1-A, O-B,DR mismatch, 1-B, O-A-DR mismatch, 1-DR,O-A,B mismatch, O-DR mismatch, other. Consequence was determined in percentages of transplants that would have the several categories of matches.

With a recipient pool of about 10,000 patients, about 5% of transplants would have 6 antigen matches; 4%, HLA identical with less than 6 antigens; and 10%, non-HLA identical but without A,B,DR mismatch. Smaller pools apply to kidneys shared only regionally. Even in the smaller pools many transplants would have no B,DR mismatch, and 80% to 90% could be matched to the extent of no DR mismatch. Secondary priorities were important, and the highest secondary priority given to longest wait resulted in acceptable dynamic stability to the recipient pool for several years.

▶ The jury is still out regarding the importance of HLA matching in organ allografting. However, HLA matching is required for many highly sensitized patients, and it may also be crucial for long-term (10-year) graft survival. Organ sharing on a national basis will provide compatible organs for some patients. Applying statistical analyses based on HLA frequencies in the United States, Mickey et al. have shown that organ sharing will achieve compatible transplants for a substantial number of patients. This effort is really worthwhile, if for no other reason than to resolve the question of the value of HLA matching in transplanation.—O. Jonasson, M.D.

Diagnosis of Renal Allograft Rejection by Macrophage Immunostaining With a CD14 Monoclonal Antibody, WT14

Bogman MJJT, Dooper IMM, van de Winkel JGJ, Tax WJM, Hoitsma AJ, Assmann KJM, Ruiter DJ, Koene RAP (Univ Hosp, Nijmegen, The Netherlands)
Lancet 1:235–238, July 29, 1989   8–10

Acute interstitial rejection (AIR) of renal allografts is associated with a rise in macrophages in the graft. The diagnostic value of immunohistologic staining of biopsy specimens with a monoclonal antibody of the DC14 cluster directed against monocyte and macrophages, WT14, was assessed in 44 patients with clinically and histologically proved AIR.

In all 44 patients an indirect immunoperoxidase technique on frozen

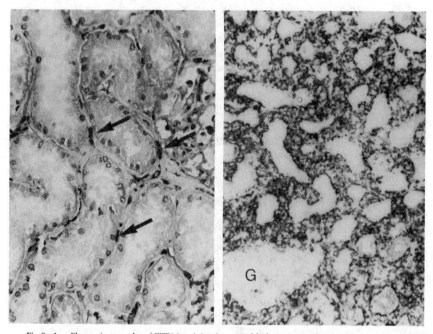

Fig 8–1.—Photomicrographs of WT14 staining in normal kidney, original magnification, ×80 (**left**), and in renal allograft with acute interstitial rejection, original magnification, ×40 (**right**). *Arrows*, positive dispersed interstitial cells with the morphology of dendritic cells; G, glomerulus. **Left,** immunoperoxidase and hematoxylin; **right,** diffuse increase of WT14-positive cells around negative tubules, immunoperoxidase without counterstain. (Courtesy of Bogman MJJT, Dooper IMM, van de Winkel JGJ, et al: *Lancet* 1:235–238, July 29, 1989.)

sections revealed a diffuse interstitial increase in WT14-positive cells. This pattern did not occur in 10 normal kidneys or in biopsy specimens from 9 patients with proved cyclosporine nephrotoxicity, 13 with chronic vascular rejection, and 60 with various other renal diseases. Staining with other monoclonal antibodies against monocytes and macrophages revealed a variable pattern, mostly weak or less specific when compared with WT14 (Fig 8–1).

In biopsy specimens from all patients with AIR, immunohistologic staining with the CD14 monoclonal antibody WT14 revealed a characteristic increase of positive peritubular cells not found in cyclosporine nephrotoxicity or nontransplanted patients with other renal disease. Thus WT14 staining appeared to be a more specific indicator of rejection than the expression of HLA-DR antigens on tubular epithelial cells, which were increased in many other lesions.

▶ In this study an important role for macrophages in accomplishing rejection was suggested by their predominance in irreversible rejections. More questions are raised about the relevance of the graft-infiltrating lymphocytes in mediating the cytotoxicity of rejection as evidence accumulates of the importance of the non-specific effect of macrophages and their products.— O. Jonasson, M.D.

The Relevance of Induced Class II HLA Antigens and Macrophage Infiltration in Early Renal Allograft Biopsies

Raftery MJ, Seron D, Koffman G, Hartley B, Janossy G, Cameron JS (UMDS, Guy's Campus, London)
Transplantation 48:238–243, August 1989   8–11

Immunohistologic analysis of early biopsy specimens may provide a better understanding of the mechanisms of alloantigen recognition and generation of the rejection response. Biopsy specimens obtained during the first week after transplantation were analyzed for cellular infiltration with lymphocytes and macrophages and the induction of class II major histocompatibility complex antigens on parenchymal cells.

Frozen sections were obtained from 14 peritransplant renal specimens and 42 specimens taken a mean of 6 days after surgery. Of the 42 post-transplant specimens, 26 were diagnosed as rejecting and 16, nonrejecting. Expression of HLA-DR antigen was strong on 8 of the 14 peritrans-

Graft Outcome in Relation to Phenotype of Cellular Infiltrate

	Lymphocytic (n = 9)	Lymphocyte/ macrophage (n = 8)	Macrophage (n = 9)
Graft losses	0	1	4
Rejection episodes	1.8	1.9	3.56
Mean creatinine	138±22	155±51	192±28

(Courtesy of Raftery MJ, Seron D, Koffman G, et al: *Transplantation* 48:238–243, August 1989.)

plant specimens, 23 of 26 rejecting specimens and 13 of 16 nonrejecting specimens. The tubular expression of HLA-DP and DQ was absent or weak. Rejecting specimens had a significantly greater infiltrate of T lymphocytes of all phenotypes and macrophages than nonrejecting ones had. The rejecting group had 4 graft losses, all caused by rejection. Further study showed that all losses were associated with macrophage-dominated infiltrates in the peritransplant specimens (table).

Immunohistologic analysis of early allograft biopsy specimens yields an accurate prognosis of subsequent graft acceptance or rejection. Early macrophage infiltration indicates a poor prognosis.

▶ The availability of a new monoclonal reagent identifying activated macrophages has demonstrated that early macrophage infiltration of an allograft carries a serious prognosis. Upregulated HLA class II antigen expression appeared to be irrelevant, because this was seen in most grafts irrespective of rejection and seemed to be a nonspecific response to injury of any kind. Many of our preconceived notions of the pathophysiology of acute rejection will need updating as we develop new technologies to study the phenomenon.—O. Jonasson, M.D.

Association of Antiidiotypic Antibody With Successful Second Transplant of a Kidney Sharing HLA Antigens With the Previous Hyperacutely Rejected First Kidney

Rodey GE, Phelan DL (Emory Univ; Atlanta; American Red Cross, Missouri-Illinois Region, St Louis)

Transplantation 48:54–57, July 1989   8–12

Immune responses partly regulate alloimmune effector responses to HLA molecules. In animal organ transplant models, long-term engraftment seems to be dependent on the development of donor-specific suppressor cells. A renal transplant recipient had successful retransplantation with a kidney having the same mismatched HLA-A2 antigen that was present on the hyperacutely rejected kidney.

Woman, 44, was studied for 18 months for the evolution of HLA antibodies and autoanti-idiotypic antibodies (AB2). After the transplanted kidney was rejected, serum from the patient was found to contain an HLA-A2 antibody that reacted with 100% of HLA-A2-positive panel cells. After several months the HLA-A2 antibody activity was lost precipitously within a 1 month. About 1 year later the patient had transplantation of another HLA-A2-positive kidney. This kidney was functioning after 2 years and had not been associated with significant rejection episodes. Before and episodically after the second transplant, the patient's sera had anti-idiotypic-like antibodies that inhibited HLA alloantibodies against HLA-A2. Auto-anti-idiotypic antibodies, specific for a putative idiotype on HLA-A2 alloantibodies, were present concurrently with other HLA alloantibodies.

In this patient the loss of a specific HLA antibody was associated temporally with the development of an AB2 with inhibitory specificity for the antibody. Anamnestic responses to donor-specific antigens are not always present in previously alloimmunized patients who are rechallenged with the same HLA antigens.

▶ It is as interesting to study why some organ transplants are successful and undergo essentially no transplant rejection as it is to study rejection phenomena. In this well-documented case report of a patient heavily presensitized to a strong transplant antigen, HLA2, Rodey and Phelam demonstrated the development of AB2 or anti-idiotypic antibodies that blocked the cytotoxic antibody present in the patient. The importance of the AB2 was clearly shown when a second HLA2+ kidney was not only not hyperacutely rejected but even seemed to escape expected milder acute rejection episodes. Anti-idiotypic antibodies specifically block the immune response.—O. Jonasson, M.D.

Cyclosporine Inhibits Endothelial Cell Prostacyclin Production
Rosenthal RA, Chukwuogo NA, Ocasio VH, Kahng KU (State Univ of New York, Brooklyn)
J Surg Res 46:593–596, June 1989   8–13

A reduction in renal blood flow may be an important early event in cyclosporine-induced nephrotoxicity. Arteriolopathy and glomerular thrombosis have been described in this disorder. Both the decline in blood flow and glomerular thrombosis may be related to a change in endothelial production of prostacyclin (PGI_2), a vasodilator that participates in the regulation of renal blood flow and acts as an inhibitor of platelet aggregation.

The effects of cyclosporine on arachidonic acid-stimulated production of PGI_2 were studied in confluent monolayers of human vein endothelial cells (HUVEC). Stimulation of HUVEC with arachidonic acid led to an increase in production of PGI_2 that was nearly 1,000% above baseline. Cyclosporine had a dose-dependent effect on production of PGI_2; concentrations of up to 0.1 μM were stimulatory, but greater concentrations inhibited production of PGI_2. Cyclosporine did not affect the growth of endothelial cells.

Short-term exposure to cyclosporine in concentrations that represent high therapeutic levels decreases production of arachidonic acid-stimulated PGI_2 by cultured HUVEC. The findings are consistent with a role for altered endothelial production of PGI_2 in the development of cyclosporine nephrotoxicity.

▶ The endothelial cells of the graft are the interface between the host and the graft. There is much interest in this boundary area, where many of the rejection-related events appear to take place. In this study cyclosporine was demonstrated to diminish prostacyclin production by cultured endothelial cells of human umbilical veins, a common in vitro model for the study of the structure and function of endothelial cells. Because prostacyclin participates in regulation of renal blood flow, the authors suggest that cyclosporine nephrotoxicity may be related to this inhibitory effect. The addition of PGE analogues may be useful in ameliorating cyclosporine nephrotoxicity.—O. Jonasson, M.D.

The Effect of Cyclosporine on the Use of Hospital Resources for Kidney Transplantation

Showstack J, Katz P, Amend W, Bernstein L, Lipton H, O'Leary M, Bindman A, Salvatierra O (Univ of California, San Francisco)
N Engl J Med 321:1086–1092, Oct 19, 1989   8–14

To learn whether the advent of cyclosporine immunosuppression has reduced hospital charges for kidney transplantation, the records of 702 patients receiving kidney transplants in 1982–1986 were reviewed. The series included 463 cadaver kidney and 239 living related donor kidney transplants. All services were priced in 1985 dollars, and multiple regression analysis was used to adjust for changing patient and hospital characteristics.

Cadaver kidney recipients had a higher in-hospital graft survival rate when receiving cyclosporine. The mean postoperative hospital stay was significantly shorter in cyclosporine-treated cadaver kidney recipients. Charges for clinical laboratory services, nuclear medicine, and dialysis all were lower with cyclosporine. Sequential cyclosporine therapy led to a shorter hospital stay and lower mean total charges than did nonsequential treatment (table) despite the fact that the sequential regimen was more expensive because of the cost of antilymphoblast globulin.

Adjusted Mean Postoperative Length of Stay and Charges for Recipients of Cadaver Kidneys According to Medication Regimen

	No Cyclosporine	Nonsequential Cyclosporine	Sequential Cyclosporine
No. of patients	141	71	251
Adjusted mean length of stay (days)	37.1	28.6 *	25.7 †‡
		1985 dollars	
Mean charges			
Room and board	16,970	13,846 §	11,716 † ‖
Ancillary services	18,353	14,974 †	12,763 †
Subtotal	35,283	28,781 *	24,438 † ‡
Pharmacy	2,673	2,103	3,487 † ‖
Total	37,997	30,925 *	27,966 †

Note: Postoperative length of stay and charges were adjusted through multiple regression analysis. Columns may not add to totals because separate estimates were derived for each comparison.
*Significantly different from the no-cyclosporine group; *P* < .001.
†Significantly different from the no-cyclosporine group; *P* < .0001.
‡Significantly different from the nonsequential group; *P* < .05.
§Significantly different from the no-cyclosporine group; *P* < .01.
‖Significantly different from the nonsequential group; *P* < .01.
(Courtesy of Showstack J, Katz P, Amend W, et al: *N Engl J Med* 321:1086–1092, Oct 19, 1989.)

Cyclosporine use is associated with lower use of resources by renal transplant patients. New medications such as cyclosporine that lower the rate of complications and improve patient outcome may also reduce the use of hospital resources.

▶ The outcome of cadaveric renal transplantation is considerably improved in patients receiving cyclosporine. Moreover, rehabilitation and return to productivity is likely. Unfortunately, this powerful immunosuppressive drug is very costly ($5,000 to $6,000 per year). Salvatierra and colleagues have demonstrated that hospital costs are reduced by at least that amount with the use of this drug—but at the patients' expense, as they must pay for their outpatient medications. Especially with the expectation of rehabilitation, a strong case can be made for inclusion of the costs of effective but expensive immunosuppressants in covered services.—O. Jonasson, M.D.

Effects of Combination Treatment With FK506 and Cyclosporine on Survival Time and Vascular Changes in Renal-Allograft-Recipient Dogs
Ochiai T, Sakamoto K, Gunji Y, Hamaguchi K, Isegawa N, Suzuki T, Shimada H, Hayashi H, Yasumoto A, Asano T, Isono K (Chiba Univ, Chiba-Shi, Japan; Sakura Natl Hosp, Japan)
Transplantation 48:193–197, August 1989   8–15

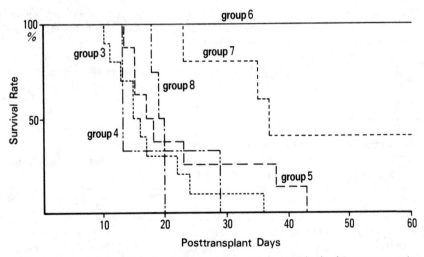

Fig 8–2.—Survival rates of renal recipient dogs that received various kinds of immunosuppressive treatments. Group 3: no immunosuppression in 10 dogs; median survival of 15.5 days. Group 4: CsA, 2.5 mg/kg/day in 3 dogs; median survival of 13 days. Group 5: FK, 0.32 mg/kg/day in 8 dogs; median survival of 17.5 days. Group 6: FK, 1.0 mg/kg/day in 5 dogs; median survival of more than 140 days. Group 7: FK 0.32 + CsA 2.5 mg/kg/day in 5 dogs; median survival of 37 days. Group 8: FK 0.32 + prednisolone 0.5 mg/kg/day in 4 dogs; median survival of 19.5 days. Statistical difference: group 3 vs. group 7, < 0.01; and group 3 vs. group 4, group 3 vs. group 5, group 3 vs. group 8, not significant. (Courtesy of Ochiai T, Sakamoto K, Gunji Y, et al: *Transplantation* 48:193–197, August 1989.)

Previous studies of the effects of FK506 in canine renal allograft recipients have shown anorexia, which generally is dose dependent, and vascular changes that actually are more prominent at lower doses. In the present study a nonanorexic, nonimmunosuppressive dose of FK506 was combined with a low dose of cyclosporine or prednisolone in beagle dogs who received renal allografts. The dose of FK506 was 0.32, or 1 mg/kg, and that of cyclosporine, 2.5 mg/kg.

The higher dose of FK506 prolonged the survival of allograft recipients, but neither the lower dose nor cyclosporine alone did so. Combined treatment with FK506 and cyclosporine at the same doses did prolong survival significantly (Fig 8−2). The frequency of vascular changes seen with the lower dose of FK506 was reduced when cyclosporine was added. The addition of prednisolone to FK506 failed to prevent the vascular changes, which included fibrinoid necrosis, thickening of the vessel wall, and round cell infiltration of the vascular wall.

These canine renal graft recipients tolerated immunosuppressive doses of FK506 well, surviving longer than 140 days. Both FK506 and cyclosporine exhibit synergism in inhibiting renal allograft rejection in the dog. Vascular changes that reflect inadequate immunosuppression can be prevented by either a high dose of FK506 or by adding cyclosporine.

▶ This new immunosuppressive drug, FK506, has received considerable press claiming dramatic results in human organ transplantation. Much of the preliminary work in large animal models has been plagued by side effects of anorexia and severe weight loss and vasculitis. Whether the canine model is appropriate for preclinical studies is debatable, but a clearer definition of the dose-response relationships and toxicity has not been achieved.

▶ ↓ In the following paper, clinical studies are reported that seem to be less complicated by side effects than occur with the primate or canine models.—O. Jonasson, M.D.

FK506 For Liver, Kidney, and Pancreas Transplantation

Starzl TE, Todo S, Fung J, Demetris AJ, Venkataramanan R, Jain A (Univ Health Ctr of Pittsburgh; Univ of Pittsburgh; VA Med Ctr, Pittsburgh)
Lancet 2:1000−1004, Oct 28, 1989   8−16

A macrolide produced by *Streptomyces tsukubaensis*, FK506, is a new immunosuppressive and cancer chemotherapeutic agent. It was given for either salvage or primary immunosuppression in 14 high-risk liver recipients; in the first 10 of these conventional immunosuppression had failed.

Salvage therapy was successful in 7 patients, and improvements in liver function were prompt (Table 1). On biopsy, findings of liver rejection were either ameliorated or eliminated. Except for 1 patient, renal function remained almost unchanged after treatment with FK506. Two patients who had graft losses after salvage therapy with FK506 and 4 new patients underwent fresh orthotopic liver transplantation while receiving

TABLE 1.—Liver Recipients Receiving Rescue Treatment:
Follow-Up to September 14, 1989

Patient	Age/ sex	Date of last liver graft	Date FK 506 started (1989)	Fate of liver graft	Serum creatinine (μmol/l) Before	After
1	28/F	June 29, '88⁺	Feb 28	Salvaged	362	115
2	38/M	Jan 1, '89*	March 25	Replaced July 2†	195	195
3	30/F	Nov 18, '87*	April 4	Salvaged	477	Dialysis
4	42/M	April 30, '89	Feb 6	Salvaged	124	141
5	38/F	Feb 12, 82	June 29	Salvaged	239	283
6	47/M	June 15, '86	Jan 7	Salvaged	248	239
7	18/F	July 18, '86*	July 8	Salvaged	141	203
8	63/F	May 8, '89	July 30	Replacement attempted Sept 5; died†	150	141
9	37/M	July 10, '89	Feb 8	Replaced Aug 28†	88	106
10	45/F	July 29, '89	Aug 10	Salvaged	133	97

*Third (patient 1), fifth (patient 2), and second (patients 3 and 7) liver grafts.
†Graft replaced because of arterial thrombosis and septic hepatic gangrene (patient 2) or because the small bile ducts had already been destroyed (patients 8 and 9).
(Courtesy of Starzl TE, Todo S, Fung J, et al: *Lancet* 2:1000–1004, Oct 28, 1989.)

FK506 plus low-dose steroids. None of these 6 patients had rejection, although 1 with preexisting cor pulmonale and coronary atherosclerosis died of myocardial infarction (Table 2). Postoperative biopsy of the 2 livers inserted at retransplantation indicated no evidence of rejection, and none of the 6 patients had signs of nephrotoxicity.

Two of 14 liver recipients received cadaveric kidneys, either from the

TABLE 2.—Fresh Transplantations

Patient	Date started (1989)	Date of fresh transplantation	Organ transplanted	Graft function (Sept 10)	Total bilirubin (μmol/l)	Creatinine (μmol/l)
1	Feb 28	March 27	Kidney	Normal	5·1	106
2	March 25	July 2	6th liver	Normal	10·2	195
3	April 4	May 21	2nd kidney	Removed June 20	12·0	—
9	Aug 2	Aug 28	2nd liver	Normal	44·5	106
11	Aug 17	Aug 17	Liver	Normal	20·5	97
	. .		Kidney	Normal		
	. .		Pancreas	Normal		
12	Aug 18	Aug 18	Liver	Died Sept 1*	18·8	106
13	Aug 24	Aug 24	Liver	Normal	6·8	61
14	Sept 3	Sept 3	Liver	Normal	32·4	124

*Myocardial infarction.
(Courtesy of Starzl TE, Todo S, Fung J, et al: *Lancet* 2:1000–1004, Oct 28, 1989.)

same donor or from a different donor. A third recipient received a pancreas as well as a kidney from the liver donor. None of these recipients had evidence of rejection of the kidney or pancreas, and no serious side effects were noted.

These findings demonstrate the impressive performance of FK506 both for salvage and for primary immunosuppression in high-risk patients undergoing liver, kidney, and pancreas transplantation. This agent is remarkably free from unwanted effects.

▶ The clinical experience in this first report of a trial of a new immunosuppressive drug is almost entirely related to the effects associated with liver allograft procedures. The kidney and pancreas experience was limited to combined procedures accompanying liver transplants, and to 1 patient receiving a pancreatic transplant. Conclusions regarding the usefulness of this drug for kidney and pancreas grafts are premature. However, the salvage and retransplant successes in liver recipients are impressive. Its combination with cyclosporine proved to be seriously nephrotoxic but, alone, FK506 appears to be well tolerated. This is somewhat surprising in view of the toxicity of the agent in animal models.— O. Jonasson, M.D.

The Effects of OKT3 Therapy on Infiltrating Lymphocytes in Rejecting Renal Allografts
Kerr PG, Atkins RC (Prince Henry's Hosp, Melbourne)
Transplantation 48:33–36, July 1989   8–17

The monoclonal antibody OKT3 has been used successfully to treat acute allograft rejection in renal transplant recipients. However, its mode of action is not completely understood. After OKT3 antibody exposure, peripheral blood T cells fail to express the CD3 antigen, but they maintain the expression of other surface antigens. It is not known whether these peripheral blood lymphocyte changes in membrane antigen expression are reflected by lymphocytes in the graft. The leukocytes infiltrating rejecting grafts were examined in 10 patients receiving OKT3 treatment for steroid-resistant renal allograft rejection.

Immunoperoxidase examination of biopsy material and flow cytometric analysis of peripheral blood lymphocytes obtained before and during treatment indicated that the total number of infiltrating leukocytes dropped after 5 days of therapy (Fig 8–3). The relative proportions of macrophages, total lymphocytes and CD4 +ve and CD8 +ve cells did not change. Marked modulation of peripheral blood lymphocytes occurred, but no evidence of modulation of intragraft lymphocytes was noted.

These findings indicate that OKT3 antibody therapy modulates the CD3 antigen from the surface of peripheral blood T lymphocytes and suggest that OKT3 antibody treatment produces a diminution of the total leukocytic infiltrate of rejecting renal allografts. However, it appears to do this nonspecifically. No evidence of modulation of the antigen from

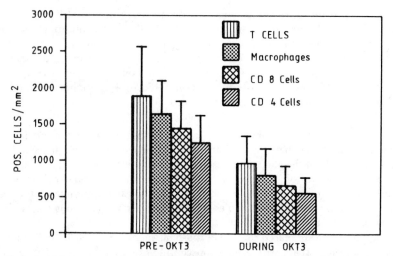

Fig 8–3.—Relative composition of the infiltrating cells in 10 rejecting renal allografts before and during OKT3 antibody therapy, expressed as the number of positive cells in 1 mm² of biopsy tissue (mean ±SD). $P < .001$ for all groups. (Courtesy of Kerr PG, Atkins RC: *Transplantation* 48:33–36, July 1989.)

the surface of intragraft lymphocytes was noted 5 days after treatment was begun, despite the marked changes of modulation of peripheral blood lymphocytes. Although OKT3 is clinically effective at ameliorating renal allograft rejection, it does not appear to modulate the CD3 antigen on intragraft lymphocytes. It may merely block the ability of peripheral T lymphocytes to respond to the foreign antigen, preventing them from homing to the graft.

► It has been assumed that OKT3 therapy affects the lymphocytic infiltrate in rejecting allografts, thereby reversing rejection. In fact, this report demonstrates that little effect is found when the graft-infiltrating lymphocytes are examined. Although the total number of infiltrating cells is reduced, the cytotoxic cell population occurs in the same distribution as was found pretreatment; the main effect of OKT3 is in modulation (removal) of the CD3 antigen recognition marker from lymphocytes in the peripheral blood. The significance of the lymphocytes in the infiltrate during rejection is not clear, and it may be that these cells are not directly responsible for the graft cell necrosis of a rejection reaction. Macrophages may be more important as mediators of the damage.— O. Jonasson, M.D.

Use of Cryopreserved Donor Bone Marrow in Cadaver Kidney Allograft Recipients
Barber WH, Diethelm AG, Laskow DA, Deierhoi MH, Julian BA, Curtis JJ (Univ of Alabama, Birmingham; Univ Hosp, Birmingham)
Transplantation 47:66–71, January 1989   8–18

Donor-specific unresponsiveness to organ allografts is still an elusive goal. In animals the use of an induction course of antilymphocyte serum beginning at the time of transplantation, followed by transfusion to the recipient of donor-specific bone marrow, can induce prolonged survival of allografts. The use of cryopreserved donor bone marrow in recipients of cadaveric kidney allografts was investigated in 40 patients assigned to a bone marrow group or a control group.

Procedure.—After routine skin preparation and surgical draping to procure cadaveric organs, bone marrow was harvested just after the initial incisions and superior retraction of the abdominal viscera were completed. About 1 L of marrow aspirate was taken from many sites. Ribs were sometimes obtained as additional sources of marrow. Rib marrow and iliac crest aspirates were filtered through wire screens to remove bony spicules. The typical yield of cells from 1 L of aspirate was 2.1×10^{10} viable nucleated cells.

The samples were placed in a cryoprotectant mix of Roswell Park Memorial Institute medium 1640, with a final concentration of 10% FCS and 10% dimethyl sulfoxide. Aliquots of 200 mL were bagged and frozen. Samples were placed in the vapor phase of liquid nitrogen for storage. Immunosuppression involved a sequential protocol using an induction course of Minnesota antilymphoblast globulin (MALG) combined with cyclosporine, azathioprine, and prednisone. The day after transplant, the bone marrow group began a 10- to 14-day course of MALG. Cryopreserved marrow was transfused 7 days after MALG was stopped. Cyclosporine was not given on the day of marrow infusion. Azathioprine therapy was discontinued, and 14 days of cyclophosphamide treatment were begun the day after marrow infusion, after which azathioprine was reinitiated. Maintenance doses for both groups included cyclosporine and azathioprine.

Nine patients in the marrow group had 11 episodes of acute rejection. The other 11 patients remained free of rejection. Seventeen rejection episodes occurred in 12 controls. The remaining 8 were free of rejection. Two patients in the marrow group and 6 in the control group received second allografts. All of these patients have functioning transplants.

These preliminary results suggest that transfusion of cryopreserved cadaveric donor bone marrow after a short course of antilymphocyte serum is safe. Such transfusion did not induce graft-vs.-host disease or allograft rejection. It may improve allograft and patient survival while allowing for reduced requirements for nonspecific immunosuppressive agents with their adverse effects.

▶ Monaco, Wood, and colleagues from Harvard have described the induction of donor-specific unresponsiveness (tolerance) in small and large animal experiments using infusion of donor's nucleated bone marrow cells. These experimental protocols have been extended to a clinical series in this bold protocol, with very impressive success.— O. Jonasson, M.D.

The Effects of Pancreas Transplantation on the Glomerular Structure of Renal Allografts in Patients With Insulin-Dependent Diabetes
Bilous RW, Mauer SM, Sutherland DER, Najarian JS, Goetz FC, Steffes MW
(Univ of Minnesota)
N Engl J Med 321:80–85, July 13, 1989   8–19

The relationship between hyperglycemia and the development of vascular complications is controversial. In diabetic patients who have undergone kidney transplantation new glomerular lesions may develop, as can be demonstrated by structural increases in mesangial and glomerular volume. Partial or whole pancreas transplantation can normalize glucose levels in diabetic patients and reverse diabetic nephropathy in laboratory animals. To determine how pancreas transplantation affects diabetic nephropathy in humans, 12 diabetic patients who underwent pancreas transplantation after receiving renal allografts were examined.

Percutaneous biopsy specimens of the renal allografts were obtained before implantation of the pancreatic grafts. Repeat biopsy specimens of the renal allograft were obtained 23 months to 10 years after successful pancreas transplantation. Before pancreas transplantation all 12 patients were taking insulin daily, and all had severe proliferative retinopathy and peripheral neuropathy.

Renal biopsy specimens obtained before pancreas transplantation revealed a normal or modestly increased mesangial volume and moderately thickened glomerular basement membrane. Renal biopsy specimens obtained at least 1.9 years after successful pancreas transplantation revealed no disease progression in any of the glomerular structures. Actually, pancreas transplant recipients had significantly smaller glomeruli and less mesangial expansion than a matched group of conventionally treated diabetic patients who had undergone renal transplantation, but not pancreas transplantation. Although evidence of improved long-term patient survival or improved renal graft function after pancreas transplantation was not provided, the finding that pancreas transplantation prevented the progression of diabetic glomerulopathy in renal allografts has important clinical implications.

▶ Pancreas transplantation does not reverse established vascular, renal, or ophthalmologic complications in late-stage diabetics. Although it improves the quality of life of these brittle patients, there has been no evidence that more objective improvements ensue. Therefore, this is an important paper demonstrating that a new kidney, transplanted into a diabetic patient, seems to be protected from the development of diabetic nephropathy through normalization of the blood glucose levels on a permanent basis. Diabetic patients who receive a kidney transplant are known to have definite histologic evidence of diabetic nephropathy within 2 years of transplantation, and progression to more advanced disease has been documented. Protection of this new organ will be an important indication for pancreas transplantation.—O. Jonasson, M.D.

Modulation of the Major Histocompatibility Complex Antigen and the Immunogenicity of Islet Allografts

Markmann JF, Jacobson JD, Kiumura H, Choti MA, Hickey WF, Fox IJ, Silvers WK, Barker CF, Naji A (Univ of Pennsylvania)
Transplantation 48:478–486, September 1989   8–20

A common feature of allograft rejection is modulation of the major histocompatibility complex antigen by parenchymal cells and "passenger leukocytes." To assess the significance of this, the fate of antigen-presenting cell (APC)-depleted pancreatic islet allografts was examined after increasing their expression of major histocompatibility complex antigens by in vitro exposure to the lymphokine interferon-γ (IFn-γ).

Pancreatic islets were isolated from Lewis rat pancreata. Most untreated grafts survived indefinitely. Grafts exposed to IFN-γ were rejected acutely. Islet cell exposure to IFN-γ was associated with increased vulnerability to allogeneic cytotoxic T lymphocyte lysis in vitro by a $CD5^+$, $CD8^+$, $CD4^-$, class I-restricted cytotoxic T lymphocyte. The IFN-γ exposure did not affect the ability of islet cells to serve as APC for T lymphocytes.

Using an in vivo model of islet allograft rejection, it was demonstrated that IFN-γ-exposed islet allografts are uniformly susceptible to immunologic rejection when nonlymphokine-exposed grafts survive indefinitely. Antigenic modulation can be a decisive factor in graft survival by augmenting the interaction of the graft antigens with cytolytic effector T lymphocytes.

▶ In these experiments the APCs were depleted from pancreatic islets by means of culture of the islets in a high oxygen environment. Under ordinary experimental conditions this would lead to survival of islet allografts when transplanted. "Upregulation" of the HLA class II antigens of the parenchymal cells of the islets was then achieved with IFN-γ, and the capability of the islet cells to also serve as APCs was demonstrated when the islets acutely rejected. The importance of the various upregulating cytokines in initiating and maintaining rejection activity cannot be underestimated.— O. Jonasson, M.D.

Extended Preservation of Human Liver Grafts With UW Solution

Todo S, Nery J, Yanaga K, Podesta L, Gordon RD, Starzl TE (Univ of Pittsburgh)
JAMA 261:711–714, Feb 3, 1989   8–21

Cold ischemia of canine and human liver allografts can be extended safely to 1 day with an infusate developed at University of Wisconsin (UW). The superior quality of the UW solution was confirmed in other laboratories with liver replacement experiments in dogs and rats. The outcomes of 185 human cadaveric liver homografts preserved for 4–24 hours in UW solution were compared with those of 180 grafts preserved in conventional Euro-Collins solution for 3–9.5 hours.

The average preservation time of the livers preserved with UW solution was almost twice that of the livers preserved with Euro-Collins solution. The grafts preserved with UW solution survived at a higher rate, resulted in equivalent rates of patient survival, and were associated with a lower rate of primary nonfunction, of need for retransplantation, and of hepatic artery thrombosis. The time of preservation of grafts preserved with UW solution to 24 hours and liver function abnormality in the first week

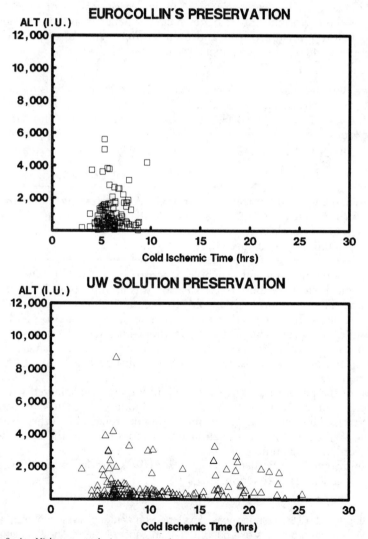

Fig 8–4.—Highest serum alanine aminotransferase values in first postoperative week after transplantation of livers preserved with UW *(bottom)* and Euro-Collins *(top)* solutions for variable periods. (Courtesy of Todo S, Nery J, Yanaga K, et al: *JAMA* 261:711–714, Feb 3, 1989.)

after surgery were not correlated. Livers preserved in Euro-Collins solution for more than 5 hours had significantly higher perturbations of hepatic function tests (Fig 8−4).

The remarkable success of the UW solution has revolutionized liver transplantation. The increased margin of safety allows more effective use of organs that can be stored safely while waiting for operating room facilities or personnel. Grafts now can be transported from places once considered too far away. There is ample time for detailed histopathologic analysis of graft biopsy specimens. The increased margin of safety also enables the performance of a better recipient hepatectomy, better hemostasis before graft placement, and even leisurely removal of part of the homograft when size discrepancies occur.

▶ After years of research and development, Belzer and colleagues at the University of Wisconsin have succeeded in developing a preservation solution that permits up to 24 hours of cold ischemia before transplantation. This has facilitated liver transplantation greatly, allowed organ sharing over longer distances, and improved early liver allograft function.—O. Jonasson, M.D.

Combined Liver and Pancreas Procurement With Belzer-UW Solution
Sollinger HW, Vernon WB, D'Alessandro AM, Kalayoglu M, Stratta RJ, Belzer FO (Univ of Wisconsin)
Surgery 106:685−691, October 1989   8−22

Combined procurement of whole pancreaticoduodenal and liver grafts is technically feasible. Belzer-UW solution was used for both aortic in situ flushing (Fig 8−5) and ex vivo cold storage in 20 consecutive multiorgan procurements that included the liver, pancreas, and kidneys. Ten hearts also were procured. The mean preservation times were 14 hours for the pancreas; 16 hours for the kidney transplanted with the pancreas; 30 hours for isolated kidneys, which were machine-perfused; and 14 hours for the liver.

All of the pancreatic transplants and all kidneys transplanted with the pancreas survived, as did 93% of isolated kidneys. The survival rate for liver transplants was 78.5%. Including organs referred to other centers, 84 of 89 procured organs functioned at 1 month. All of the hearts were functioning at this time.

Multiorgan procurement using Belzer-UW solution consistently provides excellent graft function.

▶ Although the UW solution was developed primarily for liver transplantation, the Wisconsin group has extended its use in pancreas and kidney transplantation with equally good results. The group also perfused hearts with UW solution, with excellent function reported, although extension of the preservation

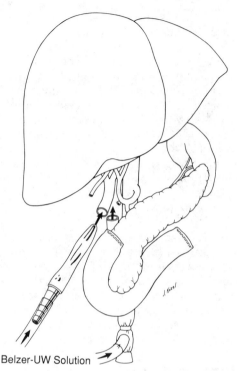

Belzer-UW Solution

Fig 8–5.—Simultaneous intra-aortic and portal flush with Belzer-UW solution. (Courtesy of Sollinger HW, Vernon WB, D'Alessandro AM, et al: *Surgery* 106:685–691, October 1989.)

period for the heart was not attempted. This will be the next step in improving short-term organ preservation.— O. Jonasson, M.D.

Intercellular Adhesion Molecule 1 on Liver Allografts During Rejection

Adams DH, Hubscher SG, Shaw J, Rothlein R, Neuberger JM (Queen Elizabeth Hosp, Birmingham, England; Univ of Birmingham; Boehringer Ingelheim Pharmaceuticals Inc, Ridgefield, Conn)
Lancet 2:1122–1125, Nov 11, 1989   8–23

Graft rejection results when host immune cells recognize donor antigens and begin an inflammatory cascade of effector cells that can damage the graft. Leukocyte adhesion to target cells and other immune cells occurs. Adhesion is mediated by several receptors on the leukocyte surface, including lymphocyte-function-associated antigen 1, which binds to intercellular adhesion molecules (ICAM) 1 and 2. The fact that ICAM-1 expression can be induced in vitro by proinflammatory cytokines suggests that it might be an important regulator of the inflammatory response. The expression of ICAM-1 in the liver after transplantation was investigated in 53 biopsy samples from 50 liver transplant recipients and 13 control samples from donor livers at transplantation.

Greater ICAM-1 expression was noted on bile ducts, endothelium, and perivenular hepatocytes in patients with acute rejection when compared with donor livers, patients with stable transplants, or patients with non-rejection complications. Patients in whom there was progression to chronic, irreversible rejection had greater expression of ICAM-1 on bile ducts and hepatocytes. After high-dose corticosteroid therapy in patients with resolving rejection, ICAM-1 expression was decreased greatly.

The induction of ICAM-1 on tissues may be important in the development of inflammatory responses and in determining which cells are the targets of immune damage. Treatment with high-dose corticosteroids reduced ICAM-1 expression, suggesting that this may be an important mode of action of these drugs.

▶ The cytotoxic cells involved in allograft rejection must bind to the target cells to be effective. The sites to which binding occurs have been identified and labeled as intercellular adhesion molecules (ICAM). Interestingly, these ICAMs are induced and expressed through the action of the cytokines, probably produced by infiltrating activated lymphocytes and macrophages. Steroids downregulate the expression of ICAMs and this may be an important component of their immunosuppressive effect.—O. Jonasson, M.D.

Efficacy of Liver Transplantation in Patients With Primary Biliary Cirrhosis
Markus BH, Dickson ER, Grambsch PM, Fleming TR, Mazzaferro V, Klintmalm GBG, Wiesner RH, Van Thiel DH, Starzl TE (Univ of Pittsburgh; Mayo Clinic and Found, Rochester, Minn; Univ of Washington; Baylor Univ Med Ctr, Dallas)
N Engl J Med 320:1709–1713, June 29, 1989   8–24

The efficacy of liver transplantation was examined in 161 patients who underwent transplantation and in patients with the same diagnosis not having transplantation. The former patients were operated on in 1980–1987 and were followed for a median of 25 months. The primary indication for liver transplantation was poor liver function in 132 patients.

Analysis using the Kaplan-Meier model indicated a substantially higher probability of survival in the recipients 3 months after liver transplantation than in nonrecipients as predicted using the Mayo model (Fig 8–6). At 2 years the Kaplan-Meier survival probability was 0.74, whereas the mean Mayo-model survival probability was 0.31. Patients at all risk levels according to the Mayo model were more likely to survive after liver transplantation. At last follow-up two thirds of the transplant recipients were working full time and another 27% part time. Only 3% of the patients were hospitalized.

Liver transplantation demonstrably improves long-term survival in patients with primary biliary cirrhosis. Survival has improved further with

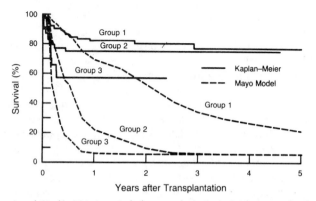

Fig 8–6.—Actual (Kaplan-Meier) survival after transplantation in 3 risk groups of patients with primary biliary cirrhosis and estimated survival without transplantation as predicted by the Mayo Model. Risk groups were formed on the basis of pretransplantation Mayo-model risk scores. Group 1 (low risk) had 98 patients with risk scores of less than 8.67; group 2 (medium risk) had 41 patients with risk scores between 8.67 and 9.93; group 3 (high risk) had 22 patients with scores of more than 9.93. (Courtesy of Markus BH, Dickson ER, Grambsch PM, et al: *N Engl J Med* 320:1709–1713, June 29, 1989.)

the use of OKT3 treatment for transplant rejection. More than 90% of patients who survive transplantation can expect to return to work, at least part time.

▶ Excellent outcomes are achieved with liver transplantation in patients with primary biliary cirrhosis. The accumulated clinical series shows essentially no long-term attrition in 5 years.

▶ ↓ This is in contrast to the next paper selected for review, in which suspected recurrence of the original disease is addressed.— O. Jonasson, M.D.

Evidence for Disease Recurrence After Liver Transplantation for Primary Biliary Cirrhosis: Clinical and Histologic Follow-up Studies
Polson RJ, Portmann B, Neuberger J, Calne RY, Williams R (King's College Hosp, London; Addenbrooke's Hosp, Cambridge, England)
Gastroenterology 97:715–725, September 1989   8–25

Primary biliary cirrhosis remains one of the most frequent indications for liver transplantation. Twenty-three patients with primary biliary cirrhosis who lived longer than a year after liver transplantation were followed. The patients, 19 women and 4 men aged 31–58 years, had been ill for a median of 6 years. All initially had marked symptomatic improvement and decreases in serum bilirubin, alkaline phosphatase, IgM, and antimitochondrial antibody levels.

Liver biopsy specimens showed changes indicating recurrence in 9 of 10 patients more than a year after transplantation. Four others had pruritus or associated abnormalities. Levels of IgM were increased in 80% of patients, and antimitochondrial antibody titers were elevated in all of the patients tested. Some patients initially given prednisone and azathioprine had histologic improvement when given cyclosporine.

Primary biliary cirrhosis can recur after liver transplantation. There may well be a constitutional abnormality in these patients that underlies disordered immune regulation.

▶ Although the early postoperative results of liver transplantation in this small series of patients with primary biliary cirrhosis were as good as those reported in the preceding paper (Abstract 8–24), late biopsies seemed to demonstrate recurrence of the disease, with increased IgM levels and antimitochondrial antibodies. Whether these troublesome findings are disease recurrence or chronic rejection—the "disappearing bile duct syndrome"—is unclear, but biopsy data on more patients over the long-term are clearly needed.—O. Jonasson, M.D.

Serial Decrease in Glomerular Filtration Rate in Long-Term Pediatric Liver Transplantation Survivors Treated With Cyclosporine
McDiarmid SV, Ettenger RB, Fine RN, Busuttil RW, Ament ME (Univ of California, Los Angeles)
Transplantation 47:314–318, February 1989   8–26

Pediatric liver transplant recipients may face lifelong use of cyclosporine A, and a balance must be found between immunosuppression and renal toxicity. The glomerular filtration rate (GFR) was calculated serially in 31 pediatric patients who survived for more than a year after liver

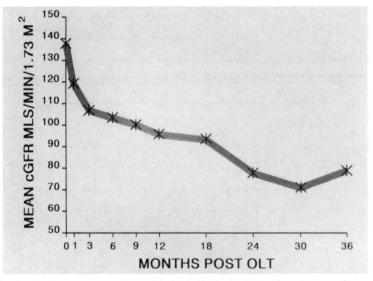

Fig 8–7.—Means and standard error of mean of serial levels of cGFR for 31 patients who survived for more than 1 year after orthotopic liver transplantation (OLT). Mean cGFR was calculated pre-OLT and at 1, 3, 6, 9, 12, 18, 24, 30, and 36 months. (Courtesy of McDiarmid SV, Ettenger RB, Fine RN, et al: *Transplantation* 47:314–318, February 1989.)

transplantation. The rate was computed (cGFR) from the Schwartz formula before orthotopic liver transplantation and at intervals of 3–6 months thereafter.

The mean difference between the preoperative cGFR and the most recent rates for all patients was 50 mL/min/1.73 m². In 55% of the patients the current value was less than 80 mL/min/m², indicating impairment in renal function. In 24 patients the cGFR continued to fall for more than 1 year after transplantation (Fig 8–7). Hypertension was more frequent in patients with a cGFR of less than 80 mL/min/1.73 m².

Renal function is significantly impaired in pediatric recipients of orthotopic liver transplants, and most patients have slowly progressive impairment. Prospective studies are needed to determine the effects of low-dose cyclosporine on renal function.

▶ Cyclosporine is unquestionably an effective immunosuppressive drug, allowing far better survival after liver transplantation than before it was available, but the side effects of nephrotoxicity are severe and long lasting. Similar data regarding progressive loss of renal function have been reported in heart transplant recipients. Hypertension is a frequent finding in recipients of any type of allograft who receive cyclosporine. The reduction in cyclosporine dose and addition of adjunctive immunosuppressive agents are required to achieve a reasonable balance between rejection and nephrotoxicity.— O. Jonasson, M.D.

Transplantation of Multiple Abdominal Viscera
Starzl TE, Rowe MI, Todo S, Jaffe R, Tzakis A, Hoffman AL, Esquivel C, Porter KA, Venkataramanan R, Makowka L, Duquesnoy R (Univ of Pittsburgh; St Mary's Hosp and Med School, London)
JAMA 261:1449–1457, March 10, 1989   8–27

Two children with the short gut syndrome and secondary liver failure underwent evisceration and en bloc transplantation of the stomach, small intestine, colon, pancreas, and liver. The procedure was standardized in Landrace pigs weighing 15–25 kg. The first patient died at operation, but the second lived longer than 6 months before dying of an Epstein-Barr virus-associated lymphoproliferative disorder that caused biliary obstruction and sepsis. This child had no evidence of graft rejection or of graft-vs.-host disease. The homografted organs remained morphologically intact throughout the 193-day survival period.

The problems of rejection and graft-vs.-host disease in multivisceral transplantation differ only quantitatively from those seen when individual organs are transplanted. Avoidance of graft-vs.-host disease depends on effective immunosuppression. There is a risk of too intensive treatment to prevent rejection and graft-vs.-host disease.

The definite function observed in the present patient is encouraging. The liver functioned well for some time despite early cholangitis and later biliary obstruction. Cautious trials of multivisceral or intestinal transplantation, or both, are expected.

Splanchnic Transplantation: An Approach to the Infant Dependent on Parenteral Nutrition Who Develops Irreversible Liver Disease

Williams JW, Sankary HN, Foster PF, Lowe J, Goldman GM (Rush-Presbyterian-St Luke's Med Ctr, Chicago)
JAMA 261:1458–1462, March 10, 1989   8–28

If cholestatic liver failure develops in an infant dependent on parenteral nutrition, death is inevitable unless life-sustaining enteric nutrition can be achieved. Liver transplantation has not seemed worthwhile in these children.

Two infants with short-bowel syndrome and liver failure associated with obligatory parenteral nutrition underwent en bloc transplantation of the liver, stomach, duodenum, pancreas, jejunum, and ileum. Nearly normal function of the small bowel and liver was achieved in the second case, despite a number of early complications, until a monoclonal malignant B cell lymphoproliferative disorder supervened.

Irradiation of the cold ischemic intestinal allograft reduces rejection in cyclosporine-treated dogs and eliminates graft-vs.-host disease after porcine pancreas and spleen transplantation. Splanchnic transplantation is technically feasible, and metabolically fragile children tolerate it well. Inclusion of the pancreas avoids pancreatic fistula formation and duodenal injury. The high risk of lymphoma is a serious problem.

▶ These 2 patients (Abstracts 8–27 and 8–28) appeared back-to-back in a single issue of *JAMA*. In both reports multiple viscera, including the liver and small bowel, were transplanted into children who were then immunosuppressed quite heavily. The 2 who survived the perioperative procedure both died of lymphoma during the first few months. A balance between immunosuppression and the risk of graft-vs.-host disease from the heavy lymphoid cell population of the small bowel was not achieved in these patients, and a monoclonal lymphoid malignancy developed. These malignancies are well known in heavily immunosuppressed patients, and it seems that children, especially those given such a heavy lymphoid tissue load, also are vulnerable to the development of the tumors. These tumors are probably related to viral infection and may yield to antiviral chemotherapy, but until these problems are resolved it is unlikely that additional infants will be subjected to this dramatic procedures.— O. Jonasson, M.D.

Oxygenated Perfluorocarbon, Recombinant Human Superoxide Dismutase, and Catalase Ameliorate Free Radical Induced Myocardial Injury During Heart Preservation and Transplantation

Bando K, Teramoto S, Tago M, Seno S, Murakami T, Nawa S, Senoo Y (Okayama Univ, Japan)
J Thorac Cardiovasc Surg 96:930–938, December 1988   8–29

Myocardial membrane peroxidation by oxygen free radicals is implicated in reperfusion injury after myocardial ischemia. Whether maintain-

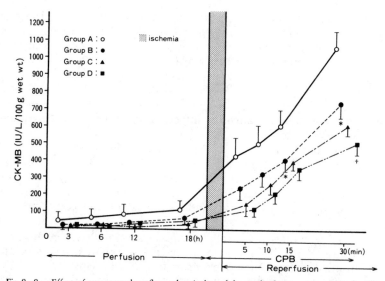

Fig 8–8.—Effect of oxygenated perfluorochemicals and free radical scavengers on level of creatine kinase MB. Values are means ± SD. *Abbreviations: CK-MB,* creatine kinase MB; *CPB,* cardiopulmonary bypass. *$P < .05$ vs. group A; †$P < .05$ vs. group B. (Courtesy of Bando K, Teramoto S, Tago M, et al: *J Thorac Cardiovasc Surg* 96:930–938, December 1988.)

ing myocardial oxygenation with an oxygenated perfluorocarbon solution could reduce or eliminate free radical-mediated functional depression after prolonged hypothermic preservation of the canine heart was investigated. Orthotopically transplanted hearts were perfused with oxygenated Collins' solution, with or without Fluosol DA and albumin. Some animals received recombinant human superoxide dismutase and bovine catalase during preservation perfusion or before and during reperfusion.

Only control hearts had significant weight gain and a decrease in passive compliance during preservation. Lactate release was reduced by Fluosol DA. Free radical generation increased during reperfusion, as did creatine kinase MB isoenzyme levels. Perfusion with perfluorochemical solution inhibited the rise in levels of thiobarbituric acid-reactive substances and in creatine kinase MB isoenzyme (Fig 8–8) and improved cardiac function during reperfusion. Exogenous free radical scavengers had similar effects when given just before and during reperfusion but not when given only during preservation.

Free-radical induced injury occurring during reperfusion after heart transplantation can be reduced by administering free radical scavengers or by perfusion with a hyperosmolar intracellular solution containing perfluorochemical. If the latter is used, adding free radical scavengers provides no further benefit.

▶ Heart transplantation is greatly impeded by the lack of an effective short-term preservation method for the heart. Deterioration of cardiac function occurs after 2–3 hours of cold ischemia, and an outer limit of 4 hours has been found to be necessary to accomplish safe cardiac transplantation. These authors tested scavengers of free oxygen radicals as well as an oxygen-carrying agent, perfluorocarbon, and demonstrated that both agents will separately improve cardiac function after cold ischemia. Application of these methods to heart preservation may be beneficial.—O. Jonasson, M.D.

Gastrointestinal Cytomegalovirus Infection in Heart and Heart-Lung Transplant Recipients
Kaplan CS, Petersen EA, Icenogle TB, Copeland JG, Villar HV, Sampliner R, Minnich L, Ray CG (Univ of Arizona)
Arch Intern Med 149:2095–2100, September 1989   8–30

Cytomegalovirus (CMV) is a significant cause of morbidity and mortality in organ transplant recipients. The use of ganciclovir, an acyclic guanine analogue that structurally resembles acyclovir, was evaluated in 10 heart and heart-lung transplant recipients who had CMV-associated gastrointestinal disease. Nine of 96 heart transplant recipients and 1 of 5 heart-lung transplant recipients were affected. Ganciclovir, 5 mg/kg, was given intravenously twice daily for at least 2 weeks.

The most common symptoms were epigastric pain, fever, nausea-vomiting, diarrhea, and gastrointestinal bleeding. The endoscopic findings were variable (table). Symptoms consistently resolved in the first week of ganciclovir therapy, and there were no new surgical complications of CMV infection in the gastrointestinal tract. Six patients continued to use the drug for 4–8 weeks.

None of the patients died of CMV infection. Gastritis began healing as early as 2 weeks after the start of treatment, and ulcers healed completely

Endoscopic Findings in Patients With Gastrointestinal Cytomegalovirus Infection	
Endoscopic Appearance	**No. of Patients**
Gastric mucosa	
Erythema	9
Erosions	7
Ulcerations	4
Nodules	3
Polyps	1
Placques	1
Hemorrhage	2
Esophagus	
Erythema	1
Nodules	1
Duodenum	
Erythema	3
Nodules	2

(Courtesy of Kaplan CS, Petersen EA, Icenogle TB, et al: *Arch Intern Med* 149:2095–2100, September 1989.)

within 12 weeks. There were no symptomatic side effects from gangiclovir. Relapses responded to retreatment with ganciclovir for 2–3 weeks. Some patients without symptoms continued to shed CMV in the urine, but treatment was not given for this reason.

Early endoscopy is indicated when a heart transplant recipient experiences gastrointestinal symptoms. Ganciclovir is well tolerated and effective in patients with CMV infection of the gastrointestinal tract.

▶ The upper gastrointestinal ulcerations in immunosuppressed transplant recipients, previously attributed to the ulcerogenic properties of steroids, are now recognized to be caused largely by invasive CMV infections. In this important clinical paper, the antiviral drug ganciclovir resolved the upper gastrointestinal lesions and promoted healing of the gastritis and mucosal ulcerations of CMV gastroduodenitis. These infections are important causes of serious morbidity and mortality in transplant recipients, and the availability of a new drug that is obviously effective is encouraging.—O. Jonasson, M.D.

9 Oncology and Tumor Immunology

Epidermal Growth Factor Receptor Gene Expression, Protein Kinase Activity, and Terminal Differentiation of Human Malignant Epidermal Cells
King I, Sartorelli AC (Yale Univ)
Cancer Res 49:5677–5681, Oct 15, 1989   9–1

Binding of epidermal growth factor (EGF) to its receptor activates protein kinase, which phosphorylates a number of cellular proteins. In addition, influx of sodium and turnover of phosphatidylinositol are observed. The number of EGF receptors is correlated inversely with the degree of epidermal cell differentiation, suggesting a role for this receptor in epidermal maturation. The gene copy number of the EGF receptor and its messenger RNA expression were measured in various EGF-resistant clones of human epidermoid carcinoma A431 cells.

Epidermal growth factor-resistant clones derived from A431 cells were capable of forming substantially more cornified envelopes in culture than was the parental line. After 6 days in culture, only 10% of parental A431 cells expressed a differentiated phenotype, compared with more than half of each of the 3 EGF-resistant variants. The EGF-resistant clones expressed fewer EGF receptors than parent cells and had a lesser capacity for EGF receptor autophosphorylation. All of the EGF-resistant variants contained fewer copies of the EGF receptor gene; no gene rearrangement was apparent in the variant cells. A corresponding reduction in EGF receptor messenger RNA was observed.

The level of EGF receptor seems to be critical in regulation of the degree of maturation of malignant epidermal cells. A reduction in EGF receptor expression leads to an increased capacity to enter the differentiation pathway. The cells may not obtain enough signals generated by the interaction between EGF and its receptor to maintain proliferative activity. Loss of control of terminal differentiation might be a reason for cells becoming tumorigenic.

► The physiologic role of EGF and the EGF receptor in growth and differentiation of epidermal cells is neatly demonstrated by these experiments, which imply that loss of control of this process leads to tumorigenesis. The failure to lose EGF receptors was associated with failure to mature and differentiate.— O. Jonasson, M.D.

Imaging of Human Tumor Xenografts With an Indium-111-Labeled Anti-Epidermal Growth Factor Receptor Monoclonal Antibody

Goldenberg A, Masui H, Divgi C, Kamrath H, Pentlow K, Mendelsohn J (Mem Sloan-Kettering Cancer Ctr, New York; Cornell Univ)
J Natl Cancer Inst 81:1616–1625, Nov 1, 1989   9–2

A wide range of human neoplasms have greater than normal expression of epidermal growth factor receptor (EGFR). Not only may this provide a potential growth advantage for these tumors, but it may serve as a relatively specific antigenic target for localizing monoclonal antibodies, which then could be used in both imaging and treatment.

The murine monoclonal antibody 225 is an IgG1 antibody that binds to the extracellular domain of human EGFR. The ^{111}In-labeled diethylenetriaminepentaacetic acid derivative of this antibody was injected intraperitoneally into nude mice with subcutaneous tumor xenografts. Uptake in A431 human vulvar squamous cell carcinoma peaked at 28% of the injected dose per gram of tumor on day 3. Excellent gamma camera images of the tumor were obtained on days 3–7. There was far less uptake of a control monoclonal antibody (KS1/4S-1) labeled with [111]In. Localization of antibody 225 was less marked in the human breast adenocarcinoma MDA 468, which contains fewer EGFRs, and there was little uptake in breast adenocarcinoma MCF-7, which has very few EGFRs.

Labeled monoclonal antibody can target the EGFR when expressed at a high level in human tumor xenografts. Labeled monoclonal antibody 225 presently is being given to patients with unresectable squamous cell lung cancer, which expresses elevated levels of EGFR.

▶ In these studies the EGFR was used as the antigen to produce monoclonal antibodies that bind and target this receptor in tumors with high concentrations of the EGFR. These monoclonal antibodies also block the physiologic effects of growth factors and may provide new approaches to specific delivery of cytotoxins.—O. Jonasson, M.D.

Leucocyte Adhesion to Cells in Immune and Inflammatory Responses

Patarroyo M, Makgoba MW (Karolinska Inst, Stockholm; Royal Postgrad Med School, London)
Lancet 2:1139–1142, Nov 11, 1989   9–3

Leukocytes interact with each other and with other cells to produce immune and inflammatory responses and to "traffic" through the body. In healthy donors' blood almost all leukocytes are separate cells, presumably because they are in the resting state. On exposure to a stimulus, leukocytes adhere to each other or to other cell types, such as vascular endothelial cells. The process is mediated by cell adhesion molecules. The adhesion is transient, and the process appears to be regulated by the state of activation of the cells.

The 2 molecular pathways of leukocyte adhesion are the binding of

CD11a-c/CD18 on leukocytes to CD54 on mononuclear leukocytes, fibroblasts, and epithelial and vascular endothelial cells and the binding of CD2 on T cells to CD58, a cell surface molecule on a variety of tissue cells. The process is essential for cytotoxicity, phagocytosis, chemotaxis, and induction of lymphocyte proliferation and differentiation that are mediated by leukocytes. Leukocyte adhesion also participates in the homing of lymphocytes into lymphoid organs and leukocyte migration from the vascular compartment to extravascular tissues. It is thus a crucial step in the development of immune and inflammatory responses.

Cell adhesion is a fundamental process required for most leukocyte functions. Stimulation of lymphoma cells with cytokines may restore expression of the adhesion molecules and cell susceptibility to growth and maturation control imposed by normal lymphocytes through cell-cell contact.

▶ Newly appreciated cell surface adhesion molecules, the "CAMs," mediate the leukocyte adhesion required for much cellular immune activity. How this system relates to the perceived lack of immune responsiveness to tumor antigens by the host's cytotoxic T cells is unclear, but activation of the adhesion molecules with adherence of cells on the vascular endothelium is undoubtedly related to the pulmonary injury mediated by lymphokines such as interleukin-2.—O. Jonasson, M.D.

Human Tumor-Infiltrating Lymphocyte (TIL) Cytotoxicity Facilitated by Anti-T-Cell Receptor Antibody
Schoof DD, Jung S-E, Everlein TJ (Brigham and Women's Hosp, Boston; Harvard Med School)
Int J Cancer 44:219–224, 1989   9–4

Tumor-infiltrating lymphocyte processes have a greater therapeutic effect in vivo than comparable lymphokine-activated killer cell immunotherapy. The in vitro cytotoxicity profile of human tumor-infiltrating lymphocytes (TIL) declines progressively during the expansion period in recombinant-interleukin-2. It is possible that TIL expanded by chronic recombinant-interleukin-2 exposure are no longer able to transduce activation signals through the T cell antigen receptor/CD3 complex. If this is true, it would mitigate the possibility of these cell populations producing cytotoxic antitumor responses after adoptive transfer.

Cytotoxicity against different tumor targets mediated by TIL in 16 consecutive tumors was characterized by an initial strong tumor-nonspecific cytotoxicity. The TIL bulk cultures became noncytotoxic against all targets with time. Noncytotoxic TIL bulk populations mediated strong cytotoxic responses when pretreated with anti-T-cell antigen receptor antibody (TcR). Anti-TcR-mediated cytotoxicity was limited to CD8$^+$ bulk populations with virtually no cytotoxicity in CD4$^+$ populations.

Despite poor in vitro antitumor cytotoxicity in short-term assays, CD8$^+$ TIL are fully competent cytotoxic effector cells when subjected to strong activation signals through the TcR complex. Adoptively transferred $CD4^+$ populations of TIL appear to have in vivo biologic functions distinct from those of $CD8^+$ populations.

▶ Tumor-infiltrating lymphoid cells may be advantageous in immunotherapy in that some of them are activated by specific tumor antigens and should have specific cytotoxicity. After the long-term clonal expansion required in tissue culture in order to provide sufficient cells for therapy, cell activation by the addition of monoclonal antibody directed toward the T cell receptor complex proved to be a very powerful adjunct. Therapeutic trials of intravenous TIL administration are underway.— O. Jonasson, M.D.

A Possible Association Between Survival Time and Transfusion in Cervical Cancer
Blumberg N, Agarwal MM, Chuang C (Univ of Rochester, NY)
Yale J Biol Med 61:493–500, November–December 1988   9–5

In an attempt to learn whether transfusion is associated with a greater risk of cancer recurrence and death, the data were reviewed concerning 130 patients operated on for cervical cancer and followed for at least 6 months. None had evidence of metastatic disease at the time of diagnosis. Multivariate stepwise logistic regression analysis was used to adjust for differences in prognostic factors.

Using the Kaplan-Meier product-limit method, transfused patients had a lower survival rate than those not transfused. The groups differed markedly in prognostic factors; however, nontransfused patients were followed considerably longer. The transfused patients were more likely to

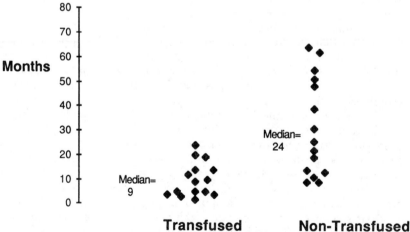

Fig 9–1.—For patients with recurrence, months from diagnosis to detection of recurrence are shown according to transfusion status. Several patients with recurrence are omitted because the exact date that recurrence was detected is not known. In 1 patient recurrence was detected at 192 weeks. (Courtesy of Blumberg N, Agarwal MM, Chuang C: *Yale J Biol Med* 61:493–500, November–December 1988.)

be anemic when diagnoses were made, but they generally had more favorable prognostic features. Nevertheless, their times to recurrence tended to be shorter (Fig 9–1), and cancer-related deaths occurred earlier than in the nontransfused group.

These findings suggest the possibility of a relationship between transfusion at the time of initial surgery and death from cervical cancer. Studies definitely are needed of the potential benefits of using white blood cell- and plasma-depleted transfusions for cancer patients who require red blood cell replacement.

▶ This report is marked by excellent statistical methodology, making the most of a set of retrospective data. By using stepwise logistic regression analysis and entering the blood transfusion variable last, the effect of transfusion on recurrence or survival could be measured. All of these studies indicate the need for a prospective randomized trial of leukocyte-depleted blood vs. whole blood or packed cell transfusions.—O. Jonasson, M.D.

Effect of Perioperative Blood Transfusion on Outcome in Patients With Surgically Resected Lung Cancer
Moores DWO, Piantadosi S, McKneally MF, for the Lung Cancer Study Group
(Albany Med College, NY; Johns Hopkins School of Medicine)
Ann Thorac Surg 47:346–351, March 1989   9–6

Because tumor antigens and histocompatibility antigens are similar, it is reasonable to believe that nonspecific immune suppression by blood transfusion might promote tumor growth. Data on 330 patients having complete resection of lung cancer, 169 of whom received blood products perioperatively, were reviewed. The mean follow-up was 3.6 years.

Transfused patients had many factors associated with more extensive disease. The average transfusion was 2.8 units. Cancer recurred in 53% of the transfused patients and in 46% of the others. The respective survival rates were 41% and 58%. Recurrence was not more likely in transfused patients after adjusting for tumor-node status and histology, but a significantly increased risk of death persisted. Similar results were obtained after adjustment with the Cox proportional hazards regression model. The adjusted risk of death from blood transfusion was about 1.6-fold, and that of recurrence was about 1.5-fold.

Perioperative blood transfusion is associated with an increased risk of recurrence and death in patients with lung cancer, even after adjusting for extent of disease. Surgeons should attempt to avoid transfusions in these patients if clinically feasible.

▶ This report represents a reasonably good statistical analysis of retrospective data from the North American Lung Cancer Study Group concerning 330 patients with non-small-cell lung cancer. Although the data were not collected with a transfusion study in mind, sufficient information was available to compare transfused and nontransfused patients. The transfused patients were adversely affected by transfusion in terms of survival and recurrence of cancer. Missing are data on previous transfusion and definitive staging, although the clinical staging data were thorough. The added risk of recurrence or death attributed to transfusion was 50%.—O. Jonasson, M.D.

Blood Transfusion and Survival After Resection of Cancers of the Breast, Colon, and Lung: The Need for Prospective Randomized Trials
Foster RS Jr, Costanza M, Foster JC, Hyman NH, Foster CB, DeMeules JE (Univ of Vermont, Burlington)
Transplant Proc 20:1125–1127, December 1988   9–7

Blood transfusions apparently have immunomodulating effects, most evident in renal transplantation, but it has been suggested that transfusions might favor the growth of micrometastases remaining after cancer surgery. This possibility was examined in a review of 3 groups of cancer patients.

Twenty-nine percent of 226 patients with primary operable invasive breast cancer had received transfusions. The numbers of overall deaths and cancer-related deaths among transfused patients were similar to those of nontransfused patients. Of 146 colon cancer patients having resection for cure, 45% had received blood. Nontransfused patients had a better rate of survival; the relative risk of cancer death for transfused patients was 2.3. Of 105 lung cancer patients who had resection for cure, 31% were given transfusions; the relative risk of death for these patients compared with nontransfused patients also was 2.3.

The available data suggest, but do not prove, that blood transfusion, possibly via an immunosuppressive mechanism, worsens the prognosis for some but not all populations of cancer patients. Prospective randomized trials are required, and it would be of interest to compare standard packed red blood cells with leukocyte- and platelet-depleted red blood cell units.

▶ This retrospective study of patients with newly diagnosed malignancies showed correlation of risk of death from cancer with number of transfusions received, for some categories of tumor. The authors correctly point out that the means to conduct prospective clinical trials with leukocyte-poor blood products are now available and that such trials should be begun. Several centers have initiated studies of this nature, and more definitive information on the possible immunosuppressive effect of whole blood infusion may soon be available.—O. Jonasson, M.D.

Perioperative Blood Transfusions Are Associated With Decreased Time to Recurrence and Decreased Survival After Resection of Colorectal Liver Metastases
Stephenson KR, Steinberg SM, Hughes KS, Vetto JT, Sugarbaker PH, Chang AE (Natl Cancer Inst, Bethesda, Md)
Ann Surg 208:679–687, December 1988   9–8

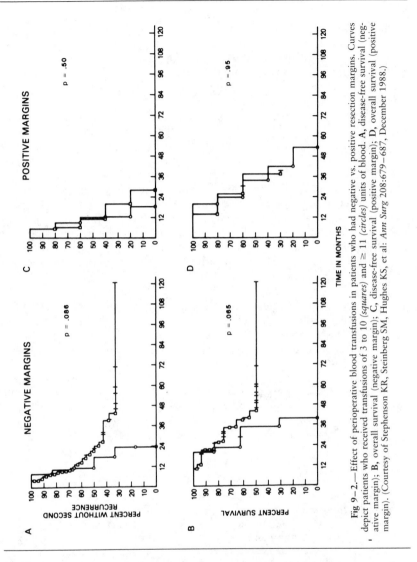

Fig 9–2.— Effect of perioperative blood transfusions in patients who had negative vs. positive resection margins. Curves depict patients who received transfusions of 3 to 10 (*squares*) and ≥ 11 (*circles*) units of blood. **A**, disease-free survival (negative margin); **B**, overall survival (negative margin); **C**, disease-free survival (positive margin); **D**, overall survival (positive margin). (Courtesy of Stephenson KR, Steinberg SM, Hughes KS, et al: *Ann Surg* 208:679–687, December 1988.)

Perioperative blood transfusions have been linked to higher rates of recurrence in patients undergoing surgery for various forms of cancer. To examine this association, retrospective studies were made of a group of patients treated surgically for isolated colorectal liver metastases. A review was made of the records of 55 patients, all of whom had received whole blood or packed red blood cells during the perioperative period. Disease-free and overall survival rates were examined in relation to a number of factors, including number of blood units received, anesthesia time, and the size and number of resected nodules.

The 5-year overall survival rate was 30%. The median time to the second recurrence was 15.5 months. When patients were grouped according to the number of blood units transfused, significant differences were apparent. The median disease-free survival for patients given 3–10 units was 19.8 months, whereas those receiving 11 or more units had recurrence at a median of 11.4 months. The median overall survival was 44.1 months for those given 3–10 units and 33.6 months when 11 or more units were given.

Intraoperative factors were examined in conjunction with units of transfused blood. Neither the number and size of metastases nor type of resection performed altered the negative effect of 11 or more transfusions on survival. But patients with positive resection margins did poorly no matter how many transfusions were given (Fig 9–2).

Each additional unit of blood lessened the time of disease-free and overall survival in patients with colorectal cancer. Studies of the effects of perioperative transfusion on survival in patients with other forms of cancer report similar results. Several explanations for the adverse effect of transfusions have been suggested, although a direct causal relationship has not been established. It seems advisable to avoid perioperative transfusions in cancer surgery whenever possible.

▶ This study is unfortunately flawed in several ways; previous transfusions, such as at the time of original operation, were not accounted for, and platelet transfusions were not included in the analysis. The effect of blood transfusion-related immunosuppression is long lasting, and it is an error to assume that it is only the transfusion at this sitting that influences outcome. Because the "transfusion effect" in transplantation is known to be carried by the nucleated cells in the blood, ignoring the platelet packs, which are really preparations of the white cells and platelets, will confound the interpretation of the results. A pronounced effect was noted and quantitated to be as much as 7% per unit transfused (increased risk of death), even in the face of these methodologic flaws.— O. Jonasson, M.D.

In Vivo Administration of Histoincompatible Lymphocytes Leads to Rapid Functional Deletion of Cytotoxic T Lymphocyte Precursors
Martin DR, Miller RG (Univ of Toronto; Ontario Cancer Inst, Toronto)
J Exp Med 170:679–690, September 1989   9–9

Studies of mice indicate that the intravenous injection of allogeneic cells can lead to specific inhibition. Specifically, lymphoid cells from a mouse previously given viable allogeneic lymphocytes mount a much reduced response of cytotoxic T lymphocytes (CTLs) against cells identical to the injected cells but not against unrelated cells. This reduction in response now has been found to result from functional deletion of CTL precursors in vivo, rather than activation of suppressor cells.

After a single injection of lymph node cells, testing showed a significant reduction in the ability to generate CTL in a mixed lymphocyte reaction (MLR) within 24 hours and a peak effect within 48 hours. The reduced response lasted for at least 11 weeks. The response of injected mice to third-party cells was unchanged. The reduction in the MLR response was reflected by a proportional decrease in the frequency of CTL precursors.

The reduction in response appears to result entirely from a functional deletion of CTL precursors. Donor F_1 cells may contain "veto" cells that, when recognized by host CTL precursors reactive against the foreign alloantigen, lead to inactivation of the CTL precursors. Induction of suppressor cells is not responsible. Both class I-restricted CTL precursors and class II-restricted helper T cells apparently are susceptible to functionally deleting antigen presentation. If this system could be manipulated to selectively delete undesired specificities from the T cell repertoire, tissue allografting would be improved and the pathogenic T cells responsible for autoimmune disorders could be inactivated.

▶ The mechanisms of the purported enhancement of transplanted organs and tumors by blood transfusions are not known; prostaglandin synthesis, suppressor cell generation, and the production of anti-idiotypic antibodies have all been advanced as mediators of the transfusion effect. In these elegant experiments the investigators propose that transfusion of viable histoincompatible lymphocytes may provide "veto cells," cells that present antigen to host lymphocytes but fail to provide the second signals required for activation of cells. The result is a deletion of the precursor cytotoxic T cells responding to that antigen and failure of the immune response.—O. Jonasson, M.D.

Experience With the Use of High-Dose Interleukin-2 in the Treatment of 652 Cancer Patients
Rosenberg SA, Lotze MT, Yang JC, Aebersold PM, Linehan WM, Seipp CA, White DE (Natl Cancer Inst, Bethesda, Md)
Ann Surg 210:474–485, October 1989   9–10

Activation of lymphocytes by specific antigen generates interleukin-2 (IL-2) receptors. The subsequent interaction of the lymphocyte with IL-2 leads to cell proliferation. In experimental animals IL-2 can mediate the rejection of cancers in lung, liver, and subcutaneous tissue. Tumor-infiltrating lymphocytes (TIL) combined with IL-2 appear to be 50–100 times more effective than lymphokine-activated killer (LAK) cells plus IL-2.

The results of treatment with high-dose IL-2 taken alone or combined with tumor necrosis factor-α (TNF), α-interferon (α-IFN), monoclonal antibodies, cyclophosphamide, LAK cells, or TIL were evaluated in 652 cancer patients receiving 1,039 courses of high-dose IL-2. Of these, 155 received IL-2 alone; 214 received IL-2 plus LAK cells; 66 received IL-2 plus TIL; 128 received IL-2 plus α-IFN; 38 received IL-2 plus TNF; 32 received IL-2 plus monoclonal antibodies; and 19 received IL-2 plus cyclophosphamide.

Objective regressions occurred in 20% to 35% of patients receiving IL-2 alone or with LAK cells. Most responses were noted in patients with metastatic renal cell cancer, melanoma, colorectal cancer, and non-Hodgkin's lymphoma (table). Eighteen patients had a complete response,

Results of Immunotherapy in Patients With Advanced Cancer

Treatment with LAK/IL-2
(number of patients)

Cancer Diagnosis	Evaluable*	CR	PR	CR + PR (%)
Renal	72	8	17	35
Melanoma	48	4	6	21
Colorectal	30	1	4	17
Non-Hodgkin's lymphoma	7	1	3	57
Sarcoma	6	0	0	—
Lung	5	0	0	—
Other†	9	0	0	—
Total	177	14	30	25

Abbreviations: CR, complete response; PR, partial response.
*Includes all treated patients except 1 lost to follow-up, 1 who died of therapy, and 35 treated in adjuvant setting.
†One patient each with cancer of breast, brain, esophagus, ovary, testes, thyroid, gastrinoma, Hodgkin's disease, unknown primary.
(Courtesy of Rosenberg SA, Lotze MT, Yang JC, et al: *Ann Surg* 210:474–485, October 1989.)

10 of whom had not had a recurrence in 18–52 months. The combination of α-IFN and IL-2 appeared more effective than cytokine alone. Additionally, IL-2 plus TIL appeared more effective than IL-2 alone.

A purely immunologic manipulation can mediate the regression of advanced cancers in certain patients. This may be a base for the development of practical, effective biologic treatments.

▶ In this report the major proponent of "adoptive immunotherapy" with cytokine and activated lymphocytes describes the extensive experience of the National Cancer Institute. It appeared to work in a few patients, with durable complete remissions in 10 and complete or partial remissions in up to 40% of those with renal cell cancer or melanoma treated with IL-2 and α-IFN at high doses. However, as pointed out by Balch in the discussion of this paper, even the TILs specifically sensitized to the host's own tumor showed a profound defect in the ability to bind or kill the tumor cells. This defect in immune response to antigen is a peculiarity of the tumor environment, and, as activation of the lymphocytes by antigen is the necessary first step before effective expansion by IL-2 can be achieved, additional methods need to be used to activate those cells. This is the area addressed in the article reviewed in Abstract 9–15.— O. Jonasson, M.D.

Tumour-Infiltrating Lymphocytes and Interleukin-2 in Treatment of Advanced Cancer

Kradin RL, Kurnick JT, Lazarus DS, Preffer FI, Dubinett SM, Pinto CE, Gifford J, Davidson E, Grove B, Callahan RJ, Strauss HW (Massachusetts Gen Hosp, Boston; Harvard Med School)
Lancet 1:577–580, March 18, 1989   9–11

Therapeutic Responses

No. (%)

	All	Melanoma	Renal cell cancer	Lung cancer
Partial response	5 (18)	3 (23)	2 (29)	0
Minor response	1 (4)	0	1 (14)	0
No response	9 (32)	4 (31)	2 (29)	3 (38)
Progression	13 (46)	6 (46)	2 (29)	5 (62)

(Courtesy of Kradin RL, Kurnick JT, Lazarus DS, et al: *Lancet* 1:577–580, March 18, 1989.)

Interleukin-2 (IL-2) enhances the growth of activated lymphocytes and their cytolytic activity against tumor cells. Activated tumor-infiltrating lymphocytes (TILs) appear to be enriched for specific cytolytic activities against their autologous tumors. They require about 100 times less IL-2 to support activity than lymphokine-activated killer cells need for activation. A trial of adoptive immunotherapy with TILs and continuous infusions of IL-2 was carried out in 28 patients with advanced non-small-cell lung cancer, malignant melanoma, or renal cell carcinoma.

The TILs were isolated and expanded from small tumor biopsy samples. The patients received autologous expanded TIL, about 10^{10}, and continuous infusions of recombinant human IL-2, $1-3 \times 10^6$ units per m^2 per 24 hours. Twenty-nine percent of the patients with renal cell cancer and 23% of those with melanoma had objective tumor responses for 3–14 months (table). Treatment produced limited toxic side effects.

These preliminary results in some chemoresistant cancers with TIL and IL-2 are promising. Further trials of this treatment approach are needed to define its role in cancer threapy.

▶ These are interesting studies. The TIL cells are clearly more effective in vitro and require far less IL-2 support to clone and during administration to patients. The effect on the tumor does not appear to be direct, however, but rather through enhancement of the host's cell-mediated immunity toward the tumor. These and other studies selected to follow in this volume describe new approaches to activation of the host immune response to tumor-associated antigens and elimination of "chemoresistant" tumors (those not amenable to conventional treatment).— O. Jonasson, M.D.

Effects of Interleukin-2 on Pulmonary and Systemic Transvascular Fluid Filtration
Harms BA, Pahl AC, Pohlman TH, Conhaim RL, Starling JR, Storm FK (Univ of Wisconsin; William S Middleton Mem VA Hosp, Madison, Wis; Univ of Washington)
Surgery 106:339–346, August 1989   9–12

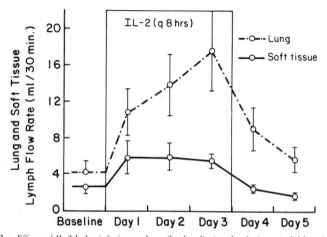

Fig 9–3.—Effects of IL-2 bolus infusion on lung *(broken line)* and soft tissue *(solid line)* lymph flow rate. Grouped peak lymph flow rate data expressed for 6 sheep as mL/30 min, mean ±SEM. (Courtesy of Harms BA, Pahl AC, Pohlman TH, et al: *Surgery* 106:339–346, August 1989.)

Interleukin-2 (IL-2) treatment for patients with advanced cancer may be limited by dose-dependent, life-threatening adverse effects such as pulmonary and systemic edema. The effects of bolus IL-2 infusion on lung and soft tissue transvascular fluid and protein filtration were examined in 6 adult sheep with chronic lung and soft tissue lymph fistulas.

The animals recuperated for 3 days after surgery, after which baseline lymph flow and hemodynamic parameters were measured. Mean aortic, pulmonary arterial, pulmonary arterial wedge, and central venous pressures were determined. Cardiac output, heart rate, and body temperature also were measured. Lymph flow was used as a quantitative measure of changes in transvascular fluid flux in lung and soft tissue. Each sheep was given an intravenous infusion of 100,000 units of IL-2 per kg every 8 hours for 3 days.

After each infusion, lung and soft tissue lymph flow rose significantly, with maximal flow occurring after 2–3 hours. A fourfold maximal increase in lung flow occurred after 72 hours of IL-2 infusion, which recovered to near baseline values within 24 hours (Fig 9–3).

Interleukin-2 increases pulmonary and systemic microvascular fluid flux. A marked increase occurs in pulmonary permeability, but not in systemic protein permeability, which does not result from changes mediated by tumor necrosis factor.

▶ These are very thorough and sophisticated studies on the mechanism(s) of toxicity of IL-2 infusion. The investigators clearly show important differences in the lung injury caused by IL-2 and that seen with endotoxin, but there are also many parallels and probably several common pathways. The major changes in the lung microvasculature observed in this animal model were largely recovered by 3 days after infusion, but the large increases in porosity of the pulmonary capillaries during IL-2 infusion at this dose rate sharply limit clinical utility.—O. Jonasson, M.D.

Antigenic Profile of Tumor Progression Stages in Human Melanocytic Nevi and Melanomas

Elder DE, Rodeck U, Thurin J, Cardillo F, Clark WH, Stewart R, Herlyn M (Hosp of the Univ of Pennsylvania; Univ of Pennsylvania; The Wistar Inst of Anatomy and Biology, Philadelphia)

Cancer Res 49:5091–5096, Sept 15, 1989   9–13

The stages of tumor progression are associated with distinct changes in morphology and biologic behavior. Cells from vertical growth phase (VGP) primary melanomas and metastases are established readily in culture, have low or no requirements for exogenous growth factors, and form permanent cell lines that are tumorigenic in nude mice. Examination was made of the in situ expression of a panel of monoclonal antibody-defined antigens on normal melanocytes and melanocytic cells from 6 histopathologically defined phases of tumor progression, ranging from normal melanocytes to highly malignant metastatic lesions.

Monoclonal antibody B 73.1 reacted exclusively with malignant cells of the last 2 stages of tumor progression, VGP primary melanoma and metastatic melanoma. All other antibodies had variable reactivity with benign proliferative lesions or radial growth phase (RGP), an early phase of primary melanoma. Two steps in tumor progression were characterized by significant quantitative alterations in the expression of antigens detected by the monoclonal antibodies. Mature nevus cells had significantly higher reactivity with the panel of monoclonal antibodies compared with normal melanocytes, and a separate panel of monocolonal antibodies discriminated between RGP and VGP primary melanoma cells. The VGP primary and metastatic melanomas were not significantly different in antigen expression.

Tumor progression of melanocytic cells in vivo appears to be accompanied by significant quantitative differences in the expression of antigens. Some of the antigens were associated with biologically aggressive malignant lesions but not with normal or premalignant melanocytic cells. The RGP primary melanoma cells were more similar antigenically to nevus cells than to VGP primary melanoma cells.

▶ This paper describes some of the problems posed by the indefinite and ubiquitous nature of tumor-associated antigens. Only one set of monoclonal antibodies was available that adequately discriminated between benign and aggressively malignant lesions, and this antibody was directed against the Fc receptor of natural killer cells, not a melanoma antigen. However, this monoclonal antibody discriminated well between indolent and aggressive tumors and might serve as the antigenic stimulus for development of anti-idiotypic antibodies to mimic the elusive and as yet undefined melanoma antigen in a technique described in the preceding paper.—O. Jonasson, M.D.

A Phase II Study of Interleukin-2 and Lymphokine-Activated Killer Cells in Patients With Metastatic Malignant Melanoma

Dutcher JP, Creekmore S, Weiss GR, Margolin K, Markowitz AB, Roper M, Parkinson D, Ciobanu N, Fisher RI, Boldt DH, Doroshow JH, Rayner AA, Hawkins M, Atkins M (Albert Einstein Cancer Ctr/Montefiore Med Ctr, New York; Loyola Univ, Maywood, Ill; Univ of Texas, San Antonio; City of Hope Cancer Research Ctr, Duarte, Calif; Univ of California, San Francisco; et al)

J Clin Oncol 7:477–485, April 1989   9–14

The medical community has long been interested in immunotherapy for melanoma. In 1985 interleukin-2 (IL-2), described as a new clinical approach to immunotherapy of malignant melanoma, was found to induce the formation of cellular precursors with the potential for development into cytotoxic cells, i.e., lymphokine-activated killer (LAK) cells. Activated autologous cells were then reinfused into patients with additional IL-2. Patient responses occurred with higher doses. A phase II trial of IL-2 and LAK cells was conducted in 36 patients wtih metastatic malignant melanoma.

Six patients responded, 1 completely and 5 partially (table). The median duration of response was 5 months. The durable complete response continued past 31 months. Response sites were lung, liver, subcutaneous nodules, and lymph nodes. Toxicity included hypotension, fluid retention with a capillary leak syndrome in most patients, and transient multiorgan dysfunction. Sixteen percent of the patients experienced adverse cardiac events.

High-dose IL-2 and LAK cells represent active immunotherapeutic treatment for patients with metastatic melanoma. Hepatic metastases, which usually do not respond to other forms of treatment, have responded to IL-2/LAK cell treatment. The toxicity of this therapy, however, is considerable.

▶ This is a report of a multicenter (National Cancer Institute IL-2/LAK Working Group) study of LAK cells and high-dose IL-2 in the treatment of melanoma. The antitumor effect was independent of the number of LAK cells administered. Enhancement of otherwise inadequate host responses is the likely mechanism of effect rather than direct tumor cell lysis by the LAK cells. The serious severe toxicity of high-dose IL-2 makes this type of treatment far less desirable than other means of stimulation of immune responses.— O. Jonasson, M.D.

Monoclonal Anti-Idiotypic Antibody Mimicking a Tumor-Associated Sialoglycoprotein Antigen Induces Humoral Immune Response Against Human Small-Cell Lung Carcinoma

Barth A, Waibel R, Stahel RA (Univ Hosp of Zurich, Switzerland)

Int J Cancer 43:896–900, 1989   9–15

Antibodies to the idiotype enhance or suppress the subsequent immune response to a certain antigen. β-Type anti-idiotypic antibodies (Ab2),

Responders

No.	Age/Sex/PS	Time to First Recurrence (mo)	Site of Disease	Tumor Bulk (cm^2)	Nonsurgical Prior Therapy	Response	Duration (mo)
1	27/M/0	6	SC	50	None	CR	31+
2	53/M/0	7	SC, adrenal, nodes	41	None	PR	13+
3	59/M/0	14	Lung, SC, nodes	48.2	None	PR	1
4	36/M/1	110	Lung	77.4	Chemotherapy, radiotherapy, immunotherapy	PR	6
5	48/M/1	106	Lower abdominal nodes, spleen, kidney, liver	135.6	None	PR	3
6	53/F/1	1	SC	8.3	Chemotherapy	PR	2
7	19/M/0	5	Lung	5.0	None	MR	2
8	53/M/0	24	SC	15.8	None	MR	2

Abbreviations: PS, performance status; *SC,* subcutaneous; *CR,* complete response; *PR,* partial response; *MR,* minor response.
(Courtesy of Dutcher JP, Creekmore S, Weiss GR, et al: *J Clin Oncol* 7:477–485, April 1989.)

which express an idiotypic determinant that mimics the structure of the antigen, are of particular interest. These "internal image" Ab2s are successful substitutes for the original antigen and can induce protective immunity against a variety of infective agents in rodents. They also elicit antitumor activity against tumor-associated antigens (TAAs) in humans. In syngeneic tumor models, Ab2 immunization significantly inhibits tumor growth. Anti-idiotypes may be superior to conventional immunization procedures when purified antigen is of limited availability, especially with most human TAAs, which are frequently complex glycolipids or glycoproteins. To obtain anti-idiotypic antibodies that might be useful as surrogates for sGP$_{90-135}$ in vaccination trials, LOU rats were immunized with LAM8 MAb. Their spleen cells were fused with Y3 rat myeloma cells. The LY8-229 hybrid was selected. Solubilized small cell carcinoma extract selectively inhibited ^{125}I-LY8-229 binding to LAM8. Serum from rodents immunized with anti-idiotypic antibody LY8-229 was reactive with antigen-positive target cell lines but not with antigen-negative control cell lines.

Induction of a specific immune responses in mice and rats by LY8-229 suggests that this antibody bears the internal image of the antigen sGP$_{90-135}$. Therefore, it might be a candidate for immunotherapy trials in patients with cancer.

▶ Induction of an effective host immune response to tumor antigens has been elusive. The TAAs are often ineffective in initiating a vigorous antibody response by the host, and antigens may be difficult to identify and obtain in the form and quantity to use therapeutically, or even experimentally. These researchers have taken an exciting new approach in which animals were strongly immunized with a monoclonal antibody (AB1) against a known TAA to produce antibodies to AB1 (anti-idiotypic antibody, AB2). This antibody reflects the TAA and is a much stronger immunogen than the tumor antigen itself. The animals responded with vigorous antibody production (AB3) that strongly inhibited the small cell lung tumor line. Experiments such as these are being conducted in several laboratories, and clinical trials have begun. I believe that this approach shows great promise.— O. Jonasson, M.D.

Augmentation of Lymphokine-Activated Killer Cell Cytotoxicity by Monoclonal Antibodies Against Human Small Cell Lung Carcinoma
Tong AW, Lee JC, Wang R-M, Ordonez G, Stone MJ (Baylor Univ Med Ctr, Dallas)
Cancer Res 49:4103–4108, Aug 1, 1989   9–16

Lymphokine-activated killer (LAK) cells are cytotoxic to tumors with or without class I major histocompatibility complex determinants on their cell surface. A better understanding of the biologic characteristics of the LAK population is needed to enhance the proficiency of LAK immunotherapy. Lymphokine-activated killer cell cytotoxicity on monoclonal antibody (MoAb)-bound tumor cells from the human small cell lung carcinoma lines H69 and H128 was analyzed.

The LAK cells were generated from normal peripheral blood mononuclear cells by incubating them with interleukin-2 for at least 3 days. The LAK cells were cytotoxic to natural killer-sensitive and killer-resistant cell lines and to freshly excised human lung and breast tumors. Cytotoxicity of LAK cells to the H69 or H128 cells was enhanced significantly by target cell preincubation with small cell lung carcinoma-reactive MoAbs 1096 or 5023.

The cytotoxicity or LAK appears to be mediated by an NKH-1 reactive large mononuclear leukocyte subpopulation. Tumor-reactive MoAbs may augment antitumor cytotoxicity through Fc binding to this large mononuclear leukocyte subset.

▶ In a preceding article (Abstract 9–4), activation of tumor-infiltrating lymphocyte cytotoxic cells was achieved with MoAbs to the T cell receptor. This study shows that a population of natural killer cells from the peripheral blood expanded by culture in IL-2 solutions (LAK cells) can also be made tumor specific and enhanced in their cytotoxicity through addition of MoAbs, this time reactive with tumor-associated antigens.—O. Jonasson, M.D.

Indomethacin-Enhanced Immunotherapy of Pulmonary Metastases Using IL-2 and IFN-α
Kim B, Warnaka P (Case Western Reserve Univ; Cleveland Metropolitan Gen Hosp)
Surgery 106:248–256, August 1989   9–17

Indomethacin occasionally produces tumor regression. Its antitumor effect may be exerted partly through blocked synthesis of PGE_2. To determine whether indomethacin might further potentiate the antitumor activity of interleukin-2 (IL-2) or a hybrid human interferon-α (IFN-α A/D), C57BL/6 female mice were studied.

The observed tumors were MCA-106, methylcholanthrene-induced sarcomas of C56BL/6 origin. Spontaneous proliferation was determined by a 4-hour tritiated thymidine incorporation assay. The mice were injected with 2.5×10^5 fresh single tumor cell suspension. Mice bearing 3-day pulmonary micrometastases of the fibrosarcoma were treated by intraperitoneal injection of saline solution, IL-2 INF-α A/D, or both. Treatments were given on 6 consecutive days.

Interleukin-2 and IL-2 plus IFN-α A/D effected 71% and 91% reductions in metastases, respectively. Indomethacin enhanced the efficacy of these 2 treatments only minimally. In mice receiving water containing indomethacin with IL-2 plus IFN treatment, median survival was prolonged by 48% compared with controls. Indomethacin combined wtih IL-2, IFN, or both, resulted in high sustained proliferative activity compared with mice not treated with indomethacin.

Indomethacin appears to augment antitumor efficacy and toxicity of immunotherapy with IFN or IL-2, or both. It may do this by sustaining proliferation of a non-T-lymphocyte population. Treatment with indomethacin and IFN was as effective as treatment with IL-2.

▶ Prostaglandins appear to have a major immunosuppressive effect and may play an important role in mediation of the "transfusion effect" in transplantation (reduces rejection) and in tumor patients (enhancement of tumor growth).

In these simple experiments with a laboratory model of pulmonary metastases, indomethacin did enhance the host immune response to the weakly antigenic tumor system, as determined by decreased metastases and increased in vitro lymphocyte activity. This work is also directed at repair of the defective process of host response to a tumor.—O. Jonasson, M.D.

Regulation of Epidermal Growth Factor Receptor by Progestins and Glucocorticoids in Human Breast Cancer Cell Lines

Ewing TM, Murphy LJ, Ng M-L, Pang GYN, Lee CSL, Watts CKW, Sutherland RL (St Vincent's Hosp, Sydney, Australia)
Int J Cancer 44:744–752, Oct 15, 1989   9–18

Epidermal growth factor (EGF) stimulates proliferation in various tissues in vitro, including human breast epithelial cells and benign breast fibroadenomas. Breast cancer cells secrete various growth factors; steroids may modulate the proliferation of breast cancer cells chiefly by regulating production of autocrine growth factor. Progestins increase the concentration of EGF receptors (EGF-R). The effects of progestins and glucocorticoids on EGF binding were studied in 10 human breast cell lines.

Five of the 10 cell lines expressed the glucocorticoid receptor. Two progesterone receptor (PR)-positive cell lines had increased binding of EGF on incubation with medroxyprogesterone acetate. Increased EGF binding also was seen in 4 PR-negative cell lines. In these, dexamethasone was a more potent inducer of EGF binding than was medroxyprogesterone acetate, which competed with dexamethasone for binding to glucocorticoid receptors in these cell lines. The increase in EGF binding was accompanied by an increase in the concentration of EGF-R.

The binding of EGF by human breast cancer cells can be regulated with both progestins and glucocorticoids acting via their respective receptors. They apparently act by promoting an increase in the level of EGF-R messenger RNA. Further studies are needed to determine the molecular basis of steroid effects on EGF binding and EGF-R gene expression in human breast cancer cells.

▶ In this and several following selections, detailed investigations of autocrine growth factor receptors on the surfaces of breast cancer cells are described. In particular, EGF and its receptor (EGF-R) have been found on breast cancer cells almost entirely in estrogen receptor-negative tumors, associated with other poor prognostic features. Growth factors, cytokines, and related soluble mediators appear to be of great importance in the establishment and proliferation of tumors; control of their production by the tumor cells involved seems feasible through a combination of receptor-related hormonal treatment schemes.—O. Jonasson, M.D.

Expression of Epidermal Growth Factor Receptors Associated With Lack of Response to Endocrine Therapy in Recurrent Breast Cancer

Nicholson S, Sainsbury JRC, Halcrow P, Chambers P, Farndon JR, Harris AL
(Univ of Newcastle upon Tyne, England)
Lancet 1:182–185, Jan 28, 1989   9–19

Epidermal growth factor (EGF) acts as a mitogen for human breast cancer cells in culture. One of the growth factors produced by these cells, TGFα, has actions similar to those of EGF and also acts via the EGF receptor (EGF-R). Expression of EGF-R appears to be related to early recurrence of and death from breast cancer.

Expression of EGF-R was related to the response to endocrine therapy in 221 women with primary operable breast cancer, followed for a median of 2 years. Initial endocrine therapy consisted of tamoxifen; second-line treatment was with low-dose aminoglutethimide and hydrocortisone. Premenopausal women had ovarian ablation before receiving tamoxifen.

Forty-five percent of the patients had recurrence. Whereas 28% of 72 patients given tamoxifen responded, only 1 of 28 patients with an EGF-R-positive tumor that did not express estrogen receptor had an objective response to tamoxifen. In all, 3 of 35 patients with EGF-R-positive tumors and 11 of 37 with EGF-R-negative tumors had objective responses. Patients with EGF-R-positive primary tumors had more rapid progression of disease. Survival after recurrence was poorer among patients with no response to endocrine therapy.

Status of EGF-R seems to be a useful marker of lack of response to endocrine therapy in women with breast cancer. Adjuvant chemotherapy might be appropriate for patients with EGF-R-positive primary tumors.

▶ Analysis of the EGF-R of excised breast tumors in this series was quite accurate in predicting response to treatment. The growth factors produced by the tumor cells (autocrine pathway) appear to have a role in breast cancer growth control. The EGF-R-positive tumors fail to respond to antiestrogen treatment.— O. Jonasson, M.D.

The Relationship Between Somatostatin, Epidermal Growth Factor, and Steroid Hormone Receptors in Breast Cancer

Reubi J-C, Torhorst J (Sandoz Research Inst, Berne; Univ of Basel, Switzerland)
Cancer 64:1254–1260, Sept 15, 1989   9–20

A small number of breast cancers, arising from tissue not known to be a target for somatostatin (SS), contain SS receptors. Epidermal growth factor receptors (EGF-Rs) are prognostic markers of patient survival and tumor invasion; they are correlated inversely with the content of estrogen receptor in breast tumors. The SS receptor content of 36 primary breast cancers was determined and correlated with the status of EGF-R and steroid receptor.

Six tumors contained SS receptors, whereas 10 contained EGF-R. None of the samples with SS receptor also had EGF-R. In contrast, all of the tumors with SS receptor contained steroid receptors as well. Receptor measurements were not related to the tumor cell growth fraction.

Breast tumors containing SS receptors appear to be relatively differentiated and to have a good prognosis. Pituitary adenomas that produce growth hormone and most endocrine gastroenteropancreatic tumors, which usually are very well differentiated, also contain SS receptors. Hormone therapy, including SS analogues, may have therapeutic value for patients wtih SS receptor-positive breast cancer. Treatment eventually may be based on assessment of tumor receptor status in each case.

▶ In contrast with the poor prognostic features associated with the expression of EGF-Rs (poorly differentiated tumors, failure to respond to antiestrogen therapy), identification of somatostatin receptors on breast tumor cells is associated with good prognostic features. Somatostatin is a regulatory peptide, with activity on many cells types and tissues.— O. Jonasson, M.D.

Immunolymphoscintigraphy for the Detection of Lymph Node Metastases From Breast Cancer
Tjandra JJ, Russell IS, Collins JP, Andrews JT, Lichtenstein M, Binns D, McKenzie IFC (Univ of Melbourne; Royal Melbourne Hosp, Parkville, Victoria, Australia)
Cancer Res 49:1600–1608, March 15, 1989   9–21

In the absence of overt distant metastases, metastases in regional lymph nodes are the major prognostic factors in breast cancer and are important indicators of the need for adjuvant therapy in breast cancer diagnosed early. Accurate assessment of axillary lymph node status currently requires axillary dissection, which is associated with morbidity. An

Comparison of Immunolymphoscintigraphy With
Clinical and Pathologic Assessment of Axillae in 26
Patients With Breast Cancer

	Pathological node positive	Assessment * node negative
Scan Result		
Positive	12	1
Negative	2	11
Clinical assessment †		
Positive	8	5
Negative	6	7

Note: Immunolymphoscintigraphy used ^{131}I-RCC-1 monoclonal antibody (400 µg) and cold iodine-labeled (blocking) Ly-2.1 monoclonal antibody.
  *Node positive implies ≥1 nodal metastases; node negative implies no nodal metastases.
  †Positive, palpable axillary lymph nodes felt to contain tumor deposits; negative, nodes not palpable, or if palpable, felt not to contain tumor deposits.
  (Courtesy of Tjandra JJ, Russell IS, Collins JP, et al: *Cancer Res* 49:1600–1608, March 15, 1989.)

alternative method of identifying node-positive patients is immunolymphoscintigraphy with subcutaneous administration of radioiodinated monoclonal antibody.

Iodine-131-labeled antibreast cancer antibody and cold iodine-labeled "blocking" antibody were injected subcutaneously into both arms of 40 patients. Scintigraphy images were obtained 16–18 hours later, using the axilla contralateral to the side of the breast cancer as the control. Results were considered positive if the amount of background-subtracted radioactive count in the axilla of interest exceeded the normal side by a ratio greater than or equal to 1.5:1. In 38 patients the findings were correlated with operative and histopathologic findings. In 26 patients examined prospectively, the method was more sensitive and specific than preoperative clinical assessment in the detection of axillary lymph node metastases (table). Combining the 2 methods resulted in improved sensitivity but deterioration in specificity. No significant complications resulted from the procedure. This novel, safe method of imaging may become a useful adjunct in the surgical management of such patients.

▶ Radio-immunoguided surgery has become quite useful in imaging tumor deposits in the abdomen and breast. If an adequate antibody can be produced with specificity for unique tumor-associated antigens, identification of tumor is often possible after inoculation of the patient with a radiolabeled antibody and application of a hand-held gamma counter. These authors suggest that radioimaging may supplant the need for axillary dissection or sampling in women with early breast cancer. This seems to be a very reasonable approach and quite reliable, at least in identifying the positive nodes not appreciated clinically.—O. Jonasson, M.D.

Promotion by Bombesin of Gastric Carcinogenesis Induced by *N*-Methyl-*N*'-nitro-*N*-nitrosoguanidine in Wistar Rats

Tatsuta M, Iishi H, Baba M, Nakaizumi A, Ichii M, Taniguchi H (Ctr for Adult Diseases, Osaka, Japan)
Cancer Res 49:5254–5257, Oct 15, 1989   9–22

Bombesin-like peptides are potent mitogens for Swiss 3T3 cells and may be autocrine growth factors for small cell lung cancer. To examine the effects of prolonged administration of bombesin on the development of gastric cancer in Wistar rats, doses of bombesin, 20 or 40 μg/kg, were given in depot form subcutaneously on alternate days after peroral administration of the carcinogen *N*-methyl-*N*'-nitro-*N*-nitrosoguanidine (MNNG) for 25 weeks.

The larger dose of bombesin led to a significant increase in the incidence of gastric cancers and in the number of cancers per rat after 1 year. The lower dose increased the number of cancers of the glandular stomach per rat but not the indicence of cancer. Neither dose influenced the histologic appearance of the lesions or depth of involvement. Bombesin also increased levels of norepinephrine in the antral and fundic regions of the stomach wall and labeling indices at the same sites. Gastrin levels and gastric acid secretion were not changed significantly.

Bombesin enhances gastric carcinogenesis in rats given MNNG. Possible explanations include a trophic effect of gastrin on the gastric mucosa, release of other peptides by bombesin, an action of bombesin on DNA synthesis and cell division, and the effect of bombesin on the sympathetic nervous system.

▶ Bombesin is a neuropeptide that is also found in the gastrointestinal tract and may be a neurotransmitter. It has been implicated as an autocrine growth factor for small cell lung cancer and has trophic effects on tumor cells and on pancreatic acinar cells. In these interesting experiments, chronic bombesin administration sharply increased the rate at which gastric cancer developed in rats when they were exposed to a potent carcinogen, while not increasing gastrin or gastric acid production. The suggestion that this is a neurologically mediated phenomenon through an increase in tissue norepinephrine concentrations in the gastric wall is interesting.— O. Jonasson, M.D.

Resection of Hepatic Metastases From Colorectal Cancer: Biologic Perspectives
Steele G Jr, Ravikumar TS (New England Deaconess Hosp, Boston; Harvard Med School)
Ann Surg 210:127–138, August 1989   9–23

Liver metastasis is a major cause of death in disseminated colorectal carcinoma. In most of these cases, however, the disease will have rapidly proliferated outside the liver. Although the percentage of patients with recurrent carcinoma of the colon and rectum who might be cured by sur-

REGISTRY OF HEPATIC METASTASES

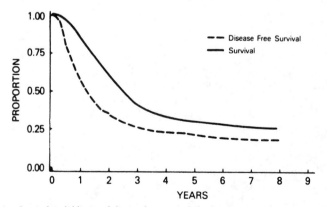

Fig 9–4.—Survival *(solid line)* and disease-free survival *(broken line)* rates for 859 patients who had hepatic resection for colorectal carcinoma metastases. (Courtesy of Steele G Jr, Ravikumar TS: *Ann Surg* 210:127–138, August 1989.)

Rules to Obtain Best Outcome
1. Resect metastases only from colorectal cancer primary
2. Resect only when no comorbid disease
3. Resect only when no extrahepatic recurrence
4. Resect three or fewer metastases (either uni- or bilobar)
5. Resect all disease (i.e., obtain tumor-free margins)

(Courtesy of Steele G Jr, Ravikumar TS: *Ann Surg* 210:127–138, August 1989.)

gical resection of the liver is small, such treatment is the only therapeutic option with any hope of cure. The surgeon must decide which patients would benefit from resection of hepatic metastases from colorectal cancer.

Ultrasound has been the most effective method of staging the liver, although lesions less than 1 cm in diameter may not be detected. Intraoperative ultrasonography now appears to be superior to preoperative CT scan, ultrasound, angiography, and intraoperative visual examination or bimanual palpation of the liver. Resection of hepatic metastases can be done safely, with a postoperative mortality rate of less than 5%. Biloma, the most frequent complication, can be handled by percutaneous placement of a pigtail catheter.

The 5-year disease-free survival in these selected patients ranges from 20% to 25%, with good expectation of a permanent cure (Fig 9–4). Failure resulting from secondary recurrences occurs within the first year in 80% to 90% of patients and usually involves the lung. An effective, adjuvant systemic therapy would benefit the 70% to 75% of patients with secondary recurrence.

It has been difficult to determine which factors predict success in resection of hepatic metastases, but there is some agreement on rules (table). Surgery is not indicated when patients have extrahepatic disease or when more than 3 metastases are evident before operation. Tumor-free surgical margins should be obtained or the patient will not be cured. Ideally, there should be no more than a 1- to 3-month delay between preoperative staging and surgical resection. Until techniques are developed that accurately distinguish between regional metastases and systemic recurrence, the surgeon must rely on clinical judgment in selecting patients for resection of hepatic metastases from colorectal cancer.

▶ The "second-look" procedure, prompted by evidence of a rising titer of carcinoembryonic antigen in the patient after resection of a colon cancer, has recently become very widely applied. The presence of metastases to the liver as the sole metastatic site lends itself to surgical resection, and new technologies in the operating room have made it possible to perform resection of hepatic metastases with a surgical mortality rate of about 5%. Yet Steele and Ravikumar calculate that, of the approximately 70,000 patients annually who have recurrence after primary resection of colon cancer, only 5,000 will be suitable candiates for operation and about 1,000 of them will survive and be cured. The evidence for effective host defense in these 1,000 survivors is striking in that even those with large deposits may be curable. The challenge is to develop a host defense system that may contain tumor development in the huge majority of patients not suitable for surgical cure.— O. Jonasson, M.D.

Endogenous Cholecystokinin Regulates Growth of Human Cholangiocarcinoma
Evers BM, Gomez G, Townsend CM Jr, Rajaraman S, Thompson JC (Univ of Texas, Galveston)
Ann Surg 210:317–323, September 1989   9–24

Cholecystokinin (CCK) modulates the growth of certain gut cancers; its exogenous administration inhibits the growth of SLU-132, a human cholangiocarcinoma possessing CCK receptors. Cholestyramine, which binds bile salts, increases the release of CCK and pancreatic growth in guinea pigs. The bile salt taurocholate inhibits the meal-stimulated release of CCK.

Whether endogenous CCK influences the growth of SLU-132 in athymic nude mice was investigated by implanting SLU-132 subcutaneously and depleting the bile salt pool by feeding 4% cholestyramine, alone or with 0.5% taurocholate. Cholestyramine significantly inhibited tumor growth and stimulated growth of the normal pancreas. Taurocholate feeding stimulated tumor growth.

Agents that alter endogenous CCK levels regulate the growth of human cholangiocarcinoma in athymic nude mice. It is possible that manipulation of endogenous gut hormone levels have a role in treating patients with certain gastrointestinal cancers. Either CCK or CCK antagonists may be used, or endogenous CCK could be manipulated by dietary supplementation or surgical procedures. This cholangiocarcinoma contains CCK receptors but is inhibited by CCK, in analogy with breast cancer.

▶ This is an interesting paper in that a known trophic hormone or growth factor for many tissues in the gastrointestinal tract, CCK, is apparently associated with retardation of growth of a tumor bearing specific receptors. As discussed in Abstract 9–18, activation of the growth factor receptor and receptor internalization precedes many intracellular events, usually associated with proliferation. The downregulation of this tumor, in contrast to the expected increase in growth rate, may indicate that hormonal or other growth factor manipulation is of potential therapeutic value.— O. Jonasson, M.D.

10 Skin, Subcutaneous Tissue, and the Hand

Ring Avulsion Injuries: Classification and Prognosis
Kay S, Werntz J, Wolff TW (The Christine M Kleinert Inst for Hand and Micro Surgery, Louisville)
J Hand Surg 14A:204–213, March 1989   10–1

The choice of treatment in ring avulsion injuries is often complicated. To decide between amputation or microvascular salvage, surgeons have considered the classification of ring avulsion injuries proposed by Urbaniak and expanded by Nissenbaum. According to this system, class III injuries, involving complete degloving or complete amputation, may best be managed by amputation. A successful outcome, with good range of motion and sensibility, is especially difficult to achieve after degloving injuries or amputation, however. To determine how the extent of the injury and its method of treatment correlated with outcome, results in 55 ring avulsion injuries, treated in a 9-year period at 1 institution, were reviewed.

Microsurgical salvage was attempted in 44 patients. Of these, 9 (20.5%) had amputation after the initial operative procedure because of vascular insufficiency. For class II injuries, those with inadequate circulation, the success rate was 86%; the rate for class III injuries was 73%. There was a lower rate of success in digits with skeletal injury (76%) than in digits without skeletal injury (91%).

Although infections occurred in 8 fingers, none was amputated because of infection. Cold intolerance was more frequent in patients with class III injuries (69%) than in those with class II injuries (26%). Total active motion of the proximal interphalangeal and distal interphalangeal joints was statistically equal for patients with classes II and III injury. Despite the effort involved in microsurgical salvage, 82% of the patients with class II injuries and 89% of those with class III injuries were satisfied with results. Primary amputation requires a second procedure in about 25% of patients and impairs finger function and appearance. But as many as 62% of patients undergoing microvascular salvage may need 1 or more additional procedures.

The present results suggest that completely amputated digits can be salvaged. A new system was developed for classifying ring avulsion injuries, taking into account the presence or absence of fracture or joint injury and whether the arterial or venous supply alone is compromised. With this more detailed classification, factors affecting prognosis may be evaluated.

▶ After ring avulsion injury, patients who have reconstruction with split-thickness skin grafts usually request amputation. Split-thickness skin does not circumferentially give a functional digit in most patients. If a full-thickness skin and subcutaneous fat graft can be used for at least part of the resurfacing procedure, achievement of function sufficient to make the procedure worthwhile may be possible.—E.E. Peacock, Jr., M.D.

Early Dynamic Splinting for Extensor Tendon Injuries
Browne EZ Jr, Ribik CA (Cleveland Clinic)
J Hand Surg [Am] 14A:72–76, January 1989   10–2

When extensor tendon injuries are splinted without motion for 3–4 weeks after repair, flexion may be limited by extensor tenodesis at the repair site. Dynamic splinting has been used to prevent this. Results in 78 patients who sustained 119 complete extensor tendon transections and had relatively tidy wounds were reviewed.

Fifty-two patients with 82 injuries underwent treatment with early passive motion by dynamic splinting in an outrigger type of splint. The splint with elastic traction provided passive extension and allowed active flexion. Motion began 3–5 days after repair and continued for 5 weeks. The goal was to flex 10 times an hour to achieve at least 70 degrees metacarpophalangeal flexion, 90 degrees of proximal interphalangeal flexion, and 50 degrees of distal interphalangeal joint flexion. The other patients had static extension splinting.

No patient treated dynamically had tendon rupture, and full extension was achieved in 77 of 82 digits. All of the patients were able to make a full fist with the wrist in functional position. Grip strength was normal in all patients with injury of the dominant hand. All patients returned to their previous work or avocation after treatment. None had secondary tendon surgery.

These results are superior to those achieved by static splinting, but a randomized study is needed. Dynamic splinting appears to be a viable option in the management of extensor tendon injuries.

▶ Prolonged immobilization after extensor tendon repair produces frequent and severe functional disability even when the tendon repair has been otherwise successful. Although I do not see the advantages of dynamic splinting, this paper is important because it emphasizes the need for early motion to protect small joints and the extensor mechanism. Modern techniques of repairing tendons, and the cautious use of active and passive motion in the first few days and thereafter, can prevent many of the disabling complications of extensor tendon repair.—E.E. Peacock, Jr., M.D.

Use of Sonography in the Early Detection of Suppurative Flexor Tenosynovitis
Schecter WP, Markison RE, Jeffrey RB, Barton RM, Laing F (Univ of California, San Francisco; San Francisco Gen Hosp)
J Hand Surg 14A:307–310, March 1989   10–3

When swelling of the finger suggests acute suppurative tenosynovitis, Kanavel's signs can confirm the diagnosis. The value of ultrasonography in early diagnosis of the condition was assessed in 18 patients (mean age, 34 years). All had at least 1 of Kanavel's signs, and all received antibiotics parenterally.

Ultrasound showed pus in the tendon sheath in 17 patients. Surgery was performed on 12 patients, all of whom had ultrasonic evidence of tendon swelling; 11 had fluid in the flexor sheath. In 8 of these patients fluid was found in the flexor sheath at operation. The 6 patients not requiring surgical drainage had full recovery after antibiotic therapy. All 18 patients recovered completely.

Sonographs can compare the affected flexor tendon with the contralateral normal tendon. In tenosynovitis the affected tendon shows a 25% or greater increase. In addition, a hypoechoic area surrounding the flexor tendon indicates pus within the flexor sheath.

In this series, patients needing drainage had a greater number of Kanavel's signs (3.6) than those not requiring surgery (2.1). Sonographic evidence of fluid in the flexor sheath and a swollen tendon may be a useful, noninvasive means of diagnosing acute suppurative tenosynovitis.

▶ This trick can be of great help. Nothing in treatment of an infected digit is more tragic than to open the flexor sheath because of a mistaken diagnosis of suppurative tenosynovitis when the correct diagnosis is surrounding cellulitis. If sonography can prevent that from happening, a major catastrophe and misdiagnosis can be averted.—E.E. Peacock, Jr., M.D.

Mycobacterium marinum Flexor Tenosynovitis

Lacy JN, Viegas SF, Calhoun J, Mader JT (Univ of Texas, Galveston)
Clin Orthop 238:288–293, January 1989   10–4

Mycobacterium marinum, identified in the past as the cause of skin lesions in swimmers, was discovered in 4 patients with flexor tenosynovitis of the hand. The organism is endogenous to both freshwater and saltwater marine life. Because it can be cultured only at 30° to 32° C, *M. marinum* has not been associated with infections in the central core structures of the body.

Man, 32, was seen with a tender cystic mass on the left thumb. He was treated a month later for wrist pain and symptoms of carpal tunnel syndrome. Symptoms persisted, the carpal tunnel syndrome progressed, and acute flexor tenosynovitis of the left thumb was noted. Surgical exploration revealed granulomatous inflammation containing acid-fast bacilli. Three weeks later the patient complained of a swollen wrist and limited finger motion. Fluid from the reopened carpel tunnel incision tested positive for *M. marinum*. After 2 weeks of antimycobacterial therapy formal flexor tenosynovectomy was performed. Four months of therapy were required before the patient was asymptomatic. He continued to receive sulfamethoxazole for 10 months and will continue with rifampin and ethambutol for 2 years.

Each of the 4 patients had a history of exposure to an aquatic environment or had sustained puncture wounds caused by shrimp or crabs. Biopsy and culture are needed for a positive diagnosis of *M. marinum.* Treatment should begin as soon as the infection is suspected; in 1 recently reported case the infection progressed to a condition requiring amputation within 6 weeks. Radical flexor tenosynovectomy and aggressive antimycobacterial chemotherapy are successful in treating *M. marinum* flexor tenosynovitis.

▶ This infection is so often overlooked that surgeons need to be reminded that it exists. The problem is access to a laboratory capable of identifying the organism. When the infection is suspected and a suitable laboratory can be found, the diagnosis is clear and treatment is reliable and effective.— E.E. Peacock, Jr., M.D.

Immediate Silastic Arthroplasty for Non-Salvageable Intraarticular Phalangeal Fractures

Nagle DJ, af Ekenstam FW, Lister GD (Akademiska Sjukhuset, Uppsala, Sweden; Northwestern Univ; Univ of Utah)
Scand J Plast Reconstr Surg 23:47–50, 1989   10–5

The treatment of traumatic nonsalvageable intra-articular fractures of the proximal interphalangeal (PIP) and metacarpophalangeal (MCP) joints may include arthrodesis, late Silastic implant arthroplasty, soft tissue interposition arthroplasty, perichondrial grafting, and free toe joint transfer. Emergency Swanson implant arthroplasty offers a viable alternative in selected patients.

Fourteen patients aged 14–49 years with nonsalvageable intra-articular fractures of 8 PIP joints and 6 MCP joints underwent emergency Silastic arthroplasty with a Swanson HP hinged implant. Operation was performed in a bloodless field using axillary block. Ten patients required repair or reconstruction of a collateral ligament, 7 of whom also underwent reconstruction of the volar plate. Motion was started on the first postoperative day; dynamic splints were applied 1–2 weeks later. Follow-up ranged from 4 months to 6 years and averaged 26 months.

The active range of motion obtained at MCP joint arthroplasties ranged from 45 degrees to 80 degrees, averaging 60 degrees. The active range of motion obtained at the PIP joint arthroplasties ranged from zero to 70 degrees, with an average of 29 degrees. None of the patients experienced deep wound infection or mechanical implant failure. Six patients were satisfied with the outcome, 3 were fairly satisfied but had some complaints, and 5 were frankly dissatisfied.

Emergency Silastic arthroplasty for nonsalvageable intra-articular phalangeal fractures maintains length and mobility, properties that are not maintained with the more traditional procedures.

▶ There is reluctance to replace small joints in the hand at the time of severe trauma because such injuries usually occur in young people, and we are not yet certain that Silastic arthroplasty is a good procedure for youngsters. The experience reported in this paper suggests that we may have been too conservative and probably should perform immediate Silastic arthroplasty, even in young patients.—E.E. Peacock, Jr., M.D.

Soft Tissue Metacarpophalangeal Reconstruction for Treatment of Rheumatoid Hand Deformity
Wood VE, Ichtertz DR, Yahiku H (Loma Linda Univ, Calif)
J Hand Surg 14A:163–174, March 1989   10–6

Silicone metacarpophalangeal joint (MP) arthroplasty offers pain relief and correction of hand deformity to patients with rheumatoid arthritis and systemic lupus erythematosus (SLE). A number of studies, however, report a high incidence of fracture in the silicone implants at long-term

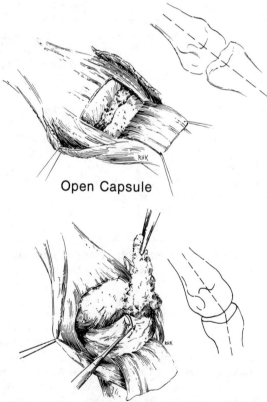

Open Capsule

Resect Synovium and Strip Palmar Plate

Fig 10–1.—After incising radial sagittal band along the central extensor tendon, the joint capsule is opened for synovectomy and freeing of palmar plate from the metacarpal neck. (Courtesy of Wood VE, Ichtertz DR, Yahiku H: *J Hand Surg* 14A:163–174, March 1989.)

follow-up. Long-term experience with soft tissue MP reconstruction without articular resection was reviewed.

The mean length of follow-up for 12 patients (16 hands) was 81 months. The mean age at surgery was 66 years and the mean disease duration, 15.9 years. Most patients were in American Rheumatoid Association class II stage 3, and all had painful, subluxated, or severely deviated MP joints. The operative procedure includes thorough synovectomy (Fig 10–1).

No immediate complications occurred, although swan-neck deformities worsened in 2 patients. Overall results were judged excellent in 6 hands, good in 7, fair in 1, and poor in 2. Except for the 2 failures the patients were satisfied with the results. Complete pain relief was reported by 88% of the patients. The operated-on hands had a mean active MP range of motion of 56 degrees and a mean proximal interphalangeal range of motion of 64 degrees. Recurrence of synovitis developed in only 1 of the operated-on MP joints.

The good results obtained with this operative technique suggest that the procedure should be performed before joint dislocation and fixed contractures occur. Many patients may be spared replacement arthroplasty, and the results of soft tissue reconstruction compare favorably with those of silicone replacement. Patients with SLE, who have less articular destruction than those with rheumatoid disease, especially may benefit from this procedure.

▶ Postoperative mobilization is the key to successful metacarpophalangeal reconstruction without replacement arthroplasty. Recurrence of disease has been a problem in the rheumatoid patient. Soft tissue reconstruction was all we had before the development of modern prosthetic joints but, in most hands, it is simpler and most effective over the long run to resect the entire diseased area and use a prosthetic spacer to maintain articulation. Ultimate stress fracture of the prosthesis is not a deterrent to replacement arthroplasty in young patients.—E.E. Peacock, Jr., M.D.

Flexor Tendon Ruptures in Patients With Rheumatoid Arthritis

Ertel AN, Millender LH, Nalebuff E, McKay D, Leslie B (Harvard Med School; Tufts-New England Med Ctr, Boston)
J Hand Surg [Am] 13A:860–866, November 1988   10–7

Rheumatoid flexor tenosynovitis, either as an isolated event or in association with dorsal tenosynovitis or joint involvement, is common, but rupture of the flexor tendon is not. Tendon ruptures in functioning joints are easily diagnosed, but the diagnosis is more difficult in stiff or unstable joints. The sites and causes of flexor tendon rupture in hands with rheumatoid arthritis were reviewed retrospectively.

From 1967 through 1984, 16 men and 20 women aged 30–74 years were treated for 115 tendon ruptures in 43 hands with rheumatoid arthritis, 1 hand with psoriatic arthritis, and 1 hand with lupus erythematosus. The average course of the disease was 9 years at the time of the initial rupture. Of 115 flexor tendon ruptures, 91 occurred at the wrist, 4 in the palm, and 20 within the digits.

Of 91 tendon ruptures at the wrist, 61 were caused by attrition of the flexor tendons on a bony spur within the carpal tunnel. Bony spurs of the scaphoid caused 44 wrist tendon ruptures. All bony spurs causing attrition ruptures at the wrist were excised, and the defects were closed either primarily or with a rotation flap. The other 30 wrist tendon ruptures were caused by direct tendon invasion of rheumatoid tenosynovitis. Invasion of the tendons by rheumatoid synovium also caused the 4 palmar and 20 digital tendon ruptures.

Although active motion was regained in 88% of the repaired tendons, motion overall was poor. Patients whose ruptures were caused by attrition had better functional results than those whose ruptures were caused by infiltrating tenosynovitis. Patients with multiple ruptures within the carpal canal had a worse prognosis, whereas those with ruptures of both tendons within the fibro-osseous canal had the worst prognosis of all.

The severity of a patient's rheumatoid arthritis had a greater long-term effect on treatment outcome than did the technical aspects of the operation itself. Because patients with isolated tendon ruptures at the wrist or palm tended to have the best functional results, early tenosynovectomy with removal of bone spurs should be the cornerstone of treatment if tendon ruptures are to be prevented.

▶ Rheumatologists are very reluctant to refer patients to surgeons for precautionary tenosynovectomy. The reason most often stated is that abnormal synovial tissue will regenerate. This is not entirely true, and even if it was, rupture of important tendons can be prevented even if some regeneration of synovial tissue occurs.—E.E. Peacock, Jr., M.D.

The Scaphoid Allograft: A New Operation for Treatment of the Very Proximal Scaphoid Nonunion or for the Necrotic, Fragmented Scaphoid Proximal Pole
Carter PR, Malinin TI, Abbey PA, Sommerkamp TG (Univ of Texas, Dallas; Baylor Univ Med Ctr, Dallas)
*J Hand Surg [Am]*14A:1–12, January 1989   10–8

In 8 patients an allograft was used to replace the proximal part of the scaphoid to avoid the frequent complications of silicone replacement arthroplasty. Four patients had true avascular necrosis; 3 had proximal pole nonunion involving less than 20% of the bone, with very small proximal fragments. One patient had severely comminuted scaphoid, trapezium, and metacarpal fractures from a gunshot wound. Follow-up ranged from 8 to 30 months.

Technique.—The proximal fragment is converted to a waist fracture by resecting the proximal half of the scaphoid and inserting a fresh-frozen, hemi-allograft.

The waist fracture lends itself to rigid internal fixation by Herbert's technique. A palmar approach is preferred. The proximal pole of the scaphoid is pinned to the capitate or radius for 8 weeks with a Kirschner wire. A short arm-thumb spica cast is maintained for 8 weeks.

Union occurred in all cases, usually within 6–12 months. Screw replacement was necessary in 2 early cases. All but 2 patients had a good clinical outcome with nearly normal motion and strength. Two early failures may have been the result of poor patient selection. No infections occurred.

Hemi-allograft replacement of the proximal scaphoid is a reliable and clinically successful procedure, but longer follow-up is necessary. The operation is used only when standard reconstruction with autogenous bone grafting is not feasible.

▶ A major weakness in the concept of bone grafting and hardware fixation of scaphoid fractures has been the realization that dead bone is a bad site for grafts and screws. An osseous allograft has not been tried in this way previously; it is a splendid idea that appears from the early results to have merit.— E.E. Peacock, Jr., M.D.

Digital Replantation at the Level of the Distal Interphalangeal Joint and the Distal Phalanx

Goldner RD, Stevanovic MV, Nunley JA, Urbaniak JR (Duke Univ)
J Hand Surg 14A:214–220, March 1989   10–9

Although replantation at the level of the distal interphalangeal (DIP) joint or distal phalanx is not essential for hand function, some patients request the procedure. Information was gathered on the success rate, costs, and patient satisfaction in replanatation at or distal to the DIP joint.

The average follow-up time for 42 cases was 6 years. Surgical and medical treatment was similar in all cases. Many patients (64%) were manual laborers who had been injured on the job. Of the attempted replantations, 34 (81%) were successful. In 4 of the failures, the decision against replantation was made during the operation. The thumb was involved in 48% of the amputations. In 79% of the hands amputation was at the DIP joint; 21% were more distal. Replantation was more successful with lacerations (89%) than with crush-avulsion injuries (69%).

Distal replantation has a number of advantages over conventional methods of skin coverage. Sensibility, length, motion, and good appearance are all maintained. Replantation is a safe procedure, usually requiring only 1 operation. Return-to-work time varies but should not be longer than that required for amputation revision. Replantation is, however, more expensive and requires a lengthy operating time and an experienced microsurgeon. Thus a number of factors should be considered before replantation of the distal digit: degree of injury, the digit involved, the patient's age, financial status, and vocation, and the surgeon's experience.

▶ As long as the average total cost of treatment is only $7,500 and the viability rate is 81%, it may be permissible to replant single digits at the DIP level. It should be pointed out, however, that the experience and costs reported in this article are not consistent with general experience throughout the country. The preponderance of experience strongly argues that replantation of a single digit, other than the thumb, at any level is not justified on a cost-effectiveness basis except under unusual circumstances.—E.E. Peacock, Jr., M.D.

11 The Breast

Screening for Breast Cancer
Eddy DM (Duke Univ)
Ann Intern Med 111:389–399, Sept 1, 1989   11–1

It was estimated that, in 1989, new primary breast cancers would be diagnosed in approximately 114,000 women in the United States, 48% of whom will eventually die of the disease. Breast cancer is the most common cause of cancer-related death in women aged 40–50 years. The probability that an average-risk woman will have breast cancer diagnosed in the next 10 years is about 130/10,000 for a 40-year-old woman, 230/10,000 for a 55-year-old woman, and 280/10,000 for a 65-year-old woman.

There is much evidence that breast cancer screening, using both mammography and breast physical examination, reduces the mortality from breast cancer in women older than 50 years of age. The results of 3 recently completed controlled clinical trials have raised doubts, however, about the effectiveness of screening in women younger than 50 years of age. Nevertheless, the long-term results of another clinical trial and an uncontrolled project suggest that breast cancer screening might also be effective for younger women.

Mathematical models based on data from controlled trials of breast cancer screening programs indicate that for women destined to have breast cancer, annual screening for 10 years with breast physical examination decreases the probability of breast cancer death by about 25/10,000 and increases life expectancy by about 20 days for women in the 3 age groups. The addition of annual mammography decreases this probability by an additional 25/10,000 and increases life expectancy by an additional 20 days. These benefits are offset by a chance for a false positive result of approximately 2,500/10,000 during the 10-year period, and the cost of screening, which may vary from about $400 to more than $2,000 for 10 annual breast examinations. The carcinogenic effect of annual mammography is small.

Current recommendations state that women older than 40 years of age who are at average risk for the development of breast cancer should have an annual breast physical examination and mammography every 1–2 years starting at age 50. Women at high risk for breast cancer should have annual mammography starting at age 40.

▶ The bottom line of this excellent study and presentation is simply that the present practice of encouraging all women to have mammograms and treating suspicious lesions by needle localization and open biopsy is not cost effective. A better way to prevent, diagnose, and treat breast cancer must be found. In my experience, the costs reported in this paper are conservative; the actual expense in many areas of the country is much greater than reported.—E.E. Peacock, Jr., M.D.

Cancellation of Preoperative Breast Localization Procedures: Analysis of 53 Cases
Meyer JE, Sonnenfeld MR, Greenes RA, Stomper PC (Brigham and Women's Hosp, Boston; Harvard Med School)
Radiology 169:629–630, December 1989   11–2

During a 1-year period, 53 women scheduled for a breast biopsy at Brigham and Women's Hospital had the biopsy canceled on the day of the procedure because the radiologist designated to do the localization

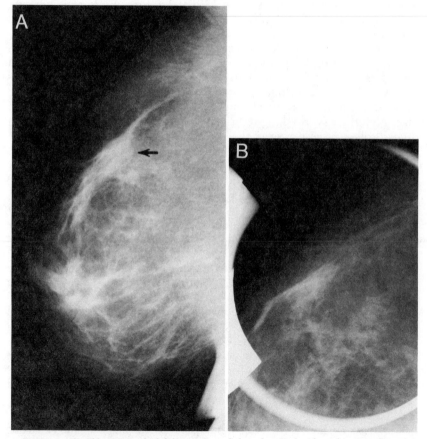

Fig 11–1.—Possible mass in the left breast. **A**, mediolateral projection showed a triangular amorphous density *(arrow)*. There was no corresponding area on the orthogonal view. **B**, with mediolateral compression spot image mass was no longer visible. (Courtesy of Meyer JE, Sonnenfeld MR, Greenes RA, et al: *Radiology* 169:629–630, December 1989.)

had found that the breast abnormalities did not warrant biopsy. In 22 patients the abnormality had disappeared or could not be duplicated in 2 projections (Fig 11–1). On ultrasound examination 13 women were found to have cysts; tangential beam radiography revealed skin calcifications in 9 women. Other reasons for cancellation of the biopsy included vascular calcifications and skin artifacts masquerading as clustered microcalcifications.

Because 8.8% of biopsies scheduled in 1 year were found to be unnecessary, the radiology department of the hospital now requires a staff radiologist to review all outside mammograms a week before the localization procedure. Radiographic follow-up is advised for many of the low-suspicion abnormalities.

If technically possible, the mass or density must be visible in 2 projections. Random or vascular calcifications should be ruled out. A tangential projection can be used to confirm suspected skin calcifications. Any solitary, well-defined mass that resembles a cyst should be examined by ultrasound and aspirated if fluid seems to be present. Further, the skin should be clean so that deodorant or powder artifacts do not appear.

▶ We probably need to cancel needle localization and biopsy of only slightly suspicious lesions on mammogram. There are too many negative biopsies. The observations reported here are a good start.—E.E. Peacock, Jr., M.D.

Residual Breast Carcinoma After Biopsy: Role of Mammography in Evaluation
Homer MJ, Schmidt-Ullrich R, Safaii H, Pile-Spellman ER, Marchant DJ, Smith TJ, Kelly K, Robert NJ (Tufts Univ; New England Med Ctr Hosps, Boston)
Radiology 170:75–77, January 1989   11–3

Patients with early-stage mammary carcinoma who choose breast conservation therapy may have residual tumor after excisional biopsy. The extent of residual tumor, and the type of further treatment required, cannot always be determined by the operative or histopathologic reports. Twenty-one cases were investigated to assess the value of postbiopsy mammography in revealing residual breast carcinoma.

All of the patients had invasive carcinoma. Because the histopathologic margins were not adequately documented at the initial operation, reexcision of the biopsy site or mastectomy was performed. Mammograms obtained at average of 2 weeks after the original excision showed residual carcinoma in 5 women (Fig 11–2). The remaining 16 mammographic findings were viewed as consistent with postsurgical changes. Histopathologic examination of reexcision biopsy or mastectomy specimens, however, revealed residual microscopic tumor in an additional 7 women. In these patients neither clinical nor mammographic evaluation was suggestive of residual carcinoma.

Inking of the specimen margin makes it possible to assess the relationship between a tumor mass and specimen margin. Because postsurgical

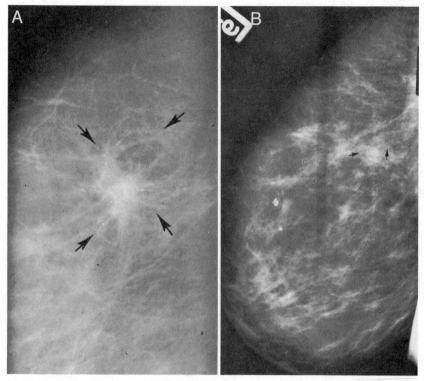

Fig 11–2.—A, prebiopsy mammogram revealed a 3-cm spiculated mass *(arrows)* with microcalcifications. **B**, postbiopsy, pretreatment mammogram showed expected surgical changes at site of excisional biopsy. Residual microcalcifications *(arrows)* were present. (Courtesy of Homer MJ, Schmidt-Ullrich R, Safaii H, et al: *Radiology* 170:75–77, January 1989.)

changes decrease the reliability of both palpation and mammography, patients whose tumor margins cannot be clearly identified histopathologically should undergo reexcision before being considered for breast conservation therapy.

▶ Using mammography to determine whether local excision is adequate is a good way to set back the progress of local treatment of small breast cancers. Wide excision of local tumors should be such that there is no need for a test that is running only about 25% positive for breast carcinoma throughout the world.—E.E. Peacock, Jr., M.D.

The Potential Value of Mammographically Guided Fine-Needle Aspiration Biopsy of Nonpalpable Breast Lesions

Masood S, Frykberg ER, Mitchum DG, McLellan GL, Scalapino MC, Bullard JB (Univ of Florida; Univ Hosp of Jacksonville, Fla)
Am Surg 55:226–231, April 1989   11–4

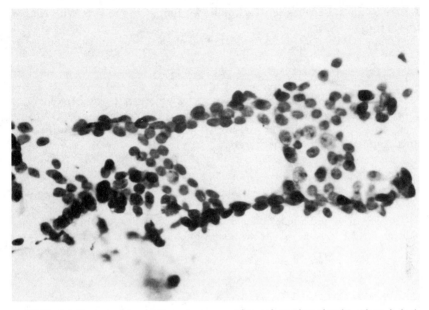

Fig 11–3.—Cytologic smear showing extensive overriding and crowding of nuclei with marked cellular material interpreted as atypical hyperplasia (hematoxylin and eosin; original magnification, ×250). (Courtesy of Masood S, Frykberg ER, Mitchum DG, et al: *Am Surg* 55:226–231, April 1989.)

The accuracy and safety of fine-needle aspiration biopsy (FNAB) for diagnosing malignancy in palpable breast lesions are established. Whether FNAB has the same attributes in diagnosing nonpalpable breast lesions was investigated. After standard needle localization of the target lesion with position confirmed by mammography, FNAB was carried out through the localizing needle. At least 6 slides were obtained. A localizing wire was inserted, and standard needle-localization, open biopsy was performed in the operating room.

In 18 of 20 women aged 37–82 years with mammographic indications for biopsy, FNAB was completed successfully. Comparison of cytologic interpretation with histologic diagnosis in these 18 patients showed agreement in 94%. The method allowed differentiation between hyperplasia with atypia (Fig 11–3) and without. No false positive results occurred, but there was 5.5% false negative results.

Fine-needle aspiration biopsy guided by mammography is reliable, safe, and cost effective in diagnosing nonpalpable breast lesions. Open biopsy may be avoided when cytologic diagnosis of malignancy is unequivocal, but open biopsy is recommended if the cytologic diagnosis is "benign" or "suspicious."

▶ The findings reported in this paper indicate that a better way is still needed to diagnose accurately any suspicious lesions seen only by mammography. Wire localization followed by open biopsy in a major operating room is too expensive and too time-consuming for the relatively low number of breast carcinomas that are found.—E.E. Peacock, Jr., M.D.

A New Surgical Localization Technique for Biopsy in Patients With Nipple Discharge

Choudhury A, Wengert PA Jr, Smith JS Jr (Polyclinic Med Ctr, Harrisburg, Pa; Milton S. Hershey Med Ctr, Hershey, Pa)
Arch Surg 124:874–875, July 1989   11–5

Because a discharge of fluid from the nipple can be associated with cancer, any persistent discharge requires further evaluation. A new technique of ductal localization for biopsy was developed that identifies the duct responsible for the discharge.

Technique.—A 30-gauge "anterior chamber" needle is used. This is a blunt-tipped, nonbeveled needle that acts like a probe. After the needle is passed into the duct, half-strength methylene blue dye (2–3 mL) is injected through it (Fig 11–4). The ducts and lobule outlined with the dye are dissected for biopsy using a circumareolar incision nearest the point of needle entry.

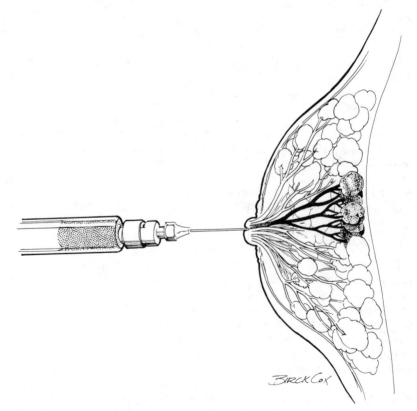

Fig 11–4.—Insertion of anterior chamber needle into duct with injection of methylene blue dye through major duct and its major tributaries. (Courtesy of Choudhury A, Wengert PA Jr, Smith JS Jr: *Arch Surg* 124:874–875, July 1989.)

In 12 patients, all of whom were found to have benign intraductal papillomas, the ductal system responsible for the bloody discharge was identified. The technique of injecting methylene blue dye into the duct is safe, effective, and can be done on an outpatient basis. In addition, this localization technique does not have the disadvantages associated with contrast mammography and cannulation of the draining duct with a lacrimal duct probe.

▶ The technique described in this paper can be helpful if no mistakes are made. The problem with methylene blue dye is that if even a single particle of the substance is introduced or spilled in the wrong place, the entire field is stained and recognition of specific tissues becomes impossible.— E.E. Peacock, Jr., M.D.

The Risk of Occult Invasive Breast Cancer After Excisional Biopsy Showing In-Situ Ductal Carcinoma of Comedo Pattern
Hardman PDJ, Worth A, Lee U (Cancer Control Agency of British Columbia, Vancouver; Univ of British Columbia)
Can J Surg 32:56–60, January 1989   11–6

Of the morphological subgroups of intraductal carcinoma, the cribriform and comedo groups are most common. Although some studies have suggested that there is little value in distinguishing between these variants, comedocarcinoma appears to have a relatively high rate of proliferation and potential for malignancy. The incidence of occult invasive ductal carcinoma in patients with a diagnosis of in situ ductal carcinoma of the predominant comedo pattern was examined.

Data from 61 patients were reviewed. In 31 women (50%), a breast lump was the presenting symptom; 25 had mammographic abnormalities, and 6 experienced nipple discharge. When biopsy specimens left doubt that diseased tissue was completely excised, wide local reexcision or total mastectomy was performed.

There were 44 total mastectomies and 13 wide local reexcisions, most performed within 1 month of the original biopsy. Residual ductal carcinoma was found in 38 women, 14 of whom had occult invasive disease. Patients with nipple discharge had the highest incidence of residual or infiltrating carcinoma. Axillary node metastases were always associated with occult invasive carcinoma at reexcision.

The high incidence of residual disease in these patients leads to the suggestions that in situ comedocarcinoma may be a kinetically active variant of intraductal disease. Because this type of breast cancer may soon progress to invasive disease, extensive local excision or total mastectomy is recommended. When conservative treatment is chosen, excision margins should be carefully examined.

▶ Although there is a good theoretical case for local excision of small carcinomas of the breast, similar reasoning does not hold for intraductal or comedocarcinoma. The generalized nature of this disease makes local excision of a single tumor dangerous. Mastectomy is probably the best procedure because of the biology and general distribution of the condition.— E.E. Peacock, Jr., M.D.

Histologic Features Predictive of an Increased Risk of Early Local Recurrence After Treatment of Breast Cancer by Local Tumor Excision and Radical Radiotherapy
Lindley R, Bulman A, Parsons P, Phillips R, Henry K, Ellis H (Westminster Hosp, London)
Surgery 105:13–20, January 1989   11–7

The histologic factors that predict local recurrence of breast cancer treated by local excision and radiation therapy have not been studied widely. Of 293 patients so treated between July 1979 and December 1984, histologic sections from 272 were available for blind review and statistical analysis by December 1986.

Pathologic features significantly associated with local recurrence, in decreasing order of significance, were as follows: more than 25% intraduct component with extensive necrosis, tumor necrosis, Bloom grade, less than 25% intraduct component with extensive necrosis, lymph node metastasis, more than 25% intraduct component, extensive inflammatory infiltrate, and lack of elastosis. The most predictive features, according to multivariate analysis, were a combination of more than 25% intraduct component and necrosis. Early local recurrence developed in 9 of 18 patients with this combination of features, increasing the risk from 10% for patients without these features to 50% for those with them.

The combination of a large intraduct component with comedonecrosis is an important indicator of prognosis in patients treated by local excision and radiation therapy. Patients with this combination should be observed closely, with regular mammography. Mastectomy might be better initial treatment for this group.

▶ Before all of the problems of local tumor excision are solved, it seems likely to me that radiotherapy will be improved on a large scale and shown to be adequate alone. Theoretically, surgery or radiation should be adequate alone; practically, there are problems with each, and it is not certain that the use of both eliminates all of the problems of each.— E.E. Peacock, Jr., M.D.

Efficacy of Peroperative Liver Function Tests and Ultrasound in Detecting Hepatic Metastasis in Carcinoma of the Breast
Clark CP III, Foreman ML, Peters GN, Cheek JH, Sparkman RS (Baylor Univ Med Ctr, Dallas)
Surg Gynecol Obstet 167:510–514, December 1988   11–8

The value of routine preoperative liver assessment in patients scheduled for treatment of operable breast carcinoma has not been determined.

In a prospective study, the benefits of ultrasound and liver function tests before mastectomy were evaluated in all breast cancer patients seen during a 2-year-period. Patients whose test results suggested hepatic metastasis underwent biopsy.

Of 220 patients with clinical stage I, II, or III cancer, liver function tests showed an abnormality, usually of the lactic dehydrogenase (LDH) level alone, in 33 patients. Abnormal sonographic findings were evident in 74 patients, but only 3 had lesions consistent with metastasis and of these 3, only 1 had confirmed metastasis. An elevated LDH level was found in the 1 patient with metastasis but not in the other 2. During follow-up for a mean of 26 months, hepatic metastases developed in 0.9% of stage I patients, 3.4% of stage II patients, and 12.5% of stage III patients. Liver enzyme levels had been normal in all of these before operation.

These results indicate that preoperative hepatic ultrasound is warranted only if there are grossly abnormal results of enzyme tests or physical examination. If metastasis is shown on ultrasound, histologic confirmation is recommended if results would change treatment.

▶ The real question, however, is whether treatment should be altered in patients who have liver metastasis, regardless of how it is discovered. The same question is yet to be answered for asymptomatic bone metastasis.—E.E. Peacock, Jr., M.D.

Immediate Breast Reconstruction: Reducing the Risks
Bailey MH, Smith JW, Casas L, Johnson P, Serra E, de la Fuente R, Sullivan M, Scanlon EF (Evanston Hosp, Evanston, Ill; Northwestern Univ)
Plast Reconstr Surg 83:845–851, May 1989   11–9

An increasing number of women are undergoing immediate reconstruction of the breast after mastectomy. The complication rate for this procedure, however, is reported to be high. To identify risk factors leading to implant loss, evaluation was made of 165 consecutive immediate breast reconstructions.

Technique.—Most patients (84%) underwent modified radical mastectomy, usually with detachment of the pectoralis minor. Complete muscle coverage is used, leaving the origin of the pectoralis muscle intact. If complete coverage of the implant is not possible, a portion of the implant remains uncovered. Depending on the amount of existing tissue coverage, a gel prosthesis is inserted or a tissue expander is used. A waiting period of at least 8 weeks is required before the expander is exchanged for the permanent prosthesis.

The average follow-up for the 157 patients was 33 weeks. Eight percent of the tumors were nonpalpable, 65% were stage I, 22% stage II, 4% stage III, and 1% stage IV. At the time of follow-up 68% of the reconstructions were complete. In the others loss of implant occurred or attempts at expansion were continuing. The implant was completely covered with muscle in 46% of the cases. Overall, the complication rate was 55%, and 18% of the implants were lost. In analyzing a number of variables, 3 emerged as significant. Complete muscle coverage was associated with an implant loss rate of only 8%, whereas the rate of loss for partial coverage was 27%. Smokers without complete muscle coverage had a 45% rate of implant loss. Further, older age was associated with a higher rate of implant loss, independent of muscle coverage. Of slightly less significance with regard to implant loss was a fourth factor—concurrent operation on the opposite breast. Clinical staging and chemotherapy were not related to reconstructive success.

Tissue expanders can be used when complete muscle coverage of the gel prosthesis is not possible. Patients are urged to stop smoking before surgery. Additional care must be taken with older women, although immediate reconstruction can be successful despite an advanced age.

▶ Loss of a gel prosthesis when immediate reconstruction is carried out occurs more often than is acceptable. Selection of patients can be used to reduce the incidence of implant extrusion. Smoking and obesity rank high as risk factors in my experience.—E.E. Peacock, Jr., M.D.

Oncological Aspects of Immediate Breast Reconstruction Following Mastectomy for Malignancy
Johnson CH, van Heerden JA, Donohue JH, Martin JH, Martin JK Jr, Jackson IT, Ilstrup DM (Mayo Clinic and Found, Rochester, Minn; Mayo Clinic, Jacksonville, Fla)
Arch Surg 124:819–824, July 1989   11–10

The immediate issues raised by reconstruction after mastectomy are whether a prosthesis interferes with the detection and treatment of recurrent disease and whether recurrence and survival rates are influenced by immediate reconstruction. Data were reviewed concerning 118 women who underwent mastectomy and immediate breast reconstruction between 1980 and 1986. Thirty-three patients received adjuvant chemotherapy after ablative surgery and 17 others received antihormonal therapy. The mean follow-up was 2½ years.

Fourteen patients had recurrent disease after a mean of 15.5 months; 7 of them had a component of local failure. No local recurrence was deep to the pectoralis major or serratus anterior muscle. No prosthesis had to be removed. The overall 5-year disease-free survival rate was 81%. Recurrences were most frequent in patients with positive axillary nodes and those with larger invasive tumors. Survival was best for patients with negative axillary nodes, even when in situ cancers were excluded. It also was better for women with estrogen receptor-positive tumors.

Immediate breast reconstruction can be offered to women having mastectomy who desire the procedure. In the authors' series, patient acceptance has been outstanding, and placement of a prosthesis has not compromised resection or interfered with adjuvant therapy or treatment of recurrent disease. Further, patient self-image is improved, and there are savings in time and money.

▶ After more than 20 years of study there seems little reason to question that immediate reconstruction following mastectomy is advisable for most women. All of the strawmen that have been raised have pretty well been knocked down.—E.E. Peacock, Jr., M.D.

12 The Head and the Neck

Surgical Treatment of Infantile Subglottic Hemangioma
Mulder JJS, van den Broek P (Radboud Univ Hosp, Nijmegen, The Netherlands)
Int J Pediatr Otorhinolaryngol 17:57–63, February 1989   12–1

A number of treatments have been proposed for infantile subglottic hemangiomas. Cryotherapy, laser therapy, and long-term steroid administration all have some degree of risk. Although surgery for this problem was previously associated with complications, new techniques make operative treatment a valuable alternative. Subglottic hemangiomas in 3 infants were removed by means of a midline cricotracheotomy.

Girl, 3½ months, had been intubated for 2 weeks after symptoms of respiratory distress developed. Swelling of subglottic soft tissue almost completely compressed the tracheal lumen (Fig 12–1). A capillary hemangioma was diagnosed at biopsy during direct laryngoscopy. Steroids were administered, but the tumor did

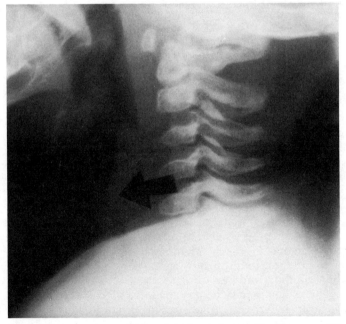

Fig 12–1.—Neck roentgenogram showing subglottic soft tissue swelling. (Courtesy of Mulder JJS, van den Broek P: *Int J Pediatr Otorhinolaryngol* 17:57–63, February 1989.)

not decrease in size. The tumor was then partially removed surgically. Although a mild stridor remained after the operation, the girl was free of respiratory symptoms 4 months later.

These tumors, located in the submucosa in all 3 infants, ranged from 0.5 cm to 1 cm in diameter. The midline cricotracheotomy allowed adequate exposure of the subglottic space. Total removal was possible in only 1 infant, but the long-term outcome appears excellent. Even in small children, laryngeal surgery can be done safely. Care in dissection of tissue under the microscope and in suturing of laryngeal and tracheal tissues is required for a successful outcome.

Nearly half of the infants with subglottic hemangioma have associated hemangiomas in other locations. Failure to diagnose the condition may result in death caused by respiratory insufficiency.

▶ Successful management of infantile subglottic hemangioma involves a high suspicion of the lesion in patients who are being treated for hemangioma or lymphangioma around the oral cavity. Unrecognized subglottic hemangioma can enlarge dangerously because venous return in adjacent lesions is ligated without the surgeon knowing that the subglottic area contains hemangioma or lymphangioma.—E.E. Peacock, Jr., M.D.

What Is the Role of Carotid Arterial Resection in the Management of Advanced Cervical Cancer?

McCready RA, Miller SK, Hamaker RC, Singer MI, Herod GT (Methodist Hosp, Indianapolis)
J Vasc Surg 10:274–280, September 1989   12–2

The incidence of malignant invasion of the carotid artery is high in patients with advanced or recurrent cervical cancer. However, there is controversy over the role of carotid artery ligation or resection in treatment of these patients. Whereas some advocate carotid artery resection in case of direct tumor invasion or if the carotid artery is encased by tumor, others are of the opinion that carotid artery resection affords little benefit because of the aggressive nature and poor prognosis of these tumors.

From 1977 through 1988, 14 men and 2 women (average age, 63 years) underwent operation for treatment of advanced cervical carcinoma. Three patients had carotid artery ligation as part of the initial treatment; the others were treated with interposition saphenous vein grafts to reconstruct the resected carotid arteries. Fifteen patients received adjunctive intraoperative irradiation to decrease the risk of recurrent disease. Since 1982, pectoralis major muscle flaps have been constructed to cover the vein grafts and protect against carotid artery blowout.

Two patients had immediate postoperative strokes, 1 of whom had excellent neurologic recovery. Another patient had a late stroke 6 months after operation and died shortly thereafter of metastatic disease. Of the 3 patients who underwent carotid artery ligation as initial treatment, postoperative transient ischemic attacks occurred in 1 with complete resolution of symptoms. The mean follow-up was 15 months. Seven patients were still alive without evidence of recurrent disease more than 1 year after carotid artery resection, 6 had died of recurrent or metastatic disease, and 2 had died of other causes.

Intraoperative irradiation appears to decrease significantly the local recurrence rate of cervical tumors. However, longer follow-up is needed to assess the effect of adjunctive therapy.

▶ The key to carotid replacement is selection of those rare individuals in whom the carotid artery alone is involved. When this is the case there is no question that modern vascular surgery can extend the limits of cure. It must be remembered, however, that isolated involvement of the carotid artery is rare; most of the time, penetration of the carotid sheath by neck cancer extends far beyond the artery and involves prevertebral fascia and other deep fascial planes more extensive than the relatively small artery.—E.E. Peacock, Jr., M.D.

Neck Dissection After Twice-A-Day Radiotherapy: Morbidity and Recurrence Rates
Parsons JT, Mendenhall WM, Cassisi NJ, Stringer SP, Million RR (Univ of Florida)
Head Neck 11:400–404, September–October 1989   12–3

Between 1978 and 1986, 56 patients with moderately advanced and advanced squamous cell carcinoma of the head and neck underwent planned unilateral radical neck dissections and 5 patients had planned bilateral radical neck dissections after high-dose, twice-daily radiotherapy with cobalt-60. A dose of 120 cGy was administered to the primary tumor site at each radiotherapy session, with a 4- to 6-hour interfraction interval. Treatments were given 5 days a week by continuous-course radiotherapy. Four patients had stage III disease and the other 57 had stage IV disease. Neck dissections were usually performed 6 weeks after completion of radiotherapy. None of the patients was lost to follow-up, and the minimum follow-up was 2 years.

Nine patients had recurrence in the neck. The overall 5-year control rate of neck disease for all 61 patients was 81%. In patients with N2–N3 disease who underwent neck dissections after twice-daily radiotherapy, significantly better control of neck disease was achieved than in those treated by radiotherapy alone during the same period (Fig 12–2). However, the 5-year control rate for patients with N1 neck disease treated by radiotherapy followed by neck dissection was somewhat lower than that for patients with N1 neck disease treated by radiotherapy alone.

Four of 53 patients who underwent planned unilateral neck dissection without flap reconstruction had wound separation, of which 2 closed spontaneously and 2 required split-thickness skin grafts. In 2 of 3 patients who underwent planned unilateral neck dissection with pectoralis

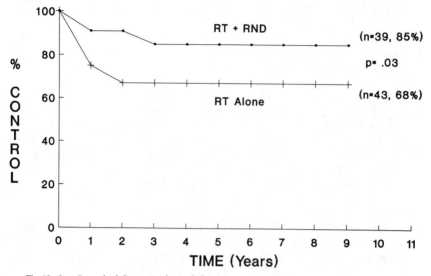

N2B, 3B

Fig 12–2.—Control of disease in the neck for 82 patients with N2B or N3B disease according to treatment technique (RT + RND = irradiation plus neck dissection). Twenty-three of 39 patients (59%) who underwent neck dissection had N3B disease vs. 26 of 43 (60%) treated by irradiation alone. (Courtesy of Parsons JT, Mendenhall WM, Cassisi NJ, et al: *Head Neck* 11:400–404, September–October 1989.)

major flap reconstruction, necrosis of the flaps developed, requiring deltopectoral flap reconstruction. In 2 of 5 patients who underwent planned bilateral radical neck dissections there were wound separations that led to carotid exposure. Both patients were treated with deltopectoral flap reconstructions.

Planned neck dissection 6 weeks after high-dose radiotherapy increases the risk of severe surgical morbidity, but the risks of the treatment sequence appear to be outweighed by the benefits of first administering intensive radiotherapy.

▶ Two important points are worthy of emphasis in this report. One is that wound healing complications do not mitigate against preoperative radiotherapy, and, even more important, radiotherapy alone is not as effective as the combination of radiation and excision of lymph nodes.—E.E. Peacock, Jr., M.D.

Transoral Carbon Dioxide Laser Ablation for Cancer, Tumors, and Other Diseases
Panje WR, Scher N, Karnell M (Univ of Chicago–Pritzker School of Medicine)
Arch Otolaryngol Head Neck Surg 115:681–688, June 1989   12–4

Oral cavity and oropharyngeal cancers can now be removed without loss of blood by use of the carbon dioxide laser. The lymphatic or hematologic spread of cancer cells does not appear to be increased by this method, and cancers of the vocal cord can be eradicated with preservation of the voice. The outcome in 71 patients who underwent transoral CO_2 laser removal of cancer was assessed, with emphasis on speech and swallowing functions.

The technique employed was excision rather than vaporization (Fig 12–3). All resections were done with a laser apparatus attached to a surgical microscope. Patients were selected on the basis of transoral accessibility of the tumor; those with bone invasion by tumor generally underwent a method other than CO_2 laser ablation. None of the wounds was reconstructed. Postoperative care consisted of prophylactic antibiotics and mouth rinses and gargles. Patients were followed for at least 2 years.

In 87% of the patients the cancers were classified as T_1 or T_2; the remaining cancers were more advanced. Squamous cell carcinoma of the oral cavity accounted for 30 of the lesions. Other malignancies included melanoma, sarcoma, lymphoma, and verrucous carcinoma. Of the patients with benign or premalignant lesions and those with T_1 or T_2 cancers, 97% had good swallowing after laser treatment. Of those with larger lesions, 21% had some swallowing impairment. Speech was unaffected in most of the patients with lower grade lesions and in all of those with benign lesions. Larger lesions with deep removal of the neoplasm that restricted motion of the tongue or jaw, or both, adversely affected speech. In these patients reconstruction of the CO_2 laser wounds and multimodality cancer therapy should be considered. On the whole, the

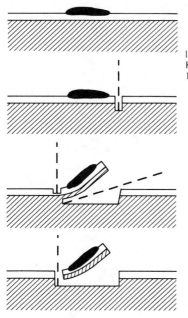

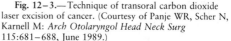

Fig. 12–3.—Technique of transoral carbon dioxide laser excision of cancer. (Courtesy of Panje WR, Scher N, Karnell M: *Arch Otolaryngol Head Neck Surg* 115:681–688, June 1989.)

CO_2 laser offers excellent preservation of function, a good cosmetic result, and cost effectiveness.

► There may or may not be advantages to using a carbon dioxide laser to remove or destroy neoplasms in the oral cavity. If there is a significant advantage, it is not apparent yet to me. Many surgeons believe that laser ablation is advantageous, so more data will be available soon. In the meantime, the danger to patients and personnel taking care of them should be emphasized. The carbon dioxide laser can zap people unintentionally and start fires accidentally, with disastrous results. Having the best equipment, and the exemplary training of everyone involved in its use, are mandatory.—E.E. Peacock, Jr., M.D.

Facial Nerve Function Following Irradiated Cable Grafts
McGuirt WF, Welling DB, McCabe BF (Wake Forest Univ; Univ of Iowa)
Laryngoscope 99:27–34, January 1989   12–5

Cable grafting is a successful method of restoring function and facial expression in patients undergoing facial nerve resection for malignant parotid tumors. The choice of cable grafting is controversial, however, when patients must undergo irradiation postoperatively. The outcome in 12 patients with postoperatively irradiated facial nerve cable grafts was reviewed in an attempt to resolve this question.

In all but 1 of the patients the graft source was the great auricular nerve. Radiation therapy consisted of more than 5,000 rad to the graft bed and was administered within 2 months of resection and grafting. Three patients died before return of function could be assessed. The other patients were evaluated for reflexes in the grafts using pontograms, axon counts, and graded function.

Function returned as early as 2 months and as late as 9 months. Earlier onset of return correlated with quality of function. Although no patient had entirely normal function, deficits were minor in 7 of the 9 patients. Those without preoperative facial nerve palsy had a better return of function.

Even when irradiation is to be carried out postoperatively, facial nerve autografting offers better results than dynamic or static slings. Benefits of the cable graft include eye protection, adequate voluntary motion, prevention of drooling, and maintenance of facial tone.

► The facial nerve is a pure motor nerve in the area where it is most frequently damaged; all pure motor nerves can be grafted successfully. Primary repair is the most effective way to reanimate the face. Secondary grafting is more difficult and the results are less rewarding.—E.E. Peacock, Jr., M.D.

The Role of Surgery in the Treatment of Squamous Cell Carcinoma of the Nasal Vestibule

Weinberger JM, Briant TDR, Cummings BJ, Wong CS (Princess Margaret Hosp, Toronto; Wellesley Hosp, Toronto)
J Otolaryngol 17:372–375, December 1988   12–6

Squamous cell carcinomas can be treated successfully by either primary radiation therapy or primary resection. At the Princess Margaret Hospital, radiation is usually the primary treatment, with surgery reserved for recurrent cancer. Data on 61 patients were reviewed to evaluate treatment and outcome in this uncommon form of cancer.

Of the patients studied, 56 received primary radiation therapy and 5 underwent primary resection. The 12 patients with recurrence after radiotherapy required partial or total rhinectomy. Cancer was controlled in 8 of these patients after surgery. Despite radiotherapy and surgery 2 patients with local and regional disease at diagnosis died. Node dissection was successful in managing late regional node metastases in 3 of 4 patients.

Small lesions can be treated by either method with a good medical outcome and cosmetic results. With larger areas of involvement, radiotherapy offers a better appearance after treatment. Bone invasion is generally a poor prognostic sign. In such cases there is a high risk of local tumor recurrence and radiation alone is often not adequate. When primary radiotherapy is combined with surgical salvage, a 90% local control rate has been achieved.

▶ Squamous cell carcinoma of the nose is treated so effectively with expert radiation, and the cosmetic deformity can be so severe following surgery, that radiation treatment clearly is the preferred form of therapy at present.—E.E. Peacock, Jr., M.D.

Preoperative Assessment of Parotid Masses: A Comparative Evaluation of Radiologic Techniques to Histopathologic Diagnosis
Byrne MN, Spector JG, Garvin CF, Gado MH (Washington Univ)
Laryngoscope 99:284–292, March 1989   12–7

The usefulness of various imaging methods was assessed in a review of 110 surgically treated parotid masses. Studies included 162 CT scans, 25 sialograms, and 10 magnetic resonance (MR) images. The MR studies included T1- and T2-weighted images and balanced images.

The findings on CT of clear borders, a homogeneous appearance, and high density strongly favored the diagnosis of a benign tumor or low-grade malignancy. Ill-defined tumor margins, heterogeneity, and high density tended to indicate a high-grade or recurrent malignancy. Mixed density was associated with lymphangioma, lymphoepithelial lesions, and sialadenitis. Sialography detected lesions in two thirds of the patients examined. Magnetic resonance imaging detected all 10 tumors. The T1-weighted images consistently showed low signal intensity, whereas most tumors had high signal intensity on T2-weighted images.

Computed tomography sialography is a sensitive means of detecting parotid mass lesions, but it may be uncomfortable and is not readily used in children. High-resolution CT readily detects parotid tumors; contrast is an effective adjunct. Use of MR imaging provides excellent soft tissue resolution. The T1-weighted images are well suited to demonstrating the tumor margins; heterogeneity is evident on T2-weighted images.

▶ Modern radiologic techniques have made preoperative diagnosis and extent of parotid tumors more accurate. Sialography is not one such technique, however. In a cost-conscious era it is even more important to avoid time-consuming, expensive techniques that have been proven to be relatively useless in the management of a difficult tumor.— E.E. Peacock, Jr., M.D.

Post-Traumatic Parotid Fistulae and Sialoceles: A Prospective Study of Conservative Management in 51 Cases
Parekh D, Glezerson G, Stewart M, Esser J, Lawson HH (Baragwanath Hosp; Univ of Witwatersrand, Johannesburg)
Ann Surg 209:105–111, January 1989   12–8

Parotid trauma usually results from injuries received in a motor vehicle accident or from an assault weapon. Acute injuries are treated by repair of the injured structures so that normal parotid function can return. Injuries that are missed when the patient is treated initially have been managed in a number of ways.

Fifty-one patients with posttraumatic parotid injuries were treated conservatively over a 3-year period. Patients in the pilot stage of the study received maintenance fluids intravenously but nothing orally for 5 days (regimen 1). Later in the study oral administration was withheld until the injury was completely healed (regimen 2). If fistulas persisted beyond 8 days, parenteral nutrition was provided.

Parotid injuries included sialoceles (58%), fistulas (30%), and effusions (15%). In 13 patients infections developed. The infections were rapidly resolved with local dressings (2) or with antibiotic therapy. One patient with a persistent sialocele was lost to follow-up. In the other 50 patients the parotid injury healed.

Regimen 1 caused a highly significant delay in healing (24 ± 4 days) compared with regimen 2 (9.4 ± 0.9 days). Delay in response to conservative management correlated with the severity of the injury as documented by sialography. Partial duct transections healed in approximately half the time of complete duct transections. Injuries to minor intraparotid ducts healed in significantly less time than injuries to major parotid ducts.

The treatment described here allows the parotid to rest and heal, because the lack of mastication and chemical stimuli minimizes parotid secretion. Conservative management is safer than radiotherapy, with its risk of secondary malignancy, or surgery, with its danger to the facial nerve. The excellent results from this therapy argue for its use as the initial treatment of choice for parotid fistulas.

▶ Conservative treatment is usually effective in a week or so. If prolonged drainage occurs, an easy solution is a single small dose of external radiation to the parotid area.—E.E. Peacock, Jr., M.D.

Early Reexploration of the Parotid Wound Following Parotidectomy
Chaffoo RAK, Fee WE Jr (US Naval Hosp, San Diego; Stanford Univ)
Am J Otolaryngol 10:38–41, January–February 1989   12–9

Several conditions may require reexploration of the parotid wound after parotidectomy. Residual malignant tissue may remain, or dysfunction of the facial nerve may be apparent. Although risks are involved in reexploration, this surgery can be safely accomplished within 3 weeks of the initial procedure. Of the 6 patients reviewed in this study, 4 had residual malignant disease and 2 had signs of neural degeneration.

Case 1.—Boy, 12 years who underwent a right "total" parotidectomy, was found to have high-grade mucoepidermoid carcinoma. Reexploration of the wound at 23 days postoperatively revealed residual parotid tissue. Surgeons performed a total parotidectomy and a modified dissection of the right side of the neck. The facial nerve was preserved. Although facial nerve weakness was observed postoperatively, its function returned completely within 8 weeks.

Case 2.—Man, 60, underwent radiotherapy for undifferentiated cancer in a left parotid mass. Facial nerve paralysis occurred after radical dissection of the left side of the neck and partial parotidectomy. Reexploration of the left parotid wound identified the main trunk of the left facial nerve and revealed the pes to be completely transected. Reconstruction was performed using a graft from the right great auricular nerve, but facial function was not recovered. Local recurrence and pulmonary metastases developed subsequently.

Early surgical reexploration of the parotid wound is feasible. In most cases, residual tissue can be removed safely without further damage to the facial nerve and, in the majority of patients, nerve function can be regained.

▶ There is not only no contraindication to early exploration of patients with suspected nerve injury, but everything argues for the earliest possible reexploration. Identification of nerve damage and the best repair of a motor nerve can be done before wound healing and scar formation take place.—E.E. Peacock, Jr., M.D.

The Pleural Osteomuscular Flap in Oropharyngeal Reconstruction
Stromberg BV (Creighton Univ, Omaha)
Laryngoscope 99:339–341, March 1989   12–10

Numerous options are available to the surgeon in oropharyngeal reconstruction, although the pectoralis major myocutaneous flap has become the most frequently chosen because of its wide application to differ-

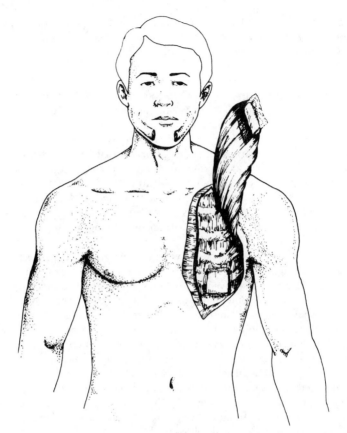

Fig 12–4.—Elevation of osteomyocutaneous flap. (Courtesy of Stromberg BV: *Laryngoscope* 99:339–341, March 1989.)

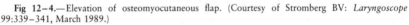

ent uses in the head and neck region. In certain cases the addition of a pleural segment to the flap is useful. When associated with the need for a rib graft, use of the pleura can provide viable tissue with a surface similar to oral mucosa.

Technique.—After the required exterior cutaneous coverage has been carefully measured, the ellipse of tissue is incised and the subcutaneous tissue raised above and below the cutaneous paddle of the flap (Fig 12–4). When the pectoralis muscle is isolated, care is taken not to remove any part of the attachment to the fifth rib. A few extra centimeters are added to the length of rib required. The pleura is entered along the lower edge of the fourth rib and divided inferiorly at the superior edge of the sixth rib. An incision may be necessary just above the clavicle to allow free guided passage of the block of tissue, pleura, rib, pectoralis major, subcutaneous tissue, and skin.

In experience with 4 patients, no difficulties were encountered in sealing the pleural cavity or removing the chest tube. Furthermore, viability was not a problem. Two patients who had had radiation had difficulty in bone healing from the rib graft to the mandibular edge, but reoperation was successful. Addition of a pleural segment can alleviate bulky flaps and difficulty with intraoral skin grafts.

▶ Lining has always been the major problem in oral cavity reconstruction. Use of the pleura is an ingenious addition to the techniques that have been advocated. Several surgical specialties are involved if a single individual is not rather broadly trained, however.—E.E Peacock, Jr., M.D.

13 The Thorax

Use of Silicone Stents in the Management of Airway Problems
Cooper JD, Pearson FG, Patterson GA, Todd TRJ, Ginsberg RJ, Goldberg M, Waters P (Univ of Toronto)
Ann Thorac Surg 47:371–378, March 1989

13–1

Previously, tracheal T tubes were used successfully in 18 patients who were treated for complex airway problems. The use of silicone rubber prostheses has been extended to include bifurcation prostheses at the carina and prostheses inserted into the main bronchi.

A total of 47 patients were treated with tracheal T tubes, including 2 treated with T-Y tubes, 2 with Y tubes, and 3 with bronchial stents. In 10 of 11 patients with malignant tumors involving the airway, T tubes were used as definitive treatment to palliate obstruction or compression of the airway. In 1 patient the T tube was placed after surgical resection of a subglottic tumor. In 2 of these 11 patients, the T-Y tube was used. The prostheses were in place for 2 weeks to 18 months (mean, 4.4 months). All patients died of their disease. Three tubes were replaced with tracheostomy tubes; no tubes were compressed by enlarging tumors, but 2 tumors progressed beyond the end of the tube.

The T tube was also used in 36 patients with benign lesions: as definitive treatment in 12, as a temporary measure before resection in 6, as an adjunct to surgery in 9, and for complications after tracheal resection in 9.

Early in the series, T tubes were inserted through a tracheostomy stoma but, more recently, the tubes have been placed endoscopically by pulling the horizontal limb out through the tracheostomy stoma. This maneuver facilitates introduction of the tube and maintains the airway during insertion. A T tube used to stent an area of tracheal stricture should remain in place for at least 9 months if subsequent extubation is anticipated. Use of the silicone stent adds another tool to the management of complicated airway problems. Its increased use is anticipated.

▶ This remarkable paper documents experiences with 47 patients who had silicone rubber stents placed in the tracheobronchial tree. These stents, originated from a silicone T tube developed by Dr. William Montgomery in 1968, have been useful in a wide variety of conditions. What is quite remarkable is the ability to leave these stents in place for years. The paper describes patients with stents in place for longer than 5 years. These findings support the recommendations of Neville, who has championed silicone tracheal prostheses for many years.—F.C. Spencer, M.D.

Evolving Management of Pectus Excavatum Based on a Single Institutional Experience of 664 Patients
Haller JA Jr, Scherer LR, Turner CS, Colombani PM (Johns Hopkins Univ)
Ann Surg 209:578–583, May 1989
13–2

Most family physicians and pediatricians do not recommend surgery in early childhood for pectus excavatum, or funnel chest. Repair should be performed between the ages of 4 years and 6 years to allow normal growth of the thorax, prevent later pulmonary and cardiac dysfunction, and improve the cosmetic appearance.

During a 40-year period, 664 patients underwent surgical correction of pectus excavatum defects. The condition was seen more often in boys (498) than in girls (166). In the past decade 5 young adults with Marfan's syndrome underwent the repair to permit median sternotomy for open-heart surgery.

Recent follow-up data were available for 460 patients. In the more recent series, more than 95% had good to excellent results. No operative deaths occurred in the entire series, and the morbidity rate was less than 5%. A modified Ravitch procedure is used. Children aged 11 years and older are now treated with temporary substernal stainless steel bar stabilization to prevent recurrence. Postoperative advances in the treatment of pectus excavatum include the use of substernal and subcutaneous drainage and subcuticular skin closure for improved cosmetic results.

Careful evaluation of chest wall growth and development should, by the age of 5 or 6 years, reveal those children with moderate or severe defects. Computed tomographic scans and pulmonary function studies also are useful in selecting patients who require repair. At surgery, 3 to 4 overgrown costal cartilages are removed, the sternum is repositioned with a transverse osteotomy, and the child's lowest ribs are used for internal support. After a mean hospital stay of 5 days, the child is asked to avoid physical contact for 6–10 weeks. Excellent long-term results can be expected.

▶ A wide range of opinions exists about the indications for operative repair of pectus excavatum. This report presents data on 664 patients treated at the Johns Hopkins Hospital over many years, concluding that the ideal age for repair is 4–6 years. This avoids the hazards of operating at an earlier age but permits correction before the deformity becomes more severe. Ninety-five percent of the patients observed during long-term follow-up have excellent results.

The approach has the additional advantage of avoiding the psychological trauma resulting from cosmetic defects during childhood, which can otherwise easily occur during the child's participation in school athletic programs.—F.C. Spencer, M.D.

Prospective Trial of the Six Hour Rule in Stab Wounds of the Chest
Kerr TM, Sood R, Buckman RF Jr, Gelman J, Grosh J (Temple Univ)
Surg Gynecol Obstet 169:223–225, September 1989
13–3

Some physicians believe that all patients with stab wounds of the chest should be admitted for 48–72 hours, whereas others believe that 6 hours of observation is adequate and that a patient without symptoms and with a normal chest roentgenogram will not have delayed complications. Data on 170 patients with stab wounds of the chest were reviewed, including those on 105 patients admitted for at least 24 hours; 18% of the patients had 2 or more thoracic stab wounds.

Four patients had delayed pneumothorax or hemothorax, all within the first 6 hours. No complications occurred at 6–24 hours, and no patient had tension pneumothorax. In addition, no patient had delayed signs of intra-abdominal injury. These findings strongly support the rule that 6 hours of observation are adequate for asymptomatic patients with stab wounds of the chest who have normal chest roentgenograms at admission.

▶ This report analyzes the management of asymptomatic stab wounds of the chest. The group of 105 patients represented about 60% of those seen over a period of 3 years. The data clearly indicate that complications seldom occurred in patients in whom the chest x-ray appearance was normal 6 hours after injury. I would be dubious of discharging such patients after 24 hours, but hospitalization in a "holding area," usually adjacent to the emergency room, for 24 hours would seem reasonable.—F.C. Spencer, M.D.

Transaxillary or Supraclavicular Decompression for the Thoracic Outlet Syndrome: A Comparison of the Risks and Benefits

Cikrit DF, Haefner R, Nichols WK, Silver D (Univ of Missouri, Columbia)
Am Surg 55:347–352, June 1989   13–4

Successful surgical management of the thoracic outlet syndrome (TOS) involves decompression of the neurovascular structures. Transaxillary first rib resection (TAR) is the most widely used technique, but exposure is difficult and the complication rate is relatively high. The supraclavicular approach (SCR) was evaluated and compared with TAR for thoracic outlet decompression in 37 patients who underwent 45 procedures for decompression of the thoracic outlet.

Procedures included 30 TARs and 15 SCRs. Most patients had multiple symptoms including arm, hand, or shoulder pain, as well as numbness, parathesias, motor weakness, and arm swelling. Neurologic symptoms were most common in the ulnar distribution. Variables analyzed were length of surgery, estimated blood loss, complications, length of hospitalization, and immediate, 2-month, and long-term relief of symptoms.

Operative time was similar for both procedures. The SCR procedure was associated with lower blood loss than was the TAR procedure. A urinary tract infection was the only complication in the SCR group. There were 21 complications in the TAR group, including pneumothorax in 13 major venous lacerations in 3, winged scapulas in 3, and pleural effusion, and wound infection in 1 each. More than 1 complication occurred in 2 patients; 9 of 13 patients with pneumothorax required chest tube placement. Significantly more patients in the TAR group required longer than 3 days of hospitalization.

All SCR patients and all but 1 TAR patient were improved or asymptomatic immediately after surgery. At 2 months postoperatively, 93% of SCR patients and 81% of TAR patients were improved or asymptomatic. At long-term follow-up, all SCR patients and 83% of TAR patients were improved or had no symptoms. No patients in the SCR group had recurrences, compared with 17% in the TAR group. The significantly higher complication rate, greater blood loss, and longer postoperative hospitalization in the TAR group suggests that SCR should be the procedure of choice in patients with thoracic outlet syndrome refractory to medical management. Benefits are comparable in both procedures, but the risk of scalenectomy are considerably less.

▶ Serious concern exists about the high frequency of complications with transaxillary resection of the first rib for the thoracic outlet syndrome. This report compares the results of 30 transaxillary resections with 15 supraclavicular scalene resections. The supraclavicular operations were virtually free of complications but resulted in equal or better outcomes at long-term follow-up (mean, 3 years). Both the simplicity and safety of the supraclavicular approach suggest that it should be considered more frequently.—F.C. Spencer, M.D.

Preoperative Chemotherapy and Irradiation for Stage III Non-Small Cell Lung Cancer
Faber LP, Kittle CF, Warren WH, Bonomi PD, Taylor SG IV, Reddy S, Lee M-S (Rush-Presbyterian-St Luke's Med Ctr, Chicago)
Ann Thorac Surg 47:669–677, May 1989   13–5

Surgical resection is the most effective treatment for non-small-cell lung carcinoma (NSCLC), but the 5-year cure rate for patients with clinical stage III disease remains no higher than 10%. Preoperative treatment that could downstage the tumor could increase long-term survival. Preoperative simultaneous chemotherapy and irradiation were administered to 85 patients with biopsy-proven clinical stage III NSCLC who were considered eligible for surgery. Preoperative treatment with cisplatin, 5-fluorouracil (5-FU), and irradiation was administered to 58 patients for 5 days every other week for 4 cycles. After treatment, 39 patients underwent resection. Cisplatin, 5-FU, and etoposide (VP-16) plus irradiation were administered to 29 patients, 23 of whom underwent thoracotomy. Overall, 60 of 62 patients who underwent thoracotomy underwent resection.

The operative mortality was 5% in the 2-drug group and 4% in the 3-drug group. Major complications occurred in 14 patients, including 4 bronchopulmonary fistulas. In the 85 patients eligible for surgery, the Kaplan-Meier median survival was estimated at 40% at 3 years. The median survival of 62 patients undergoing thoracotomy was 36.6 months. Combination preoperative chemotherapy and irradiation is feasible in patients with clinical stage III NSCLC. Toxicity and operative mortality are acceptable, but further studies may result in improved forms of treatment.

▶ Conventional surgical techniques for stage III NSCLC produce dismal results. This group analyzed the preoperative use of both chemotherapy and radiation in 85 patients who were candidates for surgical resection. Resection was performed subsequently in 60 patients, whose median survival was about 3 years. These early results are encouraging, certainly better than the disappointing results with preoperative irradiation alone.—F.C. Spencer, M.D.

A Prospective Study of Adjuvant Surgical Resection After Chemotherapy for Limited Small Cell Lung Cancer: A University of Toronto Lung Oncology Group Study

Shepherd FA, Ginsberg RJ, Patterson GA, Evans WK, Feld R, Univ of Toronto Lung Oncology Group (Toronto Gen Hosp; Mount Sinai Hosp, Toronto; Ontario Cancer Inst; Univ of Toronto)
J Thorac Cardiovasc Surg 97:177–186, February 1989   13–6

Small cell lung cancer (SCLC) accounts for approximately 25% of all bronchogenic neoplasms, but only about 5% are operated on at presentation. This is because most patients with SCLC have regional lymph node involvement, and many have hematogenous dissemination, rendering them ineligible for potentially curative operations. Although current chemotherapy combinations for SCLC achieve response rates of 80% or more, with complete clinical response in approximately 50% of patients with limited-stage disease, most patients relapse early.

Based on encouraging results obtained in a pilot study, a prospective study was undertaken of adjuvant surgical treatment after remission induction with chemotherapy in 72 patients aged 39–77 years. Of these, 21 had clinical stage I disease, 16 had stage II disease, and 35 had stage III disease. All patients underwent combination chemotherapy consisting of either cyclophosphamide, doxorubicin, and vincristine every 3 weeks for 5–6 cycles, or etoposide and cisplatin given daily for 3 days every 3–4 weeks for up to 6 cycles. Twenty-seven patients who had a complete response and 30 who had a partial response were eligible for operation.

Thirty-eight of these 57 patients underwent thoracotomy, of whom 8 required a pneumonectomy and 25 had a lobectomy. Five patients did not have resection at thoracotomy. Of the 19 remaining patients eligible for operation, 10 were randomized to radiation only, and 9 refused the operation.

There were no operative deaths. The median survival time for the 38 patients operated on was 91 weeks, and the projected 5-year survival rate was 36%. The median survival for patients with pathologic stage II tumors was 69 weeks, and for those with stage III tumors, 52 weeks. The median survival for patients with pathologic stage I tumors had not yet been reached. The median survival for the patients not operated on was 51 weeks. Thus surgery did not improve survival for patients with stage II or stage III disease. At the time of this report, 18 of the 38 surgical patients and 9 of the 34 nonsurgical patients were still alive.

Surgical therapy can contribute significantly to improved survival for patients with early-stage SCLC who have a complete or partial response to preoperative combination chemotherapy.

▶ The role of pulmonary resection in patients with SCLC is uncertain. This evaluation of 72 patients from the University of Toronto Lung Oncology Group found significant benefit after resection in patients with stage I disease but negligible benefit in those with stage II or stage III. All patients received chemotherapy beforehand. The authors concluded that the role of surgical resection in patients with SCLC is limited to the fortunate ones who can be operated on in the early stages of the disease who initially respond to chemotherapy.

However, in this group the overall survival was 35% as compared to the control group in which there were no survivors.—F.C. Spencer, M.D.

Neuroendocrine Neoplasms of the Lung: A Clinicopathologic Update
Warren WH, Faber LP, Gould VE (Rush Med College, Chicago)
J Thorac Cardiovasc Surg 98:321–332, September 1989   13–7

Data on 146 patients with pulmonary neuroendocrine tumor were reviewed. Bronchial carcinoids, which typically are central tumors, occurred in 52 patients. Resection with minimal margins usually is curative, and most patients have an excellent long-term outlook. Complete excision was possible in all but 1 of the 52 patients. The role of photoablation of carcinoid tumors is under study.

Well-differentiated neuroendocrine carcinomas, which usually are peripheral tumors, occurred in 37 patients. The prognosis after resection is less favorable than for bronchial carcinoids. Node metastases were present in 10 patients at the time of resection, but no patient had locally recurrent disease. Of 15 patients followed for 5 years or longer, 5 had metastatic disease, 2 of whom remained without symptoms for up to 4 years.

Intermediate-cell neuroendocrine carcinoma, which has an aggressive clinical course and often is mistakenly classified as large cell undifferentiated carcinoma, occurred in 15 patients. Only 4 of 10 patients with stage I tumors lived longer than 1 year and only 1 lived longer than 2 years. All patients with stage II or III disease died of metastasis within 2 years of resection.

Small-cell neuroendocrine carcinoma, which are aggressive, rapidly disseminating neoplasms, occurred in 42 patients. Patients with stage III disease, even without residual disease at the time of resection after chemotherapy or radiotherapy, usually died of metastatic disease within 2 years. Only 1 of 12 patients with stage I disease and 1 of 5 with stage II disease lived beyond 2 years.

▶ The Chicago group at Rush Medical College have had a long interest in classification of neuroendocrine neoplasms of the lung. This detailed report describes 146 such patients evaluated over a period of 20 years. Four groups were recognized, with the bronchial carcinoids being the most benign and the small cell neuroendocrine carcinomas the most lethal. The neuroendocrine term refers to the cell's ability to synthesize, store, and secrete a variety of neuropeptides. Two intermediate groups that influence prognosis were also defined—a well-differentiated neuroendocrine carcinoma and an intermediate-sized cell.—F.C. Spencer, M.D.

Management of Tumor Adherent to the Vertebral Column
DeMeester TR, Albertucci M, Dawson PJ, Montner SM (Creighton Univ, Omaha; Univ of Chicago)
J Thorac Cardiovasc Surg 97:373–378, March 1989   13–8

It is difficult for surgeons to determine whether lung tumors adherent to the vertebral column have invaded adjacent bone. In an effort to clarify principles of management, experience was evaluated with en bloc resection of tumors clinically suspected of invading the vertebral column.

Twelve patients underwent resection according to the following criteria: persistent chest wall pain, histologic diagnosis of non-small-cell lung cancer, tumor fixed to the vertebral body, disease-free costotransverse foramen, normal results at mediastinoscopy, limited bone erosion on roentgenography, and no distant organ metastasis. Tumors were fixed to the thoracic vertebra between T-1 and T-5; most were located in the apex of the chest. Patients received 3,000 rad of preoperative therapy. Three to 4 weeks later, patients underwent an en bloc resection of the posterior ribs, transverse processes, and a tangential segment of the vertebral bodies involved, as well as lobectomy or pneumonectomy.

Studies of the decalcified surgical specimens showed the tumor extending into the cortex in 2 patients, the periosteum in 6, parietal area in 3, and up to the visceral pleura in 1. Six patients are alive without evidence of recurrent tumor or arthritic pain after a follow-up of 1–11 years. Four have survived asymptomatically beyond 5 years. The overall 5- and 10-year survival rate according to the Kaplan-Meier method was 42%.

In patients with tumors adherent to the vertebral body but without roentgenographic evidence of bony erosion, en bloc removal of the lung and the involved portion of the vertebral body is necessary for complete excision. En bloc resection in these patients provides long-term survival with a good quality of life.

▶ Invasion of the vertebral column by thoracic neoplasms is usually considered a sign of inoperability. Hence this report of experiences with 12 patients is of particular interest. The involved bone was removed in a bloc with the lung. Six of the 12 patients are alive, 4 more than 5 years after operation, without evidence of recurrent tumor.—F.C. Spencer, M.D.

Metastasectomy for Soft Tissue Sarcoma: Further Evidence for Efficacy and Prognostic Indicators
Jablons D, Steinberg SM, Roth J, Pittaluga S, Rosenberg SA, Pass HI (Natl Cancer Inst, Bethesda, Md)
J Thorac Cardiovasc Surg 97:695–705, May 1989   13–9

A total of 74 patients underwent exploration for presumed metastases of high-grade soft tissue sarcoma of the head/neck, extremity, or trunk in 1982–1987. The most frequent primary tumors were synovial sarcoma, malignant fibrous histiocytoma, leiomyosarcoma, and fibrosarcoma. Initial resections had been performed in 1975–1986. The median age was 38 years; 30 patients had multiple operations for recurrences.

Median sternotomy was the most common operative approach, and the most frequent procedure was wedge resection of a peripheral nodule. There were no operative or perioperative deaths, but 8% of the patients had complications. The median postthoracotomy survival for 63 patients with confirmed sarcoma was 20.3 months. Patients who were free of disease after initial thoracotomy had a median survival of 27 months, whereas those with unresectable disease had a median survival of 9 months. Disease in the trunk carried a better outlook than tumor at other sites.

Long-term survival is possible after resecting pulmonary metastases of soft tissue sarcoma. In patients whose disease can be totally removed, the limiting factor is the amount of functioning lung tissue preserved. Patients having repeated resections should have lung function and arterial blood gases assessed preoperatively.

▶ This large report from the National Cancer Institute describes experiences with 74 patients treated over a period of 5 years. Thirty of the 74 had multiple procedures for recurrences (2 to 6 explorations). Most were performed through a median sternotomy, with a repeat sternotomy done occasionally (3 or 4 times). Wedge resection of the nodule was usually performed. Palpation often detected several more nodules than those shown by the CT scan. There were no operative deaths.

The procedure clearly is safe and beneficial. Patients rendered free of disease at initial thoracotomy had an average postthoracotomy survival time of near 27 months.—F.C. Spencer, M.D.

Intracavity Drainage for Bullous, Emphysematous Lung Disease: Experience With the Brompton Technique
Venn GE, Williams PR, Goldstraw P (Brompton Hosp, London)
Thorax 43:998–1002, December 1988   13–10

Dominant bullae are associated with advanced and generalized emphysematous lung disease. Various surgical methods have been designed to excise the dominant bullae. Although many patients benefit from surgery, it has sometimes proved difficult to equate symptomatic improvement with respiratory function improvement. Techniques using intracavitary intubation have potential advantages for patients with bullous disease.

Twenty-two procedures were done on 20 patients for relief of symptoms caused by bullous lung disease. Open intubation drainage of the bullae was used in all patients. The technique was developed initially by Monaldi for treating intrapulmonary tuberculous abscesses. This technique, as modified, involves a single stage, instilling sclerosant directly into the bulla to produce rapid contraction and fibrosis within it and inducing pleurodesis to minimize the immediate effect of any air leak in the pleural space.

Three of the 20 patients died after surgery. Death was associated with a low preoperative forced expiratory volume in 1 second (FEV_1) and higher preoperative arterial carbon dioxide tension ($PaCO_2$). Symptomatic improvement was achieved in 16 of the 17 survivors and was maintained for a median of 1.6 years. This was accompanied by objective improvement in lung function, with a 22% median improvement in FEV_1, an 11% median decrease in total lung capacity, and a 26% median decrease in residual volume. One patient's symptoms were unchanged after surgery.

This procedure is a simple method of decompressing bullae by means of a minimally invasive surgical technique. It also permits treatment of additional bullae later by closed intubation under local anesthetic. It is a suitable approach for all patients except for those with the poorest lung function.

▶ The hazards of thoracotomy and pulmonary resection in patients with bullous emphysematous disease are well known. Hence this conservative operation performed on 20 patients, with 17 survivors, is of particular interest. In brief, a 10-cm thoracotomy is performed to expose the bullae, which are opened and then secured to a large (32-French) Foley catheter that is brought through the chest wall and subsequently connected to underwater suction. This is a variation of the old Monaldi operation for lung abscess. Surprisingly enough, the bronchocutaneous fistulas closed in all patients within a short time after the Foley catheter was removed. Symptomatic improvement occurred in 16 of the 17 patients. Avoiding operation on patients whose preoperative FEV_1 is less than 500 mL is now recommended.—F.C. Spencer, M.D.

The Current Status of Surgery for Bullous Emphysema
Connolly JE, Wilson A (Univ of California, Irvine)
J Thorac Cardiovasc Surg 97:351–361, March 1989   13–11

Patients with diffuse emphysema are thought not to tolerate lung surgery well, and surgery has been recommended only when function of the

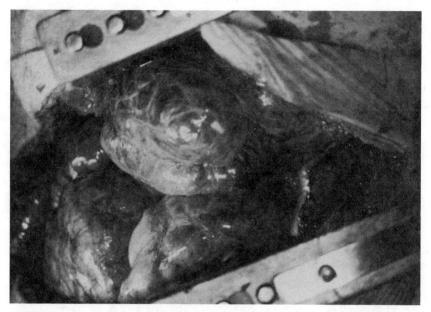

Fig 13–1.—Cotton candy-like bullae of upper lobe of left lung. Note tip of normal lower lobe on right. (Courtesy of Connolly JE, Wilson A: *J Thorac Cardiovasc Surg* 97:351–361, March 1989.)

remaining compressed lung can be improved immediately. Nineteen patients were operated on for incapacitating dyspnea. Large bullae compressing normal lung tissue are an infrequent finding, but all of the present patients had definite evidence of compression of uninvolved lung and displacement by large bullae. Bullae (Fig 13–1) were excised locally, with all normal lung tissue was preserved.

Thirty-two staged operations were performed. All 19 patients improved clinically and usually dramatically. Improvement was confirmed by preoperative and postoperative lung function testing. Initial symptomatic improvement was impressively sustained during follow-up of 3–22 years despite the fact that most of the patients continued to smoke cigarettes. Later deterioration prompted removal of contralateral bullae in some patients.

Surgery is indicated if tomography demonstrates compression of relatively normal lower lung tissue by bullae in the upper and middle lobes in a symptomatic patient. Only bullous disease is resected. Air leakage can be minimized by fine stapling and by oversewing the remaining bullae. Small narrow-based bullae may simply be ligated. Postoperative care includes underwater suction, intensive bronchial toilet, and tube thoracostomy for residual air spaces.

▶ The majority of patients with emphysema have generalized disease for which little can be done surgically. A variant, however, is described in this report. These are large bullae in the upper lobes that significantly compress the uninvolved lower lobes. The key decision is deciding if normal lung parenchyma is compressed. Pulmonary angiograms or tomograms were the best diagnostic guides. Experiences with 19 patients are presented in this report without any deaths. In the Discussion section the suggestion is made that large bullae can be collapsed and ligated, rather than excised, in hopes of avoiding the serious risk of air leak.—F.C. Spencer, M.D.

Technique of Bronchial Closure After Pneumonectomy
Sarsam MAI, Moussali H (Wythenshawe Hosp, Manchester, England)
J Thorac Cardiovasc Surg 98:220–223, August 1989   13–12

In 332 pneumonectomies performed in 1974–1984, bronchial closure was by the nontension posterior membranous flap technique. Right pneumonectomy was performed in 152 patients and left pneumonectomy in 180. The goal is to taper the trachea into the residual bronchus, leaving no stump and creating no tension on the suture line. This is achieved by using a flap from the pliable posterior membranous bronchus. The cartilaginous part must be cut flush at its origin from the carina.

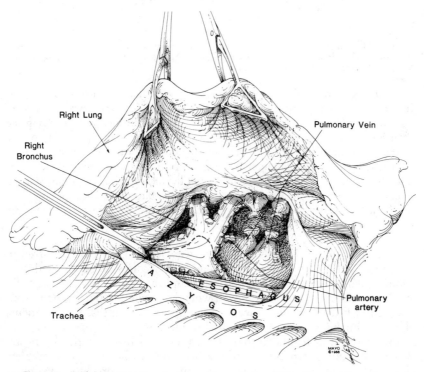

Fig 13–2.—Right pneumonectomy: exposure. (By permission of Mayo Found.; redrawn from Jack.) (Courtesy of Sarsam MAI, Moussali H: *J Thorac Cardiovasc Surg* 98:220–223, August 1989.)

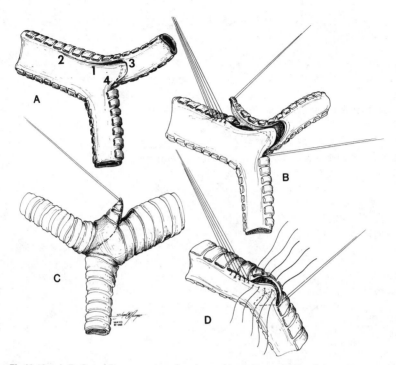

Fig 13–3.—A, B, C, and D, preparation of trachea and bronchus: surgical technique. (By permission of Mayo Found.; redrawn from Jack.) (Courtesy of Sarsam MAI, Moussali H: *J Thorac Cardiovasc Surg* 98:220–223, August 1989.)

Technique.—In a right pneumonectomy, the right main bronchus with the carina and the lower 3 cm of the trachea are dissected free; the azygos vein is retracted upward and need not be divided. It is helpful at this stage to clamp the bronchus distally and remove the specimen, as this facilitates access. Two stay sutures are inserted, 1 into the carina and the other into the trachea about 3 cm above the origin of the right main bronchus (Fig 13–2). A longitudinal incision is made at the junction of the cartilaginous and the membranous bronchus, starting at point 1 on Figure 13–3 and extending for 2 cm into the trachea (point 2) and for about 1 cm into the right main bronchus (point 3) before curving into the carina (point 4).

Mortality within 30 days of surgery was 5.1%. Empyema occurred in the pneumonectomy space in 10 patients; 2 died of sepsis within 3 months, whereas the 8 others had thoracoplasty. The 5 patients who did not have recurrent cancer were well when last seen. No patient had bronchopleural fistula during a mean follow-up of 54 months. In all patients the bronchus was closed with 2–0 chromic catgut.

Bronchopleural fistula formation was avoided in this series by posterior membranous flap closure of the bronchus without tension. Staplers have not eliminated fistula formation, and their use precludes examination of the bronchial lumen.

▶ This interesting report describes experiences with 332 pneumonectomies performed over a period of 10 years by the same group of surgeons. There were no bronchopleural fistulas despite the development of empyema in 10 patients (3% of the group). Although the popular technique of stapling is simpler and quicker, a small percentage of fistulas occurred, with serious consequences.

As I indicated in a 1972 publication (*Ann Thorac Surg* 13:288, 1972) and cited by the authors, the ideal goal is a fistula rate approaching 0, which was achieved by the authors in this interesting report.—F.C. Spencer, M.D.

Closure of Chronic Postpneumonectomy Bronchopleural Fistula Using the Transsternal Transpericardial Approach
Ginsberg RJ, Pearson FG, Cooper JD, Spratt E, Deslauriers J, Goldberg M, Henderson RD, Jones D (Univ of Toronto; Hôp Laval, Sainte-Foy, Quebec)
Ann Thorac Surg 47:231–235, February 1989   13–13

Bronchopleural fistulas occur as a complication of pneumonectomy in up to 5% of patients. Immediate reoperation is the usual treatment when the fistula develops soon after surgery. Those that occur later have been managed by a number of methods. The outcome was evaluated in 13 patients in whom the transsternal transpericardial approach was used. Chronic bronchopleural fistulas developed in these patients from 4 months to 10 years after the initial operation. The associated empyema was treated by tube thoracostomy or open window thoracostomy. A full median sternotomy was used and the affected bronchial stump dissected at the carina, isolated, and divided. If possible, the distal stump was totally excised.

In 10 patients, at follow-up ranging from 18 months to 7.5 years, the bronchial closure healed primarily and remained intact. Pneumonectomy had been performed for carcinoma in 9 patients and irreversible inflammatory disease in 4. Three patients died in the late follow-up period. Two of the 3 fistulas that recurred were quite small, and 1 closed spontaneously within 3 months.

The transsternal transpericardial approach was relatively simple and effective. No deaths or significant morbidity occurred in this series of patients. The transsternal method is especially useful when the ipsilateral transthoracic approach is not feasible for a patient or when previous attempts at closure have been unsuccessful.

▶ Postpneumonectomy bronchopleural fistula is one of the dread complications of thoracic surgery, being associated with high morbidity and mortality. This report describes experiences with 10 patients treated initially months or years following pneumonectomy. The fistula was divided using a transsternal approach, with successful results in all 10. There were no deaths.

The Discussion section describes use of the technique in the Netherlands for more than 20 years, with a high percentage of good results if the empyema was effectively treated beforehand. The transpericardial approach seems to be a valuable addition to the techniques available for this difficult problem.—F.C. Spencer, M.D.

Experience With the Grillo Pleural Wrap Procedure in 18 Patients With Perforation of the Thoracic Esophagus

Gouge TH, Depan HG, Spencer FC (New York Univ Med Ctr)
Ann Surg 209:612–619, May 1989   13–14

Perforation of the esophagus is an uncommon disease, but one that has a high mortality rate when diagnosis and treatment are delayed. Numerous surgical approaches have been tried. One of the newer methods, developed by Grillo and first reported in 1975, follows closure of the perforation with an autogenous pleural flap. Between 1975 and 1988, 14 of 18 patients seen at New York University were treated with this procedure.

The patient group included 12 men and 6 women aged 31–78 years. Perforations resulted from a variety of causes: barotrauma, forceful vomiting, balloon dilation, endoscopy, trauma, and a high-pressure gas hose accident. The esophagram performed with water-soluble contrast was the most useful diagnostic test, although the diagnosis was prompt in only 2 patients. Surgery was performed in less than 24 hours in 7 patients, between 24 and 48 hours in 5, and after more than 48 hours in 6.

The 14 patients treated by primary repair followed by reinforcement with the Grillo flap all survived, even though surgery was delayed 8 days in 1 case. The only complications were minor leaks at the suture line, which soon closed. Four patients were unable to undergo primary closure because of their advanced pathologic condition. Three of these patients died of sepsis after long periods of hospitalization.

When primary closure is possible, it seems reasonable to routinely buttress all suture repairs with autogenous tissue. This technique was successful in both prompt and delayed treatment, an important consideration because perforation of the esophagus is difficult to diagnose. When perforations are too extensive to be closed, resection and drainage is a recommended course, to be followed later by esophageal reconstruction.

▶ This report from my institution describes experiences with 18 patients treated over a period of 13 years. Only 7 were treated within the first 24 hours after perforation.

The perforation was sutured in 14 of 18 patients, after which the suture line was buttressed with a circumferential wrap of parietal pleura, as described by Grillo. All patients recovered and were discharged in good condition. In 4 other patients with extensive problems, several procedures were tried, but death ensued in 3 of them. The data indicate that a pleural flap should be used routinely after suture closure of esophageal perforations. With more extensive perforations, resection and drainage, subsequently followed by esophageal reconstruction, is probably the best choice.—F.C. Spencer, M.D.

14 Congenital Heart Disease

Total Cavopulmonary Connection: A Logical Alternative to Atriopulmonary Connection for Complex Fontan Operations: Experimental Studies and Early Clinical Experience
de Leval MR, Kilner P, Gewillig M, Bull C, McGoon DC (Hosp for Sick Children, London; Rochester, Minn)
J Thorac Cardiovasc Surg 96:682–695, November 1988   14–1

In vitro experimental studies were undertaken to clarify the hydrodynamic principles involved in the Fontan circulation. Turbulence was generated and resistance to net forward flow was increased by pulsation of a valveless chamber in a simple continuous flow circuit, emphasizing the importance of streamlining flow. These in vitro studies yielded suggestions for improving hydrodynamic designs of the Fontan circulation. Results in 20 patients using a modified approach to Fontan reconstruction were evaluated.

The patients' mean age was 6.9 years. Eleven of the children had a double-inlet ventricle, 7 had a hypoplastic systemic or pulmonary ventricle, and 2 had an absent right atrioventricular connection. The operation excludes most or all of the right atrium (total cavopulmonary connection). After end-to-end anastomosis of the superior vena cava to the undivided right pulmonary artery is performed, a composite intra-atrial tunnel, using the posterior wall of the right atrium, is constructed. The inferior vena cava is then channeled to the enlarged orifice of the transected superior vena cava, using a prosthetic patch.

Two hospital deaths and 1 late death occurred. In 1 child the pulmonary arteries remained small despite extensive reconstruction. In another, low flow velocity and serious systemic ventricular dysfunction were observed on Doppler examination. A third patient had congestive heart failure and died while awaiting a heart transplant.

The total cavopulmonary connection has a number of advantages over the atriopulmonary connection, at least for patients with a nonhypertrophied right atrium. The procedure is technically simple, the risk of arrhythmias is reduced because most of the right atrial chamber remains at low pressure, and atrial thrombosis can be minimized by the reduction of turbulence. The right atrium does not pump efficiently in a valveless atriopulmonary connection. Furthermore, incorporation of the right atrium in that circulation may in fact be detrimental. The normal functions of the right atrium, including its use as a pump and a reservoir and its roles in sinus impulse and circulatory homeostasis, should be reviewed in light of a circulation in which the right atrium does not enter into a ventricular chamber.

▶ This report describes experiences with 20 patients in whom both vena cavae were diverted to the pulmonary artery, bypassing the right atrium. This theoretically, avoids, energy losses from turbulence in a right atrial chamber. There were 2 operative deaths and 1 late death. Catheterization in 10 patients after operation confirmed favorable flow patterns. Long-term results will be of particular interest.—F.C. Spencer, M.D.

The Mustard Procedure in Infants (Less Than 100 Days of Age): Ten-Year Follow-Up
Turley K, Hanley FL, Verrier ED, Merrick SH, Ebert PA (Univ of California, San Francisco)
J Thorac Cardiovasc Surg 96:849–853, December 1988   14–2

Transposition of the great arteries (TGA) with an intact ventricular septum is a common congenital abnormality that can now be treated successfully. The Mustard procedure, used in the 1970s, has largely been replaced by the Senning intra-arterial repair and use of the arterial switch. Long-term follow-up was made after the Mustard procedure in 36 infants with TGA and an intact ventricular septum who were treated between 1975 and 1989. The infants' mean age was 46 days, and the mean weight was 3.5 kg. In the operative approach, pericardium was used for the intra-arterial baffle and patch enlargement for the new systemic atrium. The mean follow-up was 10 years.

No hospital deaths occurred. One child died at 54 months postoperatively as a result of accidental drowning. The rate of rhythm disturbance-free survival was 62%, reoperation-free survival was 89%, and pacemaker-free survival was 91%. Postoperatively, 8 patients had obstruction of the superior vena cava (SVC), 4 had tricuspid insufficiency, 3 had left ventricular outflow tract obstruction, and 2 had right ventricular dysfunction. Three, including the child who drowned, required permanent pacemakers.

Results in this unique patient group represent a benchmark against which later techniques can be judged. When performed in early infancy, the Mustard procedure results in a high rate of survival and a low incidence of late complications. The problem of superior vena cava (SVC) obstruction appears to be procedure related. No increasing incidence was seen over time, and SVC obstruction was not related to the need for a permanent pacemaker.

▶ The recurrent question in treatment of transposition in infancy is whether to perform the complex corrective arterial switch procedure or the traditional Mustard procedure with atrial baffling. This 10-year follow-up describes late results in 36 infants less than 100 days of age who had the Mustard repair before 1980. There were no early deaths, and late survival was 97%. Superior vena cava obstruction was found in 8 patients on echocardiography; 89% were free of operation at the time of the study.

These excellent results indicate the low morbidity that should be the goal of corrective operations performed in infancy.—F.C. Spencer, M.D.

Intermediate Results of the Arterial Switch Repair: A 20-Institution Study
Norwood WI, Dobell AR, Freed MD, Kirklin JW, Blackstone EH, The Congenital Heart Surgeons Society (Children's Hosp of Philadelphia; Montreal Children's Hosp; Boston Children's Hosp; Univ of Alabama, Birmingham)
J Thorac Cardiovasc Surg 96:854–863, December 1988   14–3

Arterial switch repair for transposition of the great arteries (TGA) is generally associated with better survival than atrial switch procedures. A 20-institution study undertaken between January 1985 and June 1987 enrolled 466 neonates with TGA. All neonates were less than 15 days old, and 73% were less than 48 hours old when entered into the study. Results were evaluated in the 212 who underwent arterial switch repair. The procedure was performed in 16 institutions, including 6 considered to be "low risk." The prevalence of demographic and surgical variables seemed to be the same in these 6 as in the other institutions.

The usual coronary artery anatomy was present in 67% of the patients. The 1-week, 1-year, and 2.5-year survival rates after the arterial switch repair were 82%, 79% and 78%, respectively. For the 6 low-risk institutions, survival rates after arterial switch repair for simple TGA were better than those for TGA with ventricular septal defect (VSD). The 1-week, 1-year and 2.5-year survival rates in the low-risk institutions for simple TGA were 96%, 91%, and 90%, respectively, and for TGA with VSD, 84%, 83%, and 83%, respectively. Risk factors for death in these low-risk institutions were TGA with ventricular septal defect and older age at operation (more than 14 days) in the case of simple TGA. Among the patients as a whole, freedom from reoperation for pulmonary outflow obstruction at 1 week and 1 year was 99% and 89%, respectively. Sixteen patients underwent reoperation, 12 of which were for neopulmonary outflow obstruction. Previous pulmonary artery banding and possibly, 1 institution, were identified as risk factors for reoperation.

Arterial switch repairs for TGA can be accomplished with good early results in low-risk institutions. This procedure may be more advantageous when performed early in life than at 2–3 months of age. The lack of an unfavorable effect on survival of age at repair of TGA and VSD, the risk of early pulmonary vascular disease in untreated patients with TGA and VSD, and the socioeconomic advantages of early repair argue for the primary repair of this anomaly early in life.

▶ The timing and risk of the arterial switch procedure is the key consideration in selecting an operation for transposition—choosing the corrective procedure or the atrial baffle procedure developed by Mustard. This report describes a cooperative study among 20 institutions, including 466 neonates with transposition, all younger than 2 years of age. Experiences over 2 years are described.

Six of the 20 institutions had much lower mortality rates, with 1-week, 1-year, and 2.5-year survival rates of 95%, 91%, and 90%, respectively. This clearly shows the advantages of surgical experience and technique in influencing operation. Early age was not a risk factor, suggesting that operation is best performed in the first 2 weeks of life, rather than 2 or 3 months later.—F.C. Spencer, M.D.

Current Technique of the Arterial Switch Procedure for Transposition of the Great Arteries
Bove EL (Univ of Michigan)
J Cardiac Surg 4:193–199, September 1989   14–4

The arterial switch procedure is performed under deep hypothermia and reduced flow.

Technique.—The atrial and ventricular septal defects are first repaired, the latter through the tricuspid valve. The aorta is transected about 5 mm distal to the pulmonary artery bifurcation and the pulmonary artery at the bifurcation. The distal aorta then is relocated posterior to the pulmonary artery bifurcation and joined to the proximal pulmonary artery. Excision of the coronary arteries follows. After they are reimplanted in the neo-aorta, the neo-pulmonary artery is reconstructed using a large pantaloon-shaped patch of autologous pericardium.

The arterial switch operation was done in 81 patients with transposition; operative mortality was 6%. There was only 1 death in the last 56 consecutive repairs in this series. Four patients had mild left ventricular outflow obstruction on Doppler examination. Mild supravalvar pulmonary stenosis was relatively frequent. Five patients had significant gradients requiring reoperation, but this has not occurred since use of a large patch was adopted. Five patients had mild aortic regurgitation that has not progressed. All have had normal left ventricular systolic function. No patient has arrhythmia or ischemic ECG changes. Survival after the arterial switch operation for transposition now equals or exceeds that for atrial repairs at experienced centers.

▶ This paper describes in detail the technique used in the arterial switch procedure in 81 patients at the University of Michigan. The arterial switch has been used as the procedure of choice for all suitable infants with transposition in the past 4 years. Overall mortality was 6% in this series, with only 1 death in the last 56 repairs. The original article includes some excellent illustrations.—F.C. Spencer, M.D.

Homograft Replacement of the Pulmonary Artery Bifurcation
Burczynski PL, McKay R, Arnold R, Mitchell DR, Sabino GP (Royal Liverpool Children's Hosp, England)
J Thorac Cardiovasc Surg 98:623–631, October 1989   14–5

A complete fresh homograft pulmonary artery bifurcation sterilized with antibiotics was implanted in 17 patients aged 15 months to 17 years with severe deformity or nonconfluence of the pulmonary arteries. Six patients had tetralogy of Fallot, 5 had pulmonary atresia with ventricular septal defect, and 3 had truncus arteriosus. A ventricular septal defect alone was present in 2 patients and pulmonary atresia with intact septum in 1. All but 1 of the patients had undergone palliative or corrective surgery previously.

Surgery was performed under cardiopulmonary bypass with core cooling to produce profound hypothermia. When both the valve and bifurcation were implanted, a collagen-impregnated, double-velour, knitted Dacron graft was sutured to the homograft muscle. If only the isolated bifurcation was needed, the main pulmonary artery was divided just above the valve.

Thirteen patients survived the operation, 1 of whom required reoperation for pretracheal bleeding. All of the survivors had progressively better exercise tolerance. After a mean follow-up of 16 months, 11 patients were in New York Heart Association functional class I and 2 were in class II. Four patients had trivial pulmonary regurgitation. Chest roentgenograms indicated symmetrical pulmonary perfusion in all patients, and no aneurysms occurred.

A complete adult-sized homograft has given encouraging early results in patients who require reconstruction of the pulmonary artery bifurcation.

▶ This report from Liverpool, England, describes experiences with replacement of the pulmonary artery with a pulmonary homograft in 17 children with congenital heart disease, operated on over a period of about 4 years. There were 13 survivors. Function, to date, has been satisfactory, although the mean follow-up is only 16 months. The longest is 56 months.

It is hoped that the pulmonary valve conduit will calcify less readily than the aortic homograft, first used by Ross in 1966.—F.C. Spencer, M.D.

Aortic Regurgitation After Surgical Relief of Subvalvular Membranous Stenosis: A Long-Term Follow-Up Study
Bjørn-Hansen LS, Lund O, Nielson TT, Kromann-Hansen O, Jensen FT (Skjeby Hosp/Aarhus Univ Hosp, Denmark)
Scand J Thor Cardiovasc Surg 22:275–279, 1988   14–6

Surgical correction of discrete membranous subvalvular aortic stenosis often is done in childhood. The condition is progressive and is associated with a risk of endocarditis and sudden death. In a series of 21 patients so affected, the mean age at operation was 16 years. Preoperative left-sided heart catheterization revealed associated cardiovascular anomalies in 8 patients; aortic root angiograms showed that 6 patients had moderate aortic regurgitation. Most were in New York Heart Association (NYHA) functional class II or III, and had a high peak systolic pressure gradient, left ventricular hypertrophy, or a cardiothoracic index of more than 5.50.

Common symptoms included dyspnea, angina pectoris, and syncope or presyncope.

The membrane was excised at surgery, and 5 patients underwent additional valvotomy. Twenty-one patients survived. Both deaths occurred within 30 days of surgery; 1 resulted from low cardiac output syndrome and 1 followed severe hemorrhage. At a mean follow-up of 6.7 years, all patients were in sinus rhythm and all but 6 were in NYHA class I.

Aortic regurgitation was discovered at follow-up in 8 of 13 patients who did not have regurgitation preoperatively. Those who had regurgitation had a significantly higher preoperative peak systolic pressure gradient and were seen at a significantly longer follow-up than patients with no signs of regurgitation. Regurgitation occurred in all 5 patients with valvotomy. Restenosis may also appear postoperatively and be asymptomatic; thus patients treated for subvalvular membranous stenosis should have regular check-ups with Doppler echocardiography.

▶ The association of aortic regurgitation with subvalvular aortic stenosis has long been recognized, although the mechanism is unclear. This is a long-term evaluation of 21 cases after operation for subaortic stenosis. In a long-term follow-up, 8 of 13 patients who did not have regurgitation preoperatively had signs of insufficiency on Doppler examination at some time in the next few years, with a follow-up extending to 6 years. The mechanism of the late development is unclear, but the fact that insufficiency may develop as late as 5 years after operation clearly indicated an inherent valvular abnormality rather than surgical trauma.—F.C. Spencer, M.D.

Surgical Closure of the Patent Ductus Arteriosus in the Neonatal Intensive Care Unit
Coster DD, Gorton ME, Grooters RK, Thieman KC, Schneider RF, Soltanzadeh H (Iowa Methodist Med Ctr, Des Moines)
Ann Thorac Surg 48:386–389, September 1989   14–7

The efficacy of surgical closure compared with indomethacin for treatment of patient ductus arteriosus in symptomatic neonates remains controversial. Nonsurgical mortality or morbidity occurred in 115 consecutive patent ductus closures performed in premature infants in the intensive care unit. Factors influencing the outcome were studied in 99 infants younger than 33 weeks' gestational age. All were operated on within 72 hours of diagnosis, using an extrapleural approach and metal clips.

The average age at weaning from the ventilator was about 33 weeks after conception, regardless of gestational age. The interval from surgery to weaning from total parenteral nutrition was by far longer in infants younger than 27 weeks of gestational age. Bronchopulmonary dysplasia occurred in 50% of the infants, in 12% of those at 27–30 weeks, and in 17% of infants of 30–33 weeks' gestational age. The overall incidence of necrotizing enterocolitis was 7%. No complications resulted directly from operation.

More recently, 27 infants were operated on without surgery-related morbidity or mortality. Ductus closure may be performed safely and efficiently in the neonatal intensive care unit, thereby eliminating the risks of transport.

▶ This report describes an unusually aggressive approach to closure of the patent ductus in premature infants. All patients were operated on within 72 hours of diagnosis using an extrapleural approach with metal clips. Indomethacin therapy apparently was not used. There was no surgical morbidity or mortality. Most infants were subsequently extubated at an average of 33 weeks of age. The surprising absence of any mortality or significant morbidity indicates that this approach can be seriously considered in such infants, especially if there is any contraindication to an initial trial with indomethacin.—F.C. Spencer, M.D.

Vascular Anomalies Causing Tracheosophageal Compression: Review of Experience in Children
Backer CL, Ilbawi MN, Idriss FS, DeLeon SY (Children's Mem Hosp, Chicago; Northwestern Univ)
J Thorac Cardiovasc Surg 97:725–731, May 1989   14–8

Because compression of the trachea and esophagus by vascular anomalies is uncommon, the diagnosis may be missed. The usual symptoms are stridor or noisy respiration and recurrent respiratory infections. Surgical relief of vascular rings was first reported in 1945. The outcome of treatment of this condition was studied at 1 hospital from 1947 through 1987.

Most (68%) of the 204 children who underwent surgical treatment for tracheoesophageal compression by vascular anomalies were in the first year of life. The most common finding was complete vascular rings (group I); of these patients, 61 had a double aortic arch and 52 had a right aortic arch with a left ligamentum. Nine patients (group II) had a pulmonary artery sling, 71 (group III) had innominate artery compression, and 11 (group IV) had miscellaneous anomalies.

Diagnostic methods included barium esophagography, bronchoscopy, CT, and angiography. A left thoracotomy was the operative approach in 93% of the patients in groups I, II, and IV; most (96%) patients in group II underwent right thoracotomy.

All of the operative deaths (4.9%) occurred in the first 12 years of the study period. Follow-up, at a mean of 8.5 months, was available for 159 patients. Although some (8%) experienced residual respiratory problems, most (92%) were symptom free. The best single diagnostic technique for the most common finding, complete vascular rings, is the barium swallow. Careful postoperative care is important to successful recovery, and prolonged endotracheal intubation should be avoided. Some symptoms of the condition may continue for several years after surgery.

▶ This report details an unusually extensive experience with vascular rings in infants and children, describing results in 204 patients whose mean age was

13 months. There were 113 complete vascular rings, 9 patients had a pulmonary artery sling, and 71 had innominate artery compression. The overall operative mortality was almost 5%, but there have been no operative deaths in the past 28 years, well representing the safety of operative correction. Most patients, 92%, became symptomatic, but a few had some residual respiratory problems.—F.C. Spencer, M.D.

Aneurysms After Patch Graft Aortoplasty for Coarctation of the Aorta: Long-Term Results of Surgical Management

Ala-Kulju K, Heikkinen L (Helsinki Univ Central Hosp, Finland)
Ann Thorac Surg 47:853–856, June 1989   14–9

Aneurysms sometime occur after synthetic patch repair of coarctation of the aorta in adulthood. Of 67 patients who had patch graft aortoplasty with a Dacron or Teflon graft in 1967–1978, 22 underwent reoperation between 1978 and 1988 because of aneurysm formation opposite or at the site of the graft.

Resection was performed on 19 aneurysms, and aortic continuity was reestablished with a tubular Dacron prosthesis (Fig 14–1). Femorofemoral perfusion was used in 16 of these patients and left atrium-femoral bypass in 3. In 3 patients the aneurysm was wrapped externally with a Dacron graft (Fig 14–2). There were no hospital deaths, but several patients had recurrent nerve paralysis, pneumonia/atelectasis, or, in 8 patients, bleeding requiring reoperation. A mean follow-up of 4.5 years showed no

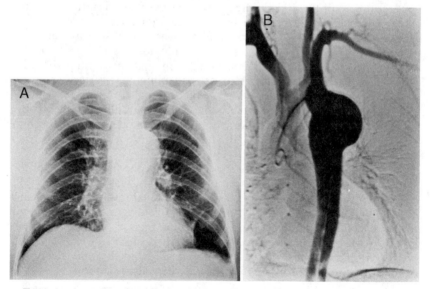

Fig 14–1.—Aneurysm at descending aorta 16 years after patch aortoplasty: **A,** standard chest roentgenogram, and **B,** aortogram. Repair was accomplished using a tubular prosthesis. (Courtesy of Ala-Kulju K, Heikkinen L: *Ann Thorac Surg* 47:853–856, June 1989.)

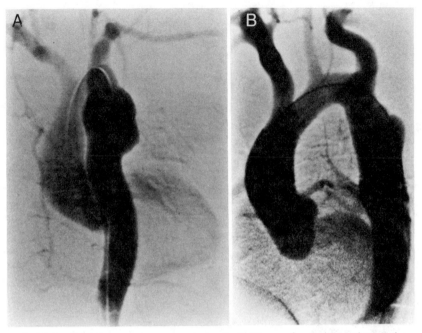

Fig 14–2.—**A** and **B**, aneurysms at coarctation repair site 18 years after patch aortoplasty. Both aneurysms were suitable for external support. (Courtesy of Ala-Kulju K, Heikkinen L: *Ann Thorac Surg* 47:853–856, June 1989.)

aneurysm formation at any site. There was no permanent neurologic disability. Two patients had a systolic gradient of 40 mm Hg or greater across the repair site but were not hypertensive.

The pathogenesis of aneurysm formation after patch graft repair of coarctation remains uncertain. Possibly, resection of the intimal ridge of the coarctation weakens the aortic wall and disposes to aneurysm formation. Hemiparesis in 2 patients probably resulted from the proximal aortic clamp causing stenosis or embolism. Patch graft aortoplasty should not be used for repair of coarctation, especially in adults. Resection with anastomosis and tubular reconstruction has given good results.

▶ This report from Helsinki describes aneurysms developing in 33% of 67 adult patients treated previously with patch graft aortoplasty for aortic coarctation. The authors suggest that the high frequency of 33% may be the highest reported in adults. Possibly it is related to the technique of intimal resection at the time of patch aortoplasty.

There were no operative deaths, but morbidity was significant: recurrent nerve paralysis in 36% and right hemiplegia, perhaps from emboli from the proximal aortic clamp, in 2 patients. The late development of the aneurysms, 16–20 years after operation, indicates the importance of permanent routine surveillance of patients who have had patch aortoplasty.—F.C. Spencer, M.D.

15 Valvular Heart Disease

The Porcine Bioprosthetic Heart Valve: Experience at 15 Years
Magilligan DJ Jr, Lewis JW Jr, Stein P, Alam M (Henry Ford Hosp, Detroit)
Ann Thorac Surg 48:324–330, September 1989   15–1

Since 1971, 980 patients at Henry Ford Hospital who received 1,081 porcine bioprosthetic valves were followed for up to 16 years. The mean patient age at operation was 55 years and the mean length of follow-up was nearly 6 years.

Patient survival, including operative deaths, was 80% at 5 years, 59% at 10 years, and 38% at 15 years. The rates of freedom from thromboembolism were 96% at 5 years, 92% at 10 years, and 89% at 15 years. There were 56 episodes of prosthetic valve endocarditis, which were fairly evenly distributed over the follow-up period. Rates of freedom from structural valve degeneration were 98% at 5 years, 71% at 10 years, and 31% at 15 years. Degeneration was related to age younger than 35 years at surgery, female sex, and a cardiac index of more than 2 L/min/m^2. Reoperation was performed 165 times for a first valve failure, and 11 patients had reoperation for a second valve failure. The overall mortality for reoperation necessitated by structural valve degeneration was 12.5%.

To date, experience with the porcine bioprosthetic valve suggests that its use be limited to older patients and those having contraindications to anticoagulation. The valve has fulfilled its promise with respect to thromboembolism, but rates of structural valve degeneration are significant.

▶ This report is from 1 of the 6 institutions participating in a collaborative study after the porcine valve was introduced in 1970–1972. The report describes experiences with more than 1,000 valves implanted at the Henry Ford Hospital in this period, with a remarkably complete follow-up of 99%. Freedom from valve degeneration for all valves was 71% at 10 years, falling sharply to 31% at 15 years. Deterioration was much more rapid in patients younger than 35 years of age.

Thromboembolism continued throughout the period of observation but was small—92% were emboli-free at 10 years and 89% at 15 years. Hence there was no increase in thromboembolism with the increased frequency of deterioration.

These data clearly indicate the probable life expectancy of porcine prostheses, unless the more recent methods of preservation sharply increase longevity.—F.C. Spencer, M.D.

Fifteen-Year Experience With 1,678 Hancock Porcine Bioprosthetic Heart Valve Replacements

Cohn LH, Collins JJ Jr, DiSesa VJ, Couper GS, Peigh PS, Kowalker W, Allred E (Harvard Med School; Brigham and Women's Hosp, Boston)
Ann Surg 210:435–443, October 1989   15–2

In all, 1,678 Hancock porcine valves were implanted in 1,533 patients at the Brigham and Women's Hospital since early 1972. There were 825 aortic, 562 mitral, and 146 double replacements in this series. Nearly all patients were in New York Heart Association functional class III or IV preoperatively. One fourth of the patients had concomitant coronary bypass surgery. The mean follow-up was 6 years.

The overall operative mortality was 6%, ranging from 4% for isolated aortic valve replacement to 10% for double valve replacement. Patients having both valve replacement and bypass grafting had a mortality of 7%; 96% of survivors were in functional class 1 or 2 after aortic replacement. Structural valve degeneration was diagnosed in 9% of aortic, 14% of mitral, and 11% of double valve replacements. Thromboembolism was relatively infrequent after aortic replacement. A total of 194 patients had secondary replacement of a porcine valve.

The Hancock porcine valve is ideal for elderly patients because structural degeneration is so infrequent in this group. It also is ideal for any patient having contraindications to long-term anticoagulation.

▶ This extensive report from Brigham and Women's Hospital in Boston describes experiences with 1,678 Hancock prostheses inserted over a period of 15 years, starting when the valves first became available for clinical use. Hence the unanswerable question is whether the porcine valves manufactured in recent years would have a better performance than the earlier models. In this series about 80% of the patients were free from reoperation at 10 years, but only 57% at 15 years. Durability was much better in older patients. The number of patients available for the 15-year evaluation, however, was naturally small. As reported by others, durability was significantly better in valves implanted in patients older than 70 years of age. More than 92% of this group had functional valves 10 years following operation, compared with 70% to 85% in younger groups.— F.C. Spencer, M.D.

A 10-Year Comparison of Mitral Valve Replacement With Carpentier-Edwards and Hancock Porcine Bioprostheses

Perier P, Deloche A, Chauvaud S, Chachques JC, Relland J, Fabiani JN, Stephan Y, Blondeau P, Carpentier A (Hôp Broussais, Paris)
Ann Thorac Surg 48:54–59, July 1989   15–3

Data on 253 patients undergoing isolated mitral valve replacement with a porcine bioprosthesis between 1975 and 1979 were reviewed. A Carpentier-Edwards valve was used in 147 patients (mean age, 54 years) and a Hancock valve was used in 106 patients (mean age, 50 years). The

2 groups were comparable clinically. The average follow-up was 7.2 years for patients given a Carpentier-Edwards valve and 6.8 years for the Hancock group. Three fourths of survivors in both groups received long-term anticoagulation.

Operative mortality was 8.8% in the Carpentier-Edwards group and 17.9% in Hancock valve group. The respective actuarial 10-year survival rates were 55% for the Carpentier-Edwards group and 50% for the Hancock group, which is not a significant difference. Valve-related deaths were comparable in the 2 groups, as were rates of thromboembolic complications and structural valve deterioration. About 60% of both groups were free of valve failure at 10 years. Twenty-nine Carpentier-Edwards recipients and 23 Hancock recipients underwent repeated surgery, usually because of structural valve deterioration. Comparable numbers of patients were free of anticoagulant-related hemorrhage during follow-up.

Comparable long-term results are achieved with the first-generation Carpentier-Edwards porcine bioprosthesis and the Hancock prosthesis in the mitral position. New methods of tissue preservation and low-pressure fixation may lessen structural valve failure.

▶ This detailed late evaluation compared results between patients with a Carpentier-Edwards porcine prosthesis and those with a Hancock porcine prosthesis. Ten years after operation the results were similar in both groups. About 94% were free from thromboembolism. The most sobering fact was that more than 30% of either type of valve required replacement during this period of time because of structural deterioration. The rate of deterioration was higher in younger adults than in older ones.—F.C. Spencer, M.D.

Ten Years' Experience With the St Jude Medical Valve Prosthesis
Arom KV, Nicoloff DM, Kersten TE, Northrup WF III, Lindsay WG, Emery RW (Minneapolis Heart Inst; St Paul Heart and Lung Ctr, Minn)
Ann Thorac Surg 47:831–837, June 1989   15–4

Data on 1,298 patients who received the St. Jude Medical prosthesis between 1977 and 1987 were reviewed. Congestive heart failure accounted for 85% of replacements. More than 25% of the group had combined valve replacement and coronary bypass grafting.

Early mortality was 5.7% and late mortality was 16.9% during some 4,300 patient-years of follow-up; 64 patients had thromboembolic episodes, 17 of which were major and 35 were permanent. Anticoagulant-related bleeding occurred in 24 patients. Other complications included valve thrombosis in 4 patients, prosthetic valve endocarditis in 7, and paravalvular leakage in 9; 10 patients were reoperated on. There were no structural valve failures. Valve-related deaths totaled 37. All but 4% of surviving patients were in New York Heart Association functional classes I or II. The actuarial estimate of freedom from all complications and from operative and valve-related death was 67% after 9 years.

Very impressive results have been achieved with the St. Jude Medical prosthesis, even in older patients and those with advanced heart disease. During this 10-year follow-up study, valve-related complications occurred at a rate of 2.7% per 100 patient-years, and deaths occurred at a rate of 0.86% per 100 patient-years. The valve has proved to be structurally durable.

▶ This report is from an institution that first used the St. Jude valve after its introduction in 1977. Experiences with 1,298 patients over a period of 10 years were reviewed. The frequency of thromboembolism was low, 1.5% per 100 patient-years, but remains a serious problem. As with all metallic prostheses, anticoagulant-related bleeding is another significant cause of morbidity. The frequency of this complication was 0.56% per 100 patient-years, and 9 of 24 patients died of this complication.

Valve thrombosis was fortunately rare, developing in only 4 patients—3 in the mitral and 1 in the tricuspid position; none developed in patients with aortic prostheses. Endocarditis was also rare, the occurrence being much less frequent than reported in some series. This developed in only 7 patients, 4 of whom were cured with antibiotics.—F.C. Spencer, M.D.

The St Jude Valve Prosthesis: Analysis of the Clinical Results in 815 Implants and the Need for Systemic Anticoagulation

Myers ML, Lawrie GM, Crawford ES, Howell JF, Morris GC Jr, Glaeser DH, DeBakey ME (Baylor College of Medicine, Houston; Methodist Hosp, Houston)
J Am Coll Cardiol 13:57–62, January 1989   15–5

The design characteristics of the St. Jude Medical valve, a bileaflet, low-profile prosthesis constructed of Pyrolite carbon, suggested that warfarin anticoagulation might be less critical in avoiding thromboembolism. Data on 785 patients who received 815 St. Jude prostheses between 1979 and 1984 were reviewed. Aortic valve replacement was performed 491 times and mitral replacement 264 times; 30 patients had double valve replacements, and 33 had St. Jude replacements of other valve types.

Operative mortality was 6.7%, ranging from 2.1% for isolated aortic valve replacement to 17.6% for mitral replacement with associated surgery. Of 5 patients having double valve replacement with associated surgery, 2 died. Seven deaths during follow-up were caused by thromboembolism; 3 were attributed to anticoagulant-related bleeding, and 2 to perivalvular leakage. Overall rates of thromboembolism were 2.6% per patient-year with warfarin, 9.2% with antiplatelet treatment, and 15.6% with no anticoagulant therapy. One patient not given anticoagulation had thrombotic obstruction of a mitral valve.

These findings confirm the clinical usefulness of the St. Jude prosthesis, but the risk of thromboembolic complications dictates the long-term use of warfarin anticoagulation. This in turn entails a significant risk of hemorrhage; antiplatelet agents alone are inadequate.

▶ In a series of 785 patients studied over a period of years, thromboembolism with anticoagulation was 2.6% per patient year, 9.2% with antiplatelet medication; and more than 15% with no anticoagulant therapy. These data well document the need for permanent anticoagulation with warfarin, even though the frequency of significant hemorrhage from anticoagulant therapy was 5.4% per patient year. Hence the basic fact is reaffirmed that all metallic prostheses require permanent anticoagulation with warfarin.—F.C. Spencer, M.D.

Viable and Nonviable Aortic Homografts in the Subcoronary Position: A Comparative Study
Bodnar E, Matsuki O, Parker R, Ross DN (Natl Heart Hosp, London)
Ann Thorac Surg 47:799–805, June 1989   15–6

The results obtained with variably treated aortic homografts in 555 hospital survivors who were followed for a mean of 5.3 years (a total of nearly 3,000 patient-years) were compared. Homografts preserved in Hanks' antibiotic solution or nutrient-antibiotic solution were given to 337 patients; 63 others received frozen homografts, and 155 received freeze-dried homografts.

The overall patient survival 20 years after surgery was 51.6%; the incidence of sudden death was low. The type of graft preservation did not influence either long-term performance or mode of homograft failure. Primary tissue failure occurred more often when valves were preserved in solution containing calf serum, but the difference was not significant. Infective endocarditis occurred at comparable rates in all groups.

Most recently, cryopreservation of aortic homografts has been preferred because of unlimited storage time. No cryopreserved valves have failed since 1988, but it also is true that valves preserved in nutrient-antibiotic solution in the same period have not failed.

▶ This remarkable study compares long-term results with aortic homografts preserved by different means: 155 were freeze-dried, 63 were frozen, and 337 were antibiotic preserved. As the authors indicate, freeze-drying was tried initially, then freezing (cryopreservation), and, subsequently, preservation in an antibiotic medium for about 6 weeks. The techniques have remained unchanged for more than a decade.

With the current interest in cryopreservation and apparent maintenance of viable fibroblasts for long periods of time, it is quite striking that these data found no long-term correlation between the method of preservation of the valve and durability. The perplexing question is whether some degree of viability in the valve is good or bad. The exciting results reported by O'Brien et al. (1) from Australia with cryopreservation suggest that continued viability of fibroblasts might be the factor responsible for a low frequency of deterioration but, to date, this possibility is unproved.—F.C. Spencer, M.D.

Reference

1. O'Brien MF, et al: Cryopreserved viable aortic valves, in Yankah AC, et al (eds): *Cardiac Valve Allografts 1962–1987.* Darmstadt, New York, Steinkopf, Springer, 1988, pp 311–322.

Freehand Homograft Aortic Valve Replacement. The Learning Curve: A Technical Analysis of the First 31 Patients
Jones EL (Emory Univ)
Ann Thorac Surg 48:26–32, July 1989   15–7

Thirty-one cryopreserved homograft valves were implanted in the aortic position in 31 patients over an 18-month period. Fourteen patients had aortic stenosis, 11 had regurgitation, and 6 had combined stenosis and regurgitation.

Technique.—The subannular sutures are placed low enough to avoid encroaching on the coronary ostia (Fig 15–1). The anterior mitral leaflet and homograft septum are trimmed to a perfect cylinder 3–4 mm wide (Fig 15–2).

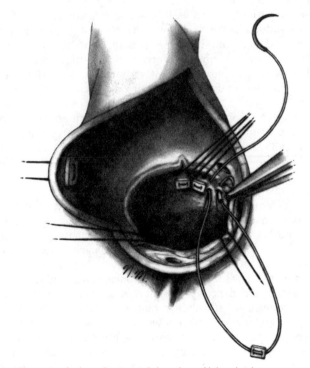

Fig 15–1.—Placement of subannular sutures below plane of left and right coronary ostia. (Courtesy of Jones EL: *Ann Thorac Surg* 48:26–32, 1989.)

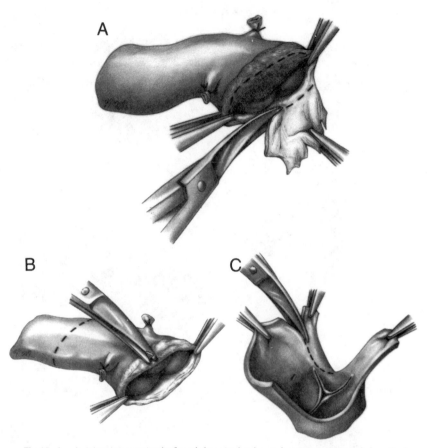

Fig 15–2.—A, trimming anterior leaflet of the mitral valve and septum 3–4 mm below the homograft leaflets. **B,** debulking the septal muscle remnant. **C,** U-shaped scallop of left and right sinuses only; thus retaining aortic wall, which orients to recipient noncoronary sinus. (Courtesy of Jones EL: *Ann Thorac Surg* 48:26–32, 1989.)

Two of the homograft sinuses are scalloped about 3 mm above the anulus in a U shape. Once oriented, the homograft is inverted to that the leaflets are external (Fig 15–3). After tying the sutures, the valve is everted from the ventricle (Fig 15–4), and tension is placed on the commissural posts to elevate the homograft commissures to about 5 mm above the top of the native commissural attachments (Fig 15–5). A second row of sutures evenly distributes the graft through the aortic circumference.

The total mortality was 3.2% in this series; the 1 death was caused by arrhythmia unrelated to the homograft valve. Explanation of the homograft was necessary in 5 patients; 4 others had diastolic murmurs probably secondary to inadequate tension setting of the homograft commissural posts.

If the transcommissural diameter of the recipient is substantially

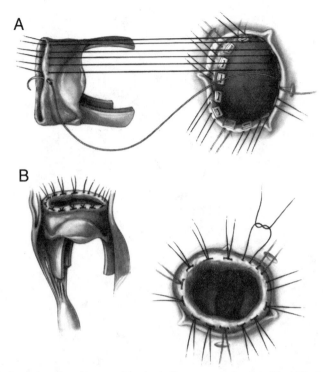

Fig 15–3.—A, inversion of homograft so that leaflets are external and readily visible. B, homograft as it appears in left ventricular cavity as sutures are tied. (Courtesy of Jones EL: *Ann Thorac Surg* 48:26–32, 1989.)

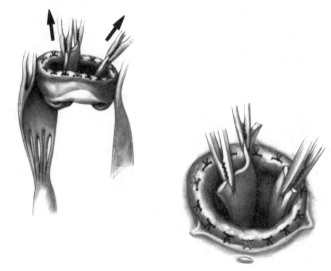

Fig 15–4.—Eversion of valve from left ventricle. (Courtesy of Jones EL: *Ann Thorac Surg* 48:26–32, 1989.)

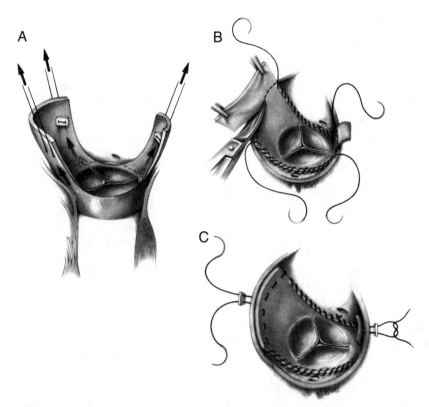

Fig 15–5.—**A,** temporary traction sutures elevate homograft commissural posts above and in line with native commissures. **B,** retention of noncoronary sinus of homograft to maintain cylindrical configuration. **C,** completion of second row of sutures, which evenly distributes homograft throughout the aortic circumference. (Courtesy of Jones EL: *Ann Thorac Surg* 48:26–32, 1989.)

greater than that of the aortic annulus or the homograft itself, another type of valve should be used. Extensive debulking of the homograft prevents excessive tissue in and around the coronary ostia. Successful implantation also depends on precise scalloping of only 2 homograft sinuses, retaining the noncoronary sinus.

▶ This useful paper describes experiences learned in the initial 31 operations for insertion of aortic homografts. With the increasing availability of homograft valves by cryopreservation, combined with their impressive performance for at least 20 years, such valves are being used more frequently, especially in children. The technical maneuvers described in this report, with excellent illustrations, should be useful to most surgeons in their initial experiences with this technique.

The authors do not recommend homograft insertion if the annulus is larger than 27 mm.—F.C. Spencer, M.D.

Composite Valve-Graft Replacement of Aortic Root Using Separate Dacron Tube for Coronary Artery Reattachment

Coselli JS, Crawford ES (Baylor College of Medicine, Houston; The Methodist Hosp, Houston)
Ann Thorac Surg 47:558–565, April 1989   15–8

The most commonly used technique for aortic root replacement comprises separate valve and graft replacement or the use of a composite valve graft. However, these conventional techniques have been associated with bleeding from the sites of reattachment, coronary artery distortion, and the late development of pseudoaneurysms at the coronary artery reattachment site. These problems have been attributed to friable inadequate aortic tissue, particularly in Marfan's syndrome, and to inaccessible suture lines. An alternative technique of direct coronary artery reattachment to a composite graft was developed subsequently.

Replacement of the aortic valve and ascending aorta was undertaken in 73 men (average age, 51) and 17 women (average age, 43). A composite valve graft was used with reattachment of the coronary ostia by a separate, smaller Dacron tube graft. Forty-one patients (46%) had an isolated composite valve-graft aortic root replacement, 26 (29%) also had various concomitant cardiac procedures, and 23 (26%) underwent repeat aortic root replacement with or without concomitant cardiac procedures.

Twenty-five patients (28%) required aortic arch replacement. Twenty-nine patients were operated on under profound hypothermia and circulatory arrest. The early survival rate was 91%. Of the 8 patients who died, 3 had undergone primary operation with isolated composite valve-graft insertion, 4 had undergone primary operation plus a concomitant procedure, and 1 died after undergoing reoperation for chronic dissection. Four of the early deaths were a result of congestive heart failure. Only 4 patients required early reoperation because of hemorrhage. There were 4 late deaths, of which 2 were caused by renal failure, 1 was a result of myocardial infarction, and 1 was of unknown causes.

Aortic root replacement with a composite valve graft and a separate, smaller Dacron tube to bridge the aortic graft and the coronary ostia is a technically simple and safe procedure that greatly reduces operative hemorrhage and virtually eliminates pseudoaneurysm formation at the coronary artery reattachment site.

▶ Aortic root replacement with a composite valve-graft traditionally includes side-to-side anastomoses between openings in the graft and the coronary ostia. In some patients this may result in hemorrhage or late formation of pseudoaneurysms. This report by Stanley Crawford and associates describes the use of a 10-mm Dacron graft in 90 patients, attaching each end of the graft to each coronary ostia as an end-to-end anastomosis and then performing a side-to-side anastomosis between the graft and the aorta. Initial results seem excellent.—F.C. Spencer, M.D.

Primary Isolated Aortic Valve Replacement: Early and Late Results

Lytle BW, Cosgro 'e DM, Taylor PC, Goormastic M, Stewart RW, Golding LAR, Gill CC, Loop FD (Cleveland Clinic Found)
J Thorac Cardiovasc Surg 97:675–694, May 1989   15–9

Aortic valve replacement was the focus of controversies about prosthesis selection, myocardial protection, cardiac surgery for the elderly, and indications for myocardial revascularization in combination with valve surgery. The recent introduction of percutaneous valvuloplasty focuses further attention on the results of aortic valve replacement. A review was made of the in-hospital results in 1,689 patients who underwent primary isolated aortic valve replacement at the Cleveland Clinic Foundation from 1972 through 1986 and late results in the 1,351 in-hospital survivors from 1972 through 1983.

Preoperative chest radiographs were available for all patients, and all but 47 underwent preoperative left heart catheterization, coronary arteriography, and left ventriculography. Aortic valve lesions were classified as stenosis, insufficiency, and mixed. Before 1975 only mechanical prostheses were used; since then, a small aortic root has been a relative indication for the use of mechanical prostheses. Most analyses were performed by dividing patients according to whether mechanical prostheses or bioprostheses were used.

There were 57 in-hospital deaths. Advanced age, preoperative blood urea nitrogen levels of more than 25 mg/100 mL, New York Heart Association function class III or IV, and preoperative atrial fibrillation were associated with increased hospital mortality. The use of cardioplegia for myocardial protection was associated with decreased hospital mortality. The survival rates were 85% at 5 years and 66% at 10 years; and the event-free survival rates were 71% at 5 years and 43% at 10 years.

Patients with bioprostheses had better survival and event-free survival rates than patients with mechanical prostheses. However, patients with bioprostheses had better results only if not receiving warfarin, and they had more reoperations and endocarditis. Patients with mechanical prostheses had more strokes, myocardial infarctions, thromboembolic events, and bleeding complications. When patients were analyzed according to age at surgery, bioprostheses were associated with improved survival and event-free survival in patients aged at least 40 years. Older patients had more thromboembolic complications, whereas younger ones had more reoperations and episodes of endocarditis. These data indicate that the 10-year outcomes after isolated aortic valve replacement are influenced both by patient-related and management-related variables.

▶ This extensive report from the Cleveland Clinic documents experiences with 1,689 aortic valve replacements over a period of 15 years. The average mortality was 3.4%. Five years and 10 years after operation survival was 85% and 66%, respectively; event-free survival rates were 71% and 43%. The use of bioprostheses resulted in better survival rates than mechanical prostheses did, 90% and 66% at 5 and 10 postoperative years vs. 81% and 61%.—F.C. Spencer, M.D.

A Comparison of Mitral Valve Reconstruction With Mitral Valve Replacement: Intermediate-Term Results

Galloway AC, Colvin SB, Baumann FG, Grossi EA, Ribakove GH, Harty S, Spencer FC (New York Univ Med Ctr)

Ann Thorac Surg 47:655–662, May 1989   15–10

Mitral valve replacement (MVR) has become a much more widely used procedure than mitral valve reconstruction. But the limitations of prosthetic mitral valves have caused renewed interest in reconstructive methods. In a comparative study, 3 patient groups were evaluated: 975 received porcine MVR, 169 mechanical MVR, and 280 Carpentier-type mitral valve reconstruction (CVR). The operative procedures were performed between 1976 and 1987. A history of cardiac surgery was more common in the mechanical MVR group (47%) than in the other 2 groups. The group having valve reconstruction was significantly younger and included fewer New York Heart Association (NYHA) class III or IV patients compared with the other 2 groups.

Overall operative mortality was 5.0% for CVR, 16.6% for mechanical MVR, and 10.6% for porcine MVR. Increased operative risk was associated with age, NYHA functional class IV status, and both previous and concomitant cardiac procedures. Actuarial 5-year survival from all cardiac-related deaths was 81.0% for CVR patients, 73.9% for those given a mechanical valve, and 73.1% for those with the porcine valve. Thus the type of valve was not predictive of operative risk or overall survival.

All groups showed excellent improvement in NYHA functional classification: 95.8% for CVR, 90.2% for the mechanical MVR, and 75.9% for the porcine MVR. Similarly good results were seen in evaluations of 5-year freedom from thromboembolic complications and from late de novo endocarditis.

Overall, the actuarial combined risk of valve-related death or complication was significantly higher with valve replacement than with valve reconstruction. Reconstruction is at least as safe as MVR and may be the preferred procedure for many patients with mitral insufficiency.

▶ A major question regarding mitral reconstruction is its influence on longevity, as thromboembolic problems are few and endocarditis rare. This retrospective analysis from my institution (NYU) compared 975 porcine replacements done since 1976, 169 mechanical replacements, and 280 Carpentier mitral reconstructions. The type of valvular procedure was individualized for each patient by the operating surgeon. Mechanical prostheses were used primarily in younger patients who could take warfarin reliably.

By the actuarial method, 5 years following the operation there was better survival with valve repair than with valve replacement. There was a virtual absence of late thromboembolic events in the first 5 years after repair. Surprisingly enough, the mechanical prostheses had a similar low frequency of thromboembolism, perhaps representing the value of precise warfarin administration, keeping the prothrombin time about 1.5 times normal. Endocarditis was virtually absent in the mitral reconstruction group but occurred with similar frequency after either type of valve replacement. With the low frequency of thromboembolism, and the virtual absence of endocarditis, a significant improvement in longevity should result if the mitral valve reconstruction is durable. Late mortality from cardiac problems in patients following successful mitral reconstruction probably reflects preoperative myocardial injury, which can be improved only by operating at an earlier stage of the disease.— F.C. Spencer, M.D.

Mitral Valve Reconstruction in the Elderly Population
Scott ML, Stowe CL, Nunnally LC, Spector SD, Moseley PW, Schumacher PD, Thompson PA (Florida Heart Inst, Orlando)
Ann Thorac Surg 48:213–217, August 1989   15–11

For 3 years the Carpentier repair has been used in elderly patients with ischemic heart disease, poor left ventricular function, and mitral valve disease. Between 1985 and 1988, the Carpentier technique was used in mitral valve reconstruction in 176 patients whose mean age was 63 years. More than half of the patients had concomitant cardiac surgical procedures. Further, 52% of the patients were aged 65 or older, with 35% being older than 70 years.

The operative mortality was 8.5% overall and 12% in patients older than 65 years. Only 3 patients having isolated mitral repair died; 4 patients required reoperation when the initial mitral repair failed. No atrial-ventricular disruptions occurred. There were 8 late deaths of the 124 patients followed; 5 of them were directly related to prolonged complications after initial mitral reconstruction. Of 101 patients followed over the long term, 93% were in New York Heart Association functional class I or II.

These results suggest that the Carpentier repair is indicated for all patients with mitral valve dysfunction, even those older than 65 years. Left ventricular function is preserved, which enhances the survival of high-risk patients. The procedure is safe and the repair is durable.

▶ This report by Scott and associates in Florida describes experiences with 176 mitral valve reconstructions, 52% of which were performed in patients over 65 years of age. The standard Carpentier techniques were used, including ring annuloplasty in 146 and quadrangular resection of the posterior leaflet in 51. Four patients required reoperation in the first year after operation because of mitral insufficiency. Results in the remainder, to date, have been very good, although detailed data regarding the frequency of mitral regurgitation are not available.

These findings represent the growing popularity of mitral valve reconstruction rather than mitral valve replacement. The data serially described in several reports from New York University reaffirm the important fact that probably 90% to 95% of patients with mitral regurgitation from nonrheumatic causes can be reconstructed successfully.— F.C. Spencer, M.D.

Effect of Surgical Reduction of Left Ventricular Outflow Obstruction on Hemodynamics, Coronary Flow, and Myocardial Metabolism in Hypertrophic Cardiomyopathy

Cannon RO III, McIntosh CL, Schenke WH, Maron BJ, Bonow RO, Epstein SE
(Natl Heart, Lung, and Blood Inst, Bethesda, Md)
Circulation 79:766–775, April 1989   15–12

The effects of reducing left ventricular (LV) outflow obstruction were examined in 20 consecutive patients, 13 of whom underwent myotomy-myectomy because of an LV gradient above 50 mm Hg basally or during isoproterenol infusion. Six patients had mitral valve replacement because the anterior basal septum was insufficiently thick. One patient had mitral replacement 5 months after myotomy-myectomy when symptoms persisted.

The outflow gradient fell from 64 mm Hg to 4 mm Hg after operation, and LV systolic pressure decreased from 186 mm Hg to 128 mm Hg. Oxygen consumption in the anterior left ventricle and septum declined. Seven patients no longer had chest pain on rapid atrial pacing after surgery. Both peak great cardiac vein flow and myocardial oxygen consumption were lower after surgery. Net lactate consumption was noted, compared with net production during pacing in the preoperative state. Postpacing LV end-diastolic pressure and pulmonary artery wedge pressure both were reduced after surgery.

Surgical relief of LV outflow obstruction favorably affects myocardial oxygen consumption and metabolism. Myocardial oxygen delivery is better matched to demand during stress. Benefit is most evident in patients who have the highest peak flow capacity preoperatively. Either less intrinsic abnormality in coronary flow delivery or less small coronary vessel disease may explain this finding.

▶ This report from the National Heart Institute in Bethesda describes impressive metabolic results following operation in a selected group of 20 patients with hypertrophic cardiomyopathy. Studies were performed about 20 months after operation. The preoperative gradient above 60 mm was reduced to 4 mm. The data clearly show impressive beneficial effects on myocardial metabolism, with overall improvement in oxygen consumption resulting from decrease in the left ventricular workload.—F.C. Spencer, M.D.

Clinical and Hemodynamic Results After Mitral Valve Replacement in Patients With Obstructive Hypertrophic Cardiomyopathy

McIntosh CL, Greenberg GJ, Maron BJ, Leon MB, Cannon RO III, Clark RE
(Natl Heart, Lung, and Blood Inst, Bethesda, Md)
Ann Thoracic Surg 47:236–246, February 1989   15–13

Fifty-eight patients with hypertrophic cardiomyopathy and no intrinsic mitral valve disease have undergone mitral valve replacement since 1983. Criteria for surgery included a septum smaller than 18 mm in the area of usual resection, atypical septal morphology, and major obstruction despite previous left ventricular myomectomy. Five patients had had a myomectomy. Optimal medical treatment had failed in all instances.

Hospital mortality was 8.6%; the 5 early deaths were related to multiorgan failure. There were 3 sudden late deaths. Low-profile mechanical prostheses and bioprostheses both were used in these cases. Of 48 patients followed, 40 were in New York Heart Association functional class I or II and 8 were in functional class III. Pulmonary wedge pressures were normal and cardiac indices were maintained 6 months after operation. The mean follow-up was 2 years. At 3 years the actuarial survival rate free of thromboembolism, anticoagulant complications, reoperation, and congestive heart failure was 68%.

Although complications such as ventricular septal defect and complete block are avoided in these cases, device-related complications do occur. Longer follow-up is needed to insure that symptomatic improvement persists. Valve replacement is indicated in selected patients with hypertrophic cardiomyopathy; others can undergo left ventricular myomectomy.

▶ Echocardiography provides a method of evaluating the thickness and contour of the ventricular septum. In this report these data were used to choose between traditional myomectomy (developed by the late Glenn Morrow) or mitral valve replacement. A long debate always existed between Morrow, who performed a myomectomy in 350 patients and believed strongly that the mitral valve should not be removed, and Cooley who frequently employed mitral valve replacement. This report describes experiences with 58 patients having mitral valve replacement. This approach was chosen when the septum was smaller than 18 mm, atypical septal morphology was present, or previous myomectomy had failed (which occurred in 25% of the series). Good results were obtained, with symptomatic improvement in 83% of the patients during a mean follow-up of 24 months.—F.C. Spencer, M.D.

16 Coronary Artery Disease

The Evolution of Medical and Surgical Therapy for Coronary Artery Disease: A 15-Year Perspective

Califf RM, Harrell FE Jr, Lee KL, Rankin JS, Hlatky MA, Mark DB, Jones RH, Muhlbaier LH, Oldham HN Jr, Pryor DB (Duke Univ)

JAMA 261:2077–2086, Apr 14, 1989   16–1

Four major randomized clinical trials have confirmed that coronary artery bypass grafting (CABG) effectively relieves angina pectoris. However, consistent evidence for improved survival was not observed in these studies. Although improved survival with CABG has been demonstrated among patients with left main coronary artery disease (CAD) and 3-vessel CAD, no statistically significant survival differences have been demonstrated for most other patient categories. An attempt was made to determine which factors are associated with improved survival after CABG.

The study population consisted of 5,809 patients treated for CAD during a 15-year period. Of these patients, 2,847 were treated medically, 2,663 underwent CABG within 6 months of initial cardiac catheterization, and 299 had at least 6 months of medical therapy before undergoing CABG.

Three factors were associated with a significant CABG survival benefit: extent of CAD, year of operation, and patient's overall medical risk. Specifically, patients with more extensive CAD had the greatest improvement in 5-year survival. Advances in surgical techniques led to progressively improved survival with CABG over time to where by 1984, 5-year survival with CABG was significantly better than 5-year survival with medical therapy for most patient categories. Patients with a poor prognosis because of older age, severe angina, or left ventricular dysfunction had a reduction in risk proportionate to their overall risk with medical therapy. Thus modern CABG yields a significant improvement in patient survival for most categories of patients with ischemic CAD. Because improved survival after CABG is not limited to select categories of patients, therapeutic recommendations for patients with CAD should be based on individual assessment of expected risks and benefits from CABG.

▶ The influence of coronary bypass on longevity has been debated for a long time. It seems clear that certain groups are significantly helped with bypass surgery and others are not.

This report evaluated more than 5,800 patients treated at Duke University over a period of 15 years. Progressive improvement in surgical results devel-

oped with time, probably reflecting both improvement in technique and in myocardial preservation. Another important factor is that the patients with the
greatest decrease in ventricular function had the best results with bypass as
compared to medical therapy. This is probably a reflection of the fact that a decrease in ventricular function is an indication of the inability of the collateral circulation to compensate for the ischemia produced by coronary artery occlusion.— F.C. Spencer, M.D.

**Improved Survival of Surgically Treated Patients With Triple Vessel Coro-
nary Artery Disease and Severe Angina Pectoris: A Report From the Cor-
onary Artery Surgery Study (CASS) Registry**
Myers WO, Schaff HV, Gersh BJ, Fisher LD, Kosinski AS, Mock MB, Holmes
DR, Ryan TJ, Kaiser GC, and Cass Investigators (Marshfield Clinic, Marshfield,
Wis)
J Thorac Cardiovasc Surg 97:487–495, April 1989   16–2

Data on patients enrolled in the National Heart, Lung, and Blood Institute's Coronary Artery Surgery Study (CASS) who had severe angina
pectoris and 3-vessel coronary artery disease were evaluated for medical-
surgical survival rates during 6-year follow-up. These patients had Canadian Cardiovascular Society class III or IV angina pectoris and stenosis of
at least 70% in either the mid or proximal segment of all 3 coronary arteries. There were 1,921 surgically treated patients and 679 medically
treated patients. This was a nonrandomized comparison. Patients were
stratified by left ventricular wall motion scores and number of proximal
coronary stenoses.

After adjustment for variables, the estimated probability of survival
at 6 years was 59% for medically treated patients and 82% for
surgically treated patients. Among patients with left ventricular wall
motion scores of 16–30, the 6-year survival rate for medically treated
patients was 30% and for surgically treated patients, 63% (table).
Patients with 3 proximal lesions had a 40% survival rate with medical
treatment and an 81% survival rate with surgical treatment. At 6
years, 90% of the surgically treated patients and 78% of the medically
treated patients with normal ventricular function were alive. If 2 or 3
proximal stenoses were present, the survival rate was significantly
better after surgical treatment than after medical treatment alone.
If there were no proximal lesions, 84% of surgically treated patients
and 67% of medically treated patients survived at 6 years. On multivariate analysis, early operation was a strong predictor of survival.

These data support the hypothesis that direct coronary artery revascularization improves survival in patients with severe angina pectoris and
3-vessel coronary disease. The findings include some patients with normal left ventricular function and those with severe proximal coronary artery stenosis.

Individual Univariate and Multivariate Cox Analyses of Stratified Variables Representing LV Function, Proximal Stenosis, and Individual Arterial Stenoses

Subgroup label	No. of valid cases in univariate analysis	No. of valid cases in Cox analysis	No. of deaths in Cox analysis	Univariate (log rank) p value	Multivariate relative risk*	95% CI for relative risk	Multivariate (Cox) p value
LV 5	600	530	49	<0.0001	0.33	0.19-0.59	0.0001
LV 6-9	833	698	102	<0.0001	0.37	0.24-0.57	<0.0001
LV 10-15	897	771	186	<0.0001	0.39	0.29-0.52	<0.0001
LV 16-30	270	255	116	<0.0001	0.38	0.25-0.58	<0.0001
PROX 0	405	357	60	<0.0001	0.44	0.26-0.74	0.0020
PROX 1	920	800	153	<0.0001	0.44	0.31-0.61	<0.0001
PROX 2	865	730	158	<0.0001	0.31	0.22-0.44	<0.0001
PROX 3	410	347	82	<0.0001	0.34	0.21-0.55	<0.0001
LAD (L, R, B)	385	336	71	<0.0001	0.51	0.31-0.86	0.0106
RCA (R, B)	375	330	57	<0.0001	0.37	0.21-0.65	0.0005
CX (R, B)	160	134	25	0.0065	0.39	0.17-0.90	0.0269
LAD, RCA (R, B)	412	350	78	<0.0001	0.23	0.14-0.38	<0.0001
LAD, CX (R, B)	202	169	39	<0.0001	0.35	0.18-0.68	0.0021
RCA, CX (R, B)	222	185	38	<0.0001	0.40	0.20-0.77	0.0063
CX (L)	29	26	3	<0.0001	NC	NC	NC
LAD, RCA, CX (R, B)	348	289	75	<0.0001	0.25	0.15-0.41	<0.0001
LAD, CX (L)	62	58	7	0.9673	NC	NC	NC

Abbreviations: LV, range of left ventricular function scores are shown; *Prox,* number of proximal stenoses; *LAD,* left anterior descending coronary artery; *RCA,* right coronary artery; *CX,* circumflex coronary artery; *L, R, B,* left or right dominant or balanced coronary artery anatomy; *NC,* not convergent; small number of events did not allow statistical modeling.

*Relative risk of death for surgical therapy vs. medical therapy.

(Courtesy of Myers WO, Schaff HV, Gersh BJ, et al: *J Thorac Cardiovasc Surg* 97:487–495, April 1989.)

▶ This important report from the Coronary Artery Surgery Study (CASS) analyzed patients with triple-vessel disease and severe angina. The data clearly showed better longevity with surgically treated patients: 82% vs. 59%. With severe left ventricular dysfunction, the difference was even greater: 63% sur-

vival for surgically treated patients vs. 30% for medically treated patients.—
F.C. Spencer, M.D.

**Coronary Angioplasty Versus Coronary Bypass: Three-Year Follow-Up of
a Matched Series of 250 Patients**
Hochberg MS, Gielchinsky I, Parsonnet V, Hussain SM, Mirsky E, Fisch D (Univ
of Medicine and Dentistry of New Jersey, Newark)
J Thorac Cardiovasc Surg 97:496–503, April 1989   16–3

In many centers percutaneous transluminal coronary angioplasty
(PTCA) has become preferred to coronary artery bypass grafting in patients with single- and double-vessel coronary artery disease. Many larger
series have confirmed the efficacy of PTCA after 6-month clinical and angiographic follow-up when compared with coronary bypass, but long-
term data are still sparse.

The clinical outcome of PTCA was compared with that of coronary
bypass after a 3-year follow-up period. The study population consisted of
125 patients who underwent PTCA and 125 who had coronary bypass
operations. Both groups had similar numbers of patients with single- or
double-vessel disease. The mean ejection fraction was 54 mm Hg in the
PTCA group and 49 mm Hg in the surgical bypass group.

Percutaneous transluminal coronary angioplasty was successful initially in 110 of the 125 patients (88%). Twelve required coronary bypass
immediately or within 48 hours, and 3 were treated medically after
PTCA failure. Four PTCA-treated patients died during hospitalization.
Coronary artery bypass grafting was successful in 124 of the 125 patients. One patient died after surgical bypass. There were 4 late deaths in
the PTCA group and 2 late deaths in the bypass group. The total early
and late mortality rate for the PTCA group was 7%, compared with 3%
for the bypass group. The difference was not statistically significant.

At the end of the 3-year study period, 76 (63%) of 121 PTCA patients
and 110 (92%) of 120 bypass patients were alive and in New York Heart
Association class I or II. This difference in symptomatic results was statistically highly significant. Furthermore, 19% of the original PTCA cohort ultimately required surgical bypass during the 3-year study period.
Therefore, if follow-up is maintained long enough, surgical bypass appears to be more effective than PTCA, even in low-risk patients with sin-
gle- or double-vessel disease.

▶ Often, uncertainty exists about choosing angioplasty over bypass. Considerations include both the short-term results and the long-term results with either
technique. This report compares a matched series of 125 patients in each
group (angioplasty vs. coronary bypass) with a 3-year follow-up. Combined
early and late mortality in the angioplasty group was 7% vs. 2.5% in the surgical group. Only 63% of the angioplasty group were in class I or II, whereas
92% of the surgical patients were in these classes. About 19% of the angioplasty patients ultimately required bypass.—F.C. Spencer, M.D.

Emergency Coronary Artery Bypass Grafting for Failed Angioplasty: Risk Factors and Outcome
Naunheim KS, Fiore AC, Fagan DC, McBride LR, Barner HB, Pennington DG, Willman VL, Kern MJ, Deligonul U, Vandormael MC, Kaiser GC (St Louis Univ; St Mary's Health Ctr, St Louis)
Ann Thorac Surg 47:816–823, June 1989   16–4

The degree of added risk involved when coronary bypass grafting is done for emergent failure of percutaneous transluminal angioplasty is uncertain. Data were reviewed on 103 patients who had emergency bypass grafting for failed angioplasty and 103 patients who had coronary bypass grafting only. The angioplasty group had a lower risk profile.

Despite more favorable risk factors in the angioplasty patients, they had a mortality of 11%, compared with 1% for the bypass group. The respective rates of perioperative infarction were 22% and 6%. Operative deaths in the angioplasty group were predicted by the left ventricular score, need for inotropic support after angioplasty, and age.

Treatment of coronary atherosclerotic disease probably will include both angioplasty and bypass grafting in a complementary, rather than a competitive, manner. Operative mortality and permanent myocardial damage are significantly more likely when bypass surgery follows failed angioplasty than when it is done electively.

▶ This report addresses the important question of the safety of performing angioplasty, with the thought that bypass can be done safely if angioplasty is unsuccessful. The study group included 103 patients undergoing emergency bypass for failed angioplasty and the identical number undergoing elective bypass. The mortality after failed angioplasty was much higher (11% vs. 1%), as was the infarction rate (22% vs. 6%). The reason for this striking difference, also observed in other studies, has never been clear. Possibly, it results from multiple embolizations from the angioplasty site.—F.C. Spencer, M.D.

Coronary Revascularization Rather Than Cardiac Transplantation for Chronic Ischemic Cardiomyopathy
Kron IL, Flanagan TL, Blackbourne LH, Schroeder RA, Nolan SP (Univ of Virginia, Charlottesville)
Ann Surg 210:348–354, September 1989   16–5

Patients with poor ventricular function are considered highly vulnerable to myocardial revascularization, and ischemic cardiomyopathy presently is the major indication for cardiac transplantation. Patients with an ejection fraction of less than 20% who are not symptomatic enough for transplantation can expect a 2-year survival after medical treatment of less than 25%.

A total of 39 patients with a mean ejection fraction of 18.3% and a mean left ventricular end-diastolic pressure of 22 mm Hg underwent coronary revascularization; 24 patients could have been candidates for cardiac transplantation. Twenty-two patients had angina, 26 had congestive failure, and 2 had ventricular arrhythmias.

All of the patients were weaned from cardiopulmonary bypass, but 5 required intra-aortic balloon pump support. One early death was related to intractable arrhythmia; 8 patients (19%) died during a mean follow-up of 21 months: 7 of arrhythmia and 1 of heart failure. The mean ejection fraction in 23 patients increased to 26% after revascularization. Three patients continued in severe heart failure, and 1 of them later had successful transplantation. Two patients are in New York Heart Association class II, and 2 others have persistent angina. The presence of angina before surgery predicted a favorable outcome.

Myocardial revascularization is a reasonable approach to ischemic cardiomyopathy given the current shortage of cardiac transplant donors. Coronary bypass surgery does not increase the risk of later cardiac transplantation.

▶ This report concerns the question of myocardial revascularization rather than cardiac transplantation for ischemic cardiomyopathy with an ejection fraction of less than 20%. The presentation was discussed by myself and others. Only 1 operative death occurred in the series of 39 patients, indicating the safety of bypass. The 3-year survival was 83%. The most important fact is that 7 of the 8 late deaths were caused by arrhythmias rather than by recurrent infarction or cardiac failure.

Control of arrhythmias, rather than resort to implantation, would seem to be the ideal goal. It is not known with certainty, but a patient with an ejection fraction of less than 20% can probably function at a limited level for many years if the revascularization done prevents further infarction and arrhythmias can be avoided.—F.C. Spencer, M.D.

Right Gastroepiploic Artery: A Third Arterial Conduit for Coronary Artery Bypass
Mills NL, Everson CT (Cardiology Ctr, New Orleans)
Ann Thorac Surg 47:706–711, May 1989   16–6

In the past 10 years the internal mammary artery (IMA) has superseded the saphenous vein to become the conduit of choice for coronary artery bypass grafting (CABG). However, with more complex CABG operations and increased numbers of reoperations, cardiac surgeons often must struggle to obtain an acceptable amount of graft material. The availability of a third conduit would be desirable.

Data on 32 men and 7 women who underwent CABG with the right gastroepiploic artery (RGEA) were reviewed; 43 concomitant IMA grafts were placed. Seven patients had extensive endarterectomies with specimens at least 6 cm long. Of 41 RGEA grafts, 15 were free grafts and 26 were pedicled grafts. Two patients had sequential RGEA grafting. In 12 patients distal anastomoses were placed to the right coronary artery; in 22, to the posterior descending artery; in 5, to the diagonal; and in 4, to the marginal circumflex branch. Postoperative angiography was performed in 28 patients.

In no patient was the RGEA unacceptable at surgery, and no patient had to be refused for RGEA grafting because of preoperative bruits high in the abdomen. Pedicled graft lengths averaged 23.7 cm. The mean length of the free grafts was 17.7 cm. The average internal diameter of pedicled RGEA grafts was 4.02 mm. Distal RGEA grafts averaged 2.14 mm in internal diameter. In 2 patients the RGEA was long enough for 2 grafts; 6 patients had no vein grafts. Of the 3 deaths in the series, none was attributable to use of the RGEA. Early postoperative cardiac catheterization showed that all RGEA grafts were patent and without kinks, but 3 free RGEA grafts had vasospasm.

Grafting with RGEA provides a third arterial conduit with artery-to-artery anastomoses of comparable size; also, the RGEA graft can be harvested simultaneously with the IMA and the saphenous vein. Other advantages are that a shorter (or no) leg incision is required, proximal anastomosis with free grafts is simple, RGEA grafting avoids bilateral IMA grafting in patients at high risk for sternal infection, and atherosclerotic ascending aortas need not be clamped. Subintimal hyperplasia and atherosclerosis of RGEA grafts are unlikely. Disadvantages are that the abdominal cavity must be entered, the graft is unavailable after gastric surgery, future abdominal procedures could damage the graft, operating time is longer, and long-term patency and adequacy of flow are uncertain at present.

▶ The RGEA is being used with increasing frequency for coronary bypass in selected patients. This report describes initial experiences with 39 patients. The gastroepiploic artery was found usable in all patients explored. The gastroepiploic artery near its origin was large, nearly 4 mm. It was used as a pedicle graft in 26 patients and was detached and connected to the aorta in 15 others. Initial results have been encouraging.

At the time of preparation of this report a literature review found that the gastroepiploic artery had been used in a total of 118 patients, summarized from a total of 7 different reports.—F.C. Spencer, M.D.

Technical Considerations for Use of the Gastroepiploic Artery for Coronary Artery Surgery
Mills NL, Everson CT (Cardiology Ctr, New Orleans)
J Cardiac Surg 4:1–9, March 1989   16–7

The right gastroepiploic artery (RGEA) may be used as an arterial graft when saphenous vein is limited or unfavorable for some reason, or in patients having reoperation, or and when an additional graft is required in the setting of severe atherosclerosis of the ascending aorta.

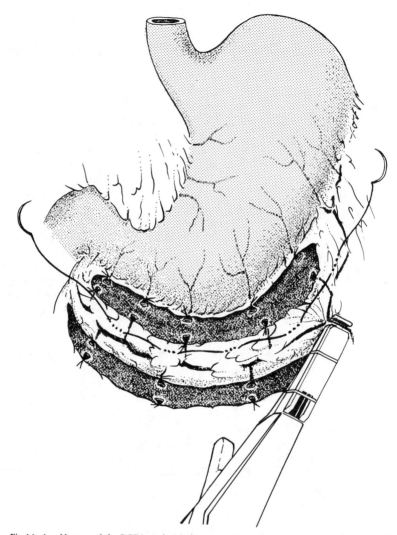

Fig 16–1.—Harvest of the RGEA graft: Marking a margin of the right gastroepiploic graft with a sterile pen or 2–0 suture as the pedicle is dissected is an important step that cannot be overemphasized. Anatomical landmarks that occur with the internal mammary graft are absent and inadvertent twist of the graft is likely. Gas-powered automatic staplers are cumbersome for RGEA harvest. All brands of clips have a tendency to catch and pull away from the thin-walled arterial branches during manipulation of the graft or the stomach. (Courtesy of Mills NL, Everson CT: *J Cardiac Surg* 4:1–9, March 1989.)

Technique.—The RGEA graft should be marked so that twisting can be avoided when it is harvested (Fig 16–1). Dissection should remain at least 1 cm from the parent artery. Papaverine in saline is introduced to prevent spasm. Various routes to the diaphragm are available (Fig 16–2). The route into the pericardial cavity may be anterior to the diaphragm or through a right anterior, middiaphragmatic, or posterior diaphragmatic window (Fig 16–3). The method of making the distal gastroepiploic anastomosis is shown in Figure 16–4. A free

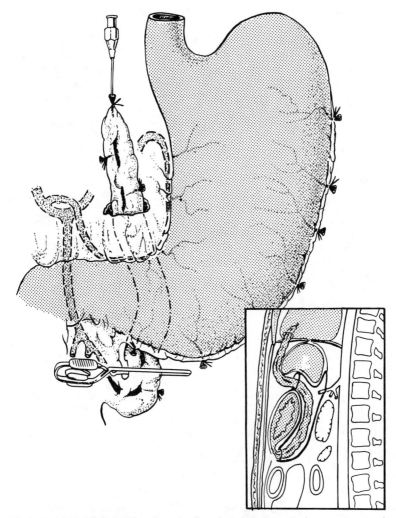

Fig 16–2.—Route of the RGEA to the pericardium through the lesser sac, lesser omentum, and over left lobe of the liver. (Courtesy of Mills NL, Everson CT: *J Cardiac Surg* 4:1–9, March 1989.)

graft is dissected like a pedicle graft except that it begins in the midpart of the stomach and is first carried over to the origin of the RGEA from the gastroduo-denal artery (Fig 16–5).

The RGEA might be the best choice for patients who lack saphenous veins of good quality. Time may be saved by harvesting grafts simulta-neously. The pedicle graft generally is thicker than an internal mammary artery graft, but this has not had adverse effects.

▶ With the astonishing durability of the internal mammary artery, there is a continuing search for other arteries that could be used for coronary bypass. At-

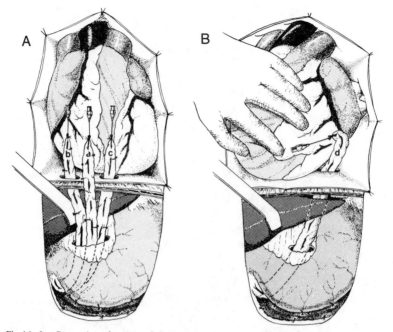

Fig 16–3.—Routes into the pericardial cavity are (**A**) anterior to the diaphragm (rarely used), (**B**) right anterior diaphragmatic window, (**C**) mid-diaphragmatic window, and (**D**) posterior diaphragmatic window. (Courtesy of Mills NL, Everson CT: *J Cardiac Surg* 4:1–9, March 1989.)

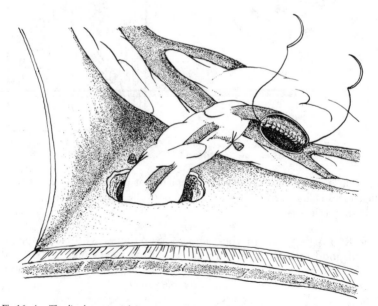

Fig 16–4.—The distal gastroepiploic anastomosis is performed with 8–0 polypropylene continuous suture that ends on the side of the anastomosis toward the surgeon. Patency in all 3 directions is assured before tying down the final sutures. (Courtesy of Mills NL, Everson CT: *J Cardiac Surg* 4:1–9, March 1989.)

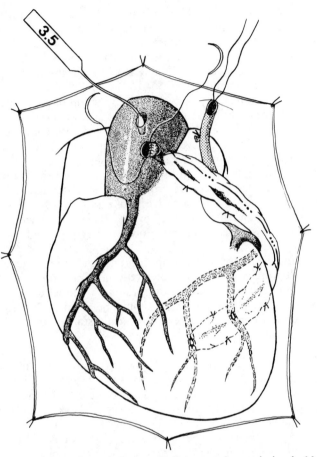

Fig 16–5.—Free RGEA grafts may be heavy and bulky compared to standard grafts. Multiple tacking sutures are required along the graft. The proximal anastomosis is performed with 6–0 polypropylene suture on a BV1 needle. Thereafter, patency is insured through an aortotomy for a subsequent saphenous vein graft when feasible. (Courtesy of Mills NL, Everson CT: *J Cardiac Surg* 4:1–9, March 1989.)

tempts years ago with radial artery grafts were disappointing, a high rate of thrombosis occurring within a year. This article on technique describes in detail the use of the gastroepiploic artery. No data are given, but the artery has been used in selected patients in a few institutions over the past few years. Preliminary results are encouraging, but long-term results will not be available for a few years.—F.C. Spencer, M.D.

Simultaneous Carotid and Coronary Disease: Safety of the Combined Approach
Cambria RP, Ivarsson BL, Akins CW, Moncure AC, Brewster DC, Abbott WM
(Massachusetts Gen Hosp, Boston; Harvard Med School)
J Vasc Surg 9:56–64, January 1989
16–8

Many centers have adopted a cautious approach toward carotid stenosis in patients who require cardiopulmonary bypass because of unacceptable operative risks. Carotid endarterectomy is performed at the time of coronary bypass grafting in selected patients. Seventy-one combined operations were done between 1978 and 1987, 51 in the past 5 years. The criterion was carotid stenosis of 75% or more.

Presently, endarterectomy is done after induction of anesthesia as veins are harvested from the leg. An indwelling shunt was used in 70% of the patients. Closure of the neck wound was delayed until completion of cardiopulmonary bypass and reversal of heparin. Shunts currently are not used if the ECG is benign after carotid clamping.

Most complications occurred in the earlier years of the study. Patients having the combined procedure from 1983 to 1987 had an operative mortality of 2% and a perioperative stroke rate of 2%. The respective figures for patients having coronary bypass surgery only were 2.2% and 0.6%. Two of 3 strokes after combined surgery occurred in the first 2 years of the study.

An individualized approach is appropriate for patients having critical carotid and coronary disease. Prophylactic endarterectomy should be limited to symptomatic or severe carotid lesions. Optimally, carotid lesions that would ordinarily be corrected should be repaired before coronary bypass surgery if coronary disease is clinically stable and if expert anesthesia is available.

▶ Despite more than a decade of study, the indications for performing carotid endarterectomy and coronary bypass at the same operation are controversial. Data suggest that carotid disease may increase the risk of stroke during coronary bypass, but this may be offset by the increased risk of stroke with combined procedures.

This report from the Massachusetts General Hospital details a decade of experience with the combined procedures, during which 71 operations were performed. Operative mortality was favorable, about 2%. Perioperative stroke ranged between 0.6% and 2%.—F.C. Spencer, M.D.

Role of Preoperative Cessation of Smoking and Other Factors in Postoperative Pulmonary Complications: A Blinded Prospective Study of Coronary Artery Bypass Patients

Warner MA, Offord KP, Warner ME, Lennon RL, Conover MA, Jansson-Schumacher U (Mayo Clinic and Found, Rochester, Minn)
Mayo Clin Proc 64:609–616, June 1989   16–9

Patients who smoke cigarettes are often advised to stop smoking before surgery to lessen their risk of postoperative pulmonary complications. To determine the effect of smoking on such complications, 200 consecutive patients undergoing elective coronary artery bypass grafting were interviewed before surgery. The patients were evaluated immediately postoperatively, at days 1 and 7, and on the day of hospital dismissal.

Of 192 patients who completed the study, 36 (18.7%) had postoperative pulmonary complications. None of the complications was fatal, and only 2 patients had a prolonged hospital stay. Pulmonary complications occurred in 33% of current smokers and in 57% of exsmokers of 8 weeks or less. Similar rates (about 11% to 12%) were found for exsmokers of more than 8 weeks, exsmokers of more than 6 months, and those who had never smoked. A logistic model predicts an increase in complication rate for the first 28 smoke-free days and a return to the current smoker rate after approximately 8 weeks; a rapid decline in the rate of complications is noted to about 3 months, and then a gradual tapering to 5 months. Thus the status of persons who never smoked was indistinguishable from that of smokers who abstained from smoking for 6 months.

Fewer smoke-free days, a lower forced expiratory volume in 1 second, and the use of enflurane were highly significant predictors of the development of postoperative pulmonary complications. Because a brief period without cigarettes does not lower postoperative the rate of respiratory complications, patients undergoing elective coronary artery bypass grafting are urged to discontinue smoking for at least 2 months before surgery.

▶ Recommending cessation of smoking before operation is a standard truism often seldom accomplished. This valuable paper studied 200 patients prospectively before elective coronary bypass. Patients who smoked within 2 months of operation had a complication rate nearly 4 times that of nonsmokers. These findings well emphasize the morbidity from smoking and the fact that pulmonary injury from smoking requires at least 2 months, possibly longer, before harmful effects recede.—F.C. Spencer, M.D.

17 Miscellaneous Cardiac Conditions and the Great Vessels

The Effect of Age on Cerebral Blood Flow During Hypothermic Cardiopulmonary Bypass
Brusino FG, Reves JG, Smith LR, Prough DS, Stump DA, McIntyre RW (Duke Univ; Wake Forest Univ)
J Thorac Cardiovasc Surg 97:541–547, April 1989   17–1

Advanced age may be a risk factor for neuropsychiatric morbidity after cardiopulmonary bypass (CPB). It was postulated that advanced age adversely modifies cerebral blood flow autoregulation by shifting the curve to the right. Persons of advanced age would be at increased risk for neuropsychiatric complications during periods of relatively low mean arterial pressure (MAP) during hypothermic CPB. To measure the effect of age on regional cerebral blood flow during nonpulsatile hypothermic CPB, cerebral blood flow was measured in 20 patients using the xenon-133 clearance method. Cerebral blood flow was measured at varying perfusion pressures in 9 patients aged 50 years or younger and in 11 patients older than 65 years. A constant pump flow rate of 1.6 L/min/m^2 was maintained at stable hypothermic conditions.

The range of MAP was 30–110 mm Hg in the younger group and 20–90 mm Hg in the older group. There was no significant difference in the MAP between the groups, nor was there a significant difference in the mean cerebral blood flow. In both groups there were poor correlations between MAP and cerebral blood flow. Repeated cerebral blood flow measurements were obtained for 12 patients to determine the effect of MAP on cerebral blood flow within an individual patient. Changes in MAP were not correlated with changes in cerebral blood flow. Age apparently does not alter cerebral blood flow. Cerebral blood flow autoregulation seems to be preserved in elderly patients during nonpulsatile hypothermic CPB.

▶ Most studies of postbypass neuropsychiatric complications find a much greater frequency in patients older than 60 years of age. The possibility exists that impairment of blood flow autoregulation in the elderly patient might render them more vulnerable to hypotensive neurologic injury.

In these carefully done studies cerebral blood flow was measured in 20 patients with a xenon-133 technique, studying 9 patients younger than 50 years and 11 older than 65. There was no significant difference in cerebral flow in the

2 groups. Cerebral blood flow was well maintained in older patients but showed little correlation with changes in perfusion pressure.—F.C. Spencer, M.D.

No Flow or Low Flow? A Study of the Ischemic Marker Creatine Kinase BB After Deep Hypothermic Procedures

Rossi R, van der Linden J, Ekroth R, Scallan M, Thompson RJ, Lincoln C (Brompton Hosp, London; Univ Hosp, Uppsala, Sweden; Inst de Cardiologia do Rio Grande do Sol, Porto Allegre, Brazil; Addenbrooke's Hosp, Cambridge Univ, England)
J Thorac Cardiovasc Surg 98:193–199, August 1989   17–2

Serial estimates of plasma creatine kinase isoenzyme BB (CK-BB) provide a measure of cerebral damage after profound hypothermia with circulatory arrest. It has been proposed that maintaining systemic perfusion at 25% of normal at normothermia will help to preserve cognitive function. Measurements of CK-BB were used to monitor 27 children with complex congenital heart malformations who required early repair. Some patients had total circulatory arrest for an average of 40 minutes, whereas others were maintained at deep hypothermia and 25% perfusion. In both groups the nasopharyngeal temperature was lowered to 15°C by topical and core cooling.

Levels of CK-BB increased in both groups of patients. The average increased from 4.3 mg/ml to 10.4 ng/mL in the circulatory arrest group, and from 2.8 ng/mL to 9.9 ng/mL in the low-flow group. The difference was not significant. Maintenance of a low level of systemic perfusion does not provide better cerebral protection than total circulatory arrest as long as moderate arrest times are used.

▶ This interesting report of experiences with 27 children operated on for complex congenital heart problems compares total hypothermic circulatory arrest for about 40 minutes with the other group in which perfusion was maintained but was reduced to 25% of normal at normothermia. The CK-BB was used as an index of cerebral injury.

The study could not demonstrate benefit from continued perfusion, as there were no neurologic problems in either group. The CK-BB level rose to a similar degree in both groups (2.5–3.0 times the initial value).

Although inconclusive, the ability to continue perfusion at a low rate seems entirely plausible and worth further investigation.—F.C. Spencer, M.D.

Coronary Sinus Versus Aortic Root Perfusion With Blood Cardioplegia in Elective Myocardial Revascularization

Fiore AC, Naunheim KS, Kaiser GC, Willman VL, McBride LR, Pennington DG, Barner HB (St Louis Univ; St Mary's Health Ctr, St Louis)
Ann Thorac Surg 47:684–688, May 1989   17–3

Recent studies have documented the ability of retrograde coronary sinus perfusion to achieve adequate preservation during global myocardial ischemia. Nevertheless, this technique has not been widely used. The efficacy of retrograde coronary sinus cardioplegia (RCSC) compared with standard aortic root cardioplegia (ARC) was evaluated in 40 patients undergoing elective coronary artery bypass grafting. They were divided equally to receive ARC or RCSC. Data recorded included sex, age, history of transmural myocardial infarction, number of vessels bypassed, and frequency of internal mammary artery grafting.

The patient groups were similar in age, ventricular function, severity of coronary artery disease, cross-clamp time, completeness of revascularization, incidence of internal mammary artery grafting, and mean infusate volume and temperature. However, the time required to deliver the initial dose of cardioplegic solution and the time to achieve arrest were prolonged in the RCSC group. Postoperatively, there were no differences between the groups in enzymatic indexes, hemodynamic parameters, or clinical outcomes. Right ventricular function was maintained equally in both groups.

The RCSC method is a safe alternative to ARC, but the procedure offers no advantage in patients scheduled for elective myocardial revascularization. However, patients with ongoing myocardial ischemia who require urgent revascularization might be better served with RCSC than with ARC. Patients with unstable angina pectoris, those requiring reoperation in the presence of stenotic bypass grafts, and patients with acute ischemia after failed balloon angioplasty all have lesions precluding optimal delivery of cardioplegia by the anterograde route. Retrograde cardioplegia might be a more effective method of myocardial preservation in these patients.

▶ Uncertainty exists about the physiologic benefits and limitations of RCSC as compared with conventional antegrade cardioplegia. This report compared experiences with 20 patients receiving antegrade cardioplegia with 20 patients receiving retrograde infusions. A similar dose, 10 cc/kg, was given to each group. This required slightly over 2 minutes to infuse in the antegrade group and more than 6 minutes in the retrograde group. Clamp times were slightly less than 80 minutes. Coronary sinus pressure was kept below 40 mm.

The results were very similar, as no deaths or major complications occurred in either group. Hence the conclusion was reached that the results seemed identical without any particular advantages or disadvantages of the retrograde method.—F.C. Spencer, M.D.

Studies of Retrograde Cardioplegia: I. Capillary Blood Flow Distribution to Myocardium Supplied by Open and Occluded Arteries
Partington MT, Acar C, Buckberg GD, Julia P, Kofsky ER, Bugyi HI (Univ of California, Los Angeles)
J Thorac Cardiovasc Surg 97:605–612, April 1989   17–4

The distribution of blood cardioplegic solutions delivered retrograde or antegrade was studied using radioactive microspheres in open-chest dogs. The microspheres were mixed with a blood cardioplegic solution and administered into the coronary sinus or the proximal aorta, with the left anterior descending coronary artery open or occluded. Nutritive flow was represented by the proportion of delivered 15-μm microspheres trapped in myocardial capillaries.

Nutritive flow averaged 65% during retrograde infusions and 87% with antegrade cardioplegia. Flow to all left ventricular regions was comparable with the left anterior descending coronary artery open. With both methods the subendocardial muscle was preferentially hyperperfused. Flow to muscle supplied by the occluded coronary vessel was preserved better with retrograde than with antegrade cardioplegia. In the latter instance flow was redistributed away from subendocardial muscle. Although left ventricular flow was markedly reduced during retrograde infusion, septal cooling was better than with antegrade cardioplegia. Right ventricular nutritive flow was maintained only by antegrade cardioplegia.

Retrograde coronary sinus perfusion of cardioplegic solution provides excellent nutritive flow to the left ventricular myocardium, even if coronary occlusion is present. The septum may be protected by flow through venovenous collaterals. Retrograde cardioplegia alone may not adequately protect the right ventricle.

▶ The major handicap to myocardial preservation with antegrade cardioplegia is a maldistribution that occurs with coronary disease. The retrograde method avoids maldistribution from obstructive disease. These experimental studies with radioactive microspheres found the retrograde method a superior means of preservation in the presence of acute coronary occlusion. Calculations indicated that the small flow with the retrograde method was large enough to supply the oxygen needs of the cold arrested heart, said to be less than 5% of those in the beating working heart.—F.C. Spencer, M.D.

Studies of Retrograde Cardioplegia: II. Advantages of Antegrade/Retrograde Cardioplegia to Optimize Distribution in Jeopardized Myocardium
Partington MT, Acar C, Buckberg GD, Julia PL (Univ of California, Los Angeles)
J Thorac Cardiovasc Surg 97:613–622, April 1989   17–5

Antegrade was compared with retrograde cardioplegic delivery in canine hearts subjected to temporary coronary ligation to simulate acute myocardial jeopardy. The left anterior descending coronary artery was ligated for 15 minutes before cardiopulmonary bypass was started. During 1 hour of aortic clamping, multidose cold blood cardioplegia at 6°C was administered. Dogs received cardioplegia either antegrade via the aortic root or retrograde via the coronary sinus; some animals were treated by both routes.

Antegrade cardioplegia produced excellent right ventricular cooling and permitted complete functional recovery of the right ventricle. However, muscle supplied by the left anterior descending artery was not cooled, and global left ventricular function recovered to only 38% after ischemia. Retrograde cardioplegia produced homogeneous cooling and allowed nearly normal recovery of global and regional left ventricular function. Right ventricular cooling, however, was variable, and right ventricular function did not recover consistently. The best protection was obtained by combined retrograde/antegrade cardioplegia. In this circumstance left and right ventricular global function recovered by 90% to 95%.

Combined retrograde and antegrade cardioplegia may allow the safe use of internal mammary grafts when myocardial tissue is in jeopardy. The initial infusion is antegrade. The aortic infusion line then is clamped, the vent is opened, and retrograde cardioplegia is delivered via the coronary sinus.

▶ These studies evaluated 3 different methods of cardioplegia: antegrade, retrograde, and combined. In the presence of acute coronary occlusion the antegrade method provided insufficient protection. The retrograde method produced inconsistent right ventricular preservation. Hence the combination of antegrade and retrograde was used and found to provide the best form of protection in the presence of acute occlusion.—F.C. Spencer, M.D.

Antegrade/Retrograde Blood Cardioplegia to Ensure Cardioplegic Distribution: Operative Techniques and Objectives
Buckberg GD (Univ of California, Los Angeles)
J Cardiac Surg 4:216–238, September 1989   17–6

The limitations of antegrade cardioplegia can be countered to some degree by retrograde cardioplegia via the coronary sinus or right atrium. A technique of antegrade/retrograde blood cardioplegia involving rapid transatrial cannulation of the coronary sinus was evaluated. This allows safe and rapid retrograde cardioplegia and avoids right heart isolation.

Technique.—The Retroplegia cannula contains a special stylet with a low-pressure, self-inflating and self-deflating balloon that can rapidly be placed in the coronary sinus using a simple atrial mattress suture. Usually only 10–15 seconds are required. Retrograde cardioplegia is delivered at 200–250 mL/min, with a coronary sinus pressure of 30–50 mm Hg. Retrograde balloon inflation during antegrade infusion may improve the distribution of antegrade cardioplegia. Cardioplegia is never given simultaneously by the 2 routes; antegrade cardioplegia is always given first. Furosemide administered just after the start of bypass promotes excretion of potassium in the cardioplegic solution. Topical hypothermia is helpful if there is total reliance on retrograde cardioplegia. Cold induction is used at elective surgery if the ejection fraction is reasonable. Warm reperfusion is given for 3–5 minutes to limit reperfusion injury, or for 20 minutes if evolving infarction is present. Extended warm reperfusion is delivered only antegrade into the graft supplying the infarcted segment.

This technique has been used in 116 patients, most having coronary bypass grafting or valve replacement. Mortality was 1.7%; both deaths occurred in high-risk patients with extending infarction.

▶ At this time the role of antegrade cardioplegia vs. retrograde cardioplegia is undergoing close evaluation. This article details the current concepts of combining antegrade and retrograde cardioplegia by Buckberg. The article is of particular interest because Buckberg has been the pioneer investigator studying methods of cardioplegia for several years.—F.C. Spencer, M.D.

Experiments With a Bowl of Saline: The Hidden Risk of Hypothermic-Osmotic Damage During Topical Cardiac Cooling

Robicsek F, Duncan GD, Rice HE, Robicsek SA (Charlotte Mem Hosp and Med Ctr, Charlotte, NC)
J Thorac Cardiovasc Surg 97:461–466, March 1989   17–7

Topical cardiac hypothermia has developed as an effective means of myocardial protection during aortic cross-clamping. But external cooling of the heart is not without risk. Hypothermic and cold-osmotic damage can affect the blood, myocardium, and phrenic nerve. Such complications occur because of a lack of knowledge about the characteristics of cold normal saline solution.

Several experiments were performed using saline slush as it is commonly prepared in operating rooms, with either salted ice or a freezer machine as the cooling medium. Stirred and unstirred saline solution and saline slush were compared to study the supercooling phenomenon—cooling of the solution below 0°C without ice formation.

The temperature of unfrozen saline solution may drop well below the freezing point. If the liquid and solid phases of the solution are separated, the components become, respectively, a highly hyperosmotic liquid saline solution and a highly hypo-osmotic ice. Tests against freshly drawn heparinized human blood showed that the melt of the "edge ice" from the bowl of the freezer machine had severe hemolytic effects.

Possible results of topical cooling include paralysis of the phrenic nerve, which can lead to respiratory distress and even death. The heart muscle and red blood cells also may be damaged by changes in the temperature or balance of the solution. These possibilities should be taken into account during the application of topical cardiac hypothermia.

▶ This short report clearly emphasizes the dangers from the use of iced saline and slush. With the use of slush the hazards are considerably greater than those that develop simply by lowering the temperature a few degrees.

At New York University, we studied the problem prospectively in 133 patients, finding a greater percentage of phrenic nerve palsy (1). Since this report in 1987 the use of iced slush has been virtually abandoned.— F.C. Spencer, M.D.

Reference

1. Esposito RA, Spencer FC: *Ann Thorac Surg* 43:303, 1987.

Use of the Pierce-Donachy Ventricular Assist Device in Patients With Cardiogenic Shock After Cardiac Operations
Pennington DG, McBride LR, Swartz MT, Kanter KR, Kaiser GC, Barner HB, Miller LW, Naunheim KS, Fiore AC, Willman VL (St Louis Univ Hosp)
Ann Thorac Surg 47:130–135, January 1989   17–8

Various systems have been developed for mechanical circulatory support of patients with cardiogenic shock after cardiotomy. At St Louis University Hospital the best results have been obtained with the Pierce-Donachy ventricular assist device (VAD), a paracorporeal pneumatic sac-type device. Its cannula system allows cannulation of the left ventricle, the left and right atria, and the aorta or pulmonary artery. During a 7-year period, 30 patients were supported with this device. The patients chosen for treatment had severe postcardiotomy ventricular failure and had not responded to drugs or to the intra-aortic balloon. In 20 patients the VAD was inserted because they could not be weaned from cardiopulmonary bypass. Support continued for a mean period of 3.6 days.

Fourteen patients had no improvement in cardiac function and died of bleeding, biventricular failure, or multiple-organ failure. Improved cardiac function was achieved in 16 patients. Fifteen patients were weaned from the VAD and 11 were discharged from the hospital. Better results, both in weaning from VAD and in survival, were obtained in the later years of the study. Six of the 16 patients who received biventricular support were long-term survivors.

Complications included biventricular failure (83%) and bleeding (73%). Survival was negatively affected by perioperative myocardial infarction, renal failure, and infection. The 8 survivors from this group of 30 patients are leading active lives. Ventricular function is normal or nearly normal in half of these patients. Survival rates should continue to improve with the Pierce-Donachy VAD.

▶ The Pierce-Donachy pneumatic assist device, one of the best engineered pumps for left heart support, has been increasingly used as a bridge to transplantation. This report from St. Louis describes experiences with 30 patients over a period of 8 years, with the late survival rate ranging between 35% and 45%. It is puzzling that the survival rate is about the same as that obtained with the roller pump, a simpler but more traumatic type of left ventricular pump.— F.C. Spencer, M.D.

Technique and Results With a Roller Pump Left and Right Heart Assist Device

Rose DM, Connolly M, Cunningham JN Jr, Spencer FC (New York Univ; Maimonides Med Ctr, Brooklyn; State Univ Hosp, Brooklyn)

Ann Thorac Surg 47:124–129, January 1989   17–9

Ventricular assist devices have had increasing success in patients with profound heart failure after cardiac surgery. One such device is a roller pump type that is inexpensive, easy to use, and relatively effective. The results of a 10-year experience with roller pump-driven left and right heart assist devices were assessed. The left heart assist device was used in 72 patients. Of these, 57 were unable to discontinue cardiopulmonary bypass and 15 underwent cardiac arrest with-in 12 hours postoperatively. In the latter group the device was inserted to wean the patients from cardiopulmonary bypass. Seven patients required a right heart assist device. In addition, 5 patients in profound cardiogenic shock after acute myocardial infarction received a percutaneous left heart assist device.

Within 1–4 days, 30 patients (42%) were weaned from the left heart assist device. Left heart function gradually returned in these patients. Forty-two patients did not survive the immediate preoperative period; 9 died within 21–90 days postoperatively, and 2 late deaths occurred, both of cardiac causes. Eleven of 19 long-term survivors were in New York Heart Association functional class I. All 5 patients with the right heart assist device died. Two were weaned from the device but died in the early postoperative period, 1 at 10 days of pneumonia and the other at 5 days of multisystem failure and sepsis. No patient could be weaned from the percutaneous left heart assist device; all in this group were extremely ill.

Further refinements of all ventricular assist devices should lead to increased rates of survival. The roller pump type of device now achieves reasonably good results in patients with severe postoperative heart failure.

▶ This report from my institution (NYU) summarizes experiences over the past decade with a roller pump left heart assist device. Among 72 patients, 30 were weaned from the device and 21 (30%) survived. A similar type of ventricular assist was used in 7 patients with right heart failure, none of whom survived.

The roller pump, the simplest of all forms of left ventricular assist, has the advantage of being available quickly in the operating room. This may be the critical factor in survival, because prompt use of a left heart assist may prevent extensive subendocardial edema and necrosis. Delay in using such support may lead to irreversible injury. This theoretical possibility is proposed because the results with the relatively crude roller pump are about the same as those with the more complex sophisticated assist heart devices.—F.C. Spencer, M.D.

Postoperative Bleeding in Cardiovascular Surgery: Does Heparin Rebound Really Exist?

Gundry SR, Drongowski RA, Klein MD, Coran AG (Univ of Michigan Hosps; Univ of Maryland)
Am Surg 55:162–165, March 1989   17–10

Heparin, commonly used as an anticoagulant during cardiovascular procedures, is thought to be released hours after cardiopulmonary bypass, resulting in heparin rebound. To treat this condition additional doses of protamine are given to neutralize any residual circulating heparin. The postoperative presence of heparin, however, has been measured only by biologic clotting tests. To determine whether heparin rebound actually exists, a test for plasma heparin, the azure A assay, was used in 27 patients.

In all 27 patients heparinization was reversed after completion of cardiopulmonary bypass with 1 mg of protamine sulfate per 1 mg of sodium heparin activity as measured by the Hepcon unit. Blood samples were tested before and for 8 hours after bypass to determine prothrombin time, partial prothrombin time, thrombin clotting time, activated clotting time, and the azure A plasma heparin content.

Control azure A ratios below 90% of baseline were found in only 5 patients (19%). Four occurred in the first bypass hour, thus indicating unreversed heparin rather than rebound. Of 252 samples of blood tested, only 1 drawn at any time except immediately after bypass contained measurable heparin. Activated clotting time prolongation occurred in 5 patients but was not associated with detection of heparin by the azure A assay. Twelve patients had abnormal partial prothrombin times, and 21 of 22 patients tested had abnormal prothrombin times during the early postoperative period.

Protamine titration tests appear to be an inaccurate measure of the presence of heparin. Although many patients have significant abnormalities after bypass that are detected by coagulation studies, these abnormalities do not correlate with the presence of heparin. Bleeding rates were similar, whether or not coagulation abnormalities existed. True heparin rebound appears to be rare, and the administration of protamine to prevent this condition is usually not warranted.

▶ Abnormal bleeding after cardiac surgery, with associated abnormalities of coagulation, has been associated with bypass surgery since its inception. Fortunately, the frequency and severity of postoperative bleeding have greatly decreased. The question of heparin rebound has long existed.

This interesting report describes studies with the azure A assay in 27 patients. This test, which measures heparin chemically rather than biologically, is said to be far more reliable than other techniques. The references cited are all by Gundry, the principal author of this report. In these studies heparin rebound was extremely rare, but elevation of the prothrombin time (PT) and the partial thromboplastin time (PTT) was not unusual. The conclusion was that these abnormalities are common and do not predict the presence of unreversed heparin.—F.C. Spencer, M.D.

Randomized Clinical Trial of Fibrin Sealant in Patients Undergoing Resternotomy or Reoperation After Cardiac Operations: A Multicenter Study

Rousou J, Levitsky S, Gonzalez-Lavin L, Cosgrove D, Magilligan D, Weldon C, Hiebert C, Hess P, Joyce L, Bergsland J, Gazzaniga A (Baystate Med Ctr, Springfield, Mass; Univ of Illinois, Chicago; Cleveland Clinic Found; Henry Ford Hosp, Detroit; Maine Med Ctr, Portland; et al)
J Thorac Cardiovasc Surg 97:194–203, February 1989   17–11

Fibrin sealant has been used in cardiovascular surgery in Europe for about 10 years, but it is not currently approved for general use in the United States. A multicenter clinical study was approved by the Food and Drug Administration to evaluate the efficacy and safety of fibrin sealant as a topical hemostatic agent in patients undergoing repeat cardiac surgery and in those requiring emergency resternotomy for postoperative bleeding.

Eleven centers and 333 patients participated in the study. When a hemostatic agent was required during surgery, patients were randomly assigned to receive either fibrin sealant or a conventional topical hemostatic agent. The agent's efficacy was evaluated by the number of bleeding episodes controlled within 5 minutes. Patients in the fibrin-sealant group were compared with historical matched controls for postoperative blood loss, blood products received, need for resternotomy, and length of hospital stay. This group was also compared with historical nonmatched controls for the incidence of resternotomy and mortality.

Fibrin sealant had a 92.6% success rate in controlling bleeding within 5 minutes of application; conventional topical agents had only a 12.4% success rate. Fibrin sealant also quickly controlled 82% of bleeding episodes not initially controlled by conventional agents. High-volume postoperative blood loss was significantly less in patients treated with fibrin sealant than in matched controls. Resternotomy rates after reoperation were also significantly lower in the fibrin-sealant group than in nonmatched historical controls. There were no significant differences in length of hospital stay or in blood products received between the fibrin-sealant group and matched historical controls. There were no differences in mortality between the fibrin-sealant group and nonmatched historical controls. In the fibrin-sealant group there were no instances of adverse reactions, transmissions of viral infection, or HIV seroconversion.

Fibrin sealant is safe and extremely effective in controlling localized bleeding during cardiac surgery. Fibrin sealant reduces postoperative blood loss and decreases the incidence of emergency resternotomy.

▶ Considerable uncertainty exists in the United States about the usefulness of fibrin sealant during cardiac operations. Much of the uncertainty stems from the fact that its routine use has not been approved by the Food and Drug Administration (FDA) because of the risk of hepatitis. The use of fibrin sealant was reported in Europe by Spangler in 1976 and subsequently popularized by Borst in Hanover, Germany.

This randomized, multicenter trial compared 164 patients in whom fibrin sealant was used with 169 controls. The results demonstrated a high degree of efficacy of the fibrin sealant, judged to be 93% effective in controlling bleeding as compared to 12% with conventional topical agents. No adverse reactions were documented. These encouraging results should lead to wider use of this agent in the United States. Approval by the FDA would greatly enhance its more widespread application.— F.C. Spencer, M.D.

Reoperative Median Sternotomy
Garrett HE Jr, Matthews J (The Cardio Vascular Ctr, Inc, Memphis)
Ann Thorac Surg 48:305, August 1989   17–12

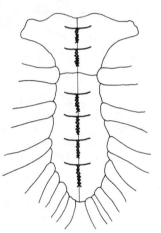

A

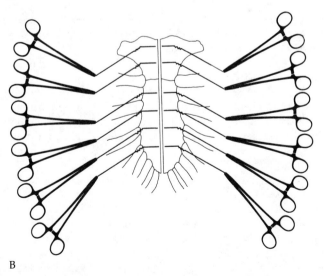

B

Fig 17–1.—**A,** previous sternal wires are exposed through a midline incision. **B,** wires are untwisted or cut but not removed. An oscillating saw may then be used to divide the sternum. The wires provide a barrier to the saw and are removed after the sternum is divided. (Courtesy of Garrett HE Jr, Matthews J: *Ann Thorac Surg* 48:305, August 1989.)

When the chest is reentered through a median sternotomy, mortality generally is increased, chiefly because of an increased risk of death on the day of surgery. Accidents at the time of reentry may be very important, especially if the right ventricle, aorta, or graft is adherent to the posterior sternal table. A simple procedure was developed that avoids many potential accidents (Fig 17–1).

Technique.—The sternal wires are cut or untwisted, but are not removed. An oscillating saw then is used to divide the sternum while applying upward traction to the wires. This elevates the sternum away from the mediastinal contents, and the wires serve as a barrier to progress of the saw. After the bone is divided throughout its length, the wires can be removed and mediastinal dissection carried out.

This technique has been used in 50 consecutive patients without adverse incident.

▶ This brief article on surgical technique was selected for its simplicity and theoretical attraction. As the authors indicate, traction on the divided ends of the sternal wires from the preceding operation elevates the sternum away from the heart and also protects from the saw inadvertently entering the underlying myocardium, the main cause of operative hemorrhage during resternotomy.

Although experiences thus far are small—only 50 patients—evaluation of the technique by others should quickly provide sufficient data to evaluate the probable merit. The key concept is the application of upward traction on the sternum while the sternum is divided by the saw. The intact wires provide an additional safeguard.—F.C. Spencer, M.D.

Primary Treatment of the Infected Sternotomy Wound With Muscle Flaps: A Review of 211 Consecutive Cases
Nahai F, Rand RP, Hester TR, Bostwick J III, Jurkiewicz MJ (Emory Univ)
Plast Reconstr Surg 84:434–441, September 1989   17–13

In 1976 Lee et al. offered the first alternative to open granulation for patients whose sternotomy wound infections failed to resolve on catheter irrigation; the greater omentum was transposed. The results of primary flap closure were reviewed in 211 consecutive patients having sternal wound infections in 1978–1987; 35 other patients had local wound care. The predominant infecting organisms were *Staphylococcus aureus* and *Staphylococcus epidermidis*.

Mortality was 5.3%; all survivors had a healed wound. Of the 377 flaps created, 212 were pectoralis major turnover and rotation-advancement flaps. In 145 patients a rectus abdominis flap was used. The omentum was transposed in 8 patients. An attempt at single-stage wound coverage succeeded in 95% of 139 patients. When 2 stages were necessary, 93% of the patients had primary healing. The flap survival rate was 99.2%. Osteomyelitis or costochondritis developed in 12 patients, and

25 others had postoperative drainage not requiring reoperation. Abdominal wall competency was compromised in 3.3% of the patients.

Use of a single muscle to close the wound is preferred when possible, and the single pectoralis turnover flap is an appropriate first choice. The rectus abdominis flap also may be used, even after both internal mammaries are harvested. Another option is use of a composite bipedicled pectoralis-rectus unit. The omentum provides useful tissue with which to treat a sternal wound. Also, the latissimus dorsi can be transferred subpectorally.

▶ This excellent report summarizes experiences with muscle flaps over a period of 10 years during which 211 patients were treated. This is the institution where the concept was developed by Jurkiewicz. The results were impressive: a 5% mortality; ability to perform the entire procedure of débridement and muscle flap in one operation in about 72% of patients; and an average hospitalization of about 15 days.

These overall results are significantly better than those reported from our institution by Grossi in 1985. The ability to débride an infected sternum, apply muscle flaps, and then close the wound in two thirds of the patients is remarkable biologically and apparently reflects the ability of viable muscle to combat infection.—F.C. Spencer, M.D.

Omental Pedicle Grafting in the Treatment of Postcardiotomy Sternotomy Infection

Lovich SF, Iverson LIG, Young JN, Ennix CL Jr, Harrell JE Jr, Ecker RR, Lau G, Joseph P, May IA (Samuel Merritt Hosp, Oakland, Calif)
Arch Surg 124:1192–1194, October 1989   17–14

Postcardiotomy sternal infection occurred in 20 (2%) of 1,007 patients who had cardiac surgery in a 28-month period in 1985–1987. The incidence was tenfold greater than in the previous 33 months. Cultures of specimen from 5 patients were sterile, but those from 12 others yielded staphylococci. In 3 a variety of organisms grew. Infections became less frequent subsequently after prophylaxis was changed to cefuroxime.

Attempts to rewire the sternum are not warranted. If gross purulence is absent, primary closure is carried out using muscle flaps, as in 2 of the present patients, or omental pedicle grafts, which were used in 17 patients. One patient died before closure was attempted. Either primary skin closure of split-thickness skin grafting is undertaken when infection is controlled. All 19 patients had primary wound healing. There were no cardiopulmonary complications.

Early definitive treatment of sternal osteomyelitis can provide a satisfactory outcome. In this series, omental pedicle grafts were used in most of the patients to good effect.

▶ This report describes experiences in the treatment of 20 sternal infections after 1,007 cardiac operations. In 17 patients the omentum was mobilized and placed into the sternotomy defect after débridement; muscle flaps were used in 2 patients. Only 1 death occurred. Rewiring of the infected sternum after débridement was not attempted.

Omentum provides an alternative source of viable tissue for the treatment of an infected sternum and is perhaps simpler to use than muscle flaps. Further observation will be of particular interest.—F.C. Spencer, M.D.

Delayed Primary Closure After Sternal Wound Infection
Johnson JA, Gall WE, Gundersen AE, Cogbill TH (Wisconsin Heart Inst; Gundersen/Lutheran Med Ctr, La Crosse, Wis)
Ann Thorac Surg 47:270–273, February 1989   17–15

Twenty-five sternal wound infections were treated in a 30-month period, 24 of them (2.7%) after 883 operations under cardiopulmonary bypass. Infection occurred most often within 2 weeks of median sternotomy. The most frequent infecting organism was *Staphylococcus aureus*.

Four patients with sternal infection died, 3 of unrelated complications. One patient with steroid-dependent rheumatoid arthritis died of persistent sepsis related to sternal infection. Eighteen patients had delayed primary closure a mean of 9 days after incision and drainage. Fifteen of them had an uneventful course, but 2 patients required reoperation for sternal dehiscence and 1 had a superficial infection. In 3 patients the sternal wound was closed with pectoralis muscle flaps; the necrotic sternum would not have held sutures. The mean hospital stay after delayed primary closure was 2 weeks.

Delayed primary closure eliminates potentially undrained spaces and permits active débridement with dressing changes. Bleeding from mediastinal vessels is less likely to occur. Closure may be done if purulent drainage is absent, the tissue surfaces are clean, and wound cultures are negative. The cosmetic results are excellent.

▶ The morbidity and mortality associated with sternotomy infections is well known. The efficacy of muscle flap closure, pioneered by Emory University, has produced excellent results. Our institution has long favored initial treatment with débridement and antibiotic drainage, achieving a success rate between 50% and 75%. This unusual report describes successful results in a group of 21 patients, using a delayed primary closure in 18. This was effective even though it was performed from 5 to 27 days after the initial drainage procedure and all cultures were positive at the time of operation. Further data with this simple approach will be most interesting.—F.C. Spencer, M.D.

Delayed Sternal Closure: A Lifesaving Maneuver After Early Operation for Complex Congenital Heart Disease in the Neonate
Odim JNK, Tchervenkov CI, Dobell ARC (Montreal Children's Hosp)
J Thorac Cardiovasc Surg 98:413–416, September 1989   17–16

Early repair of complex congenital heart anomalies can entail life-threatening respiratory and hemodynamic compromise when the sternum is closed. Sternal closure may be postponed to avoid death in this setting. Nine critically ill neonates were managed in this way when, in a 12-month period, a total of 100 patients had intracardiac surgery. Three of the neonates had hemodynamic compromise and ventilatory failure, 3 had respiratory compromise, and 3 required mediastinal reexploration for bleeding caused by coagulopathy.

Silicone elastomer sheeting was sutured to the skin edges in place of sternal closure. Definitive closure was done in the intensive care unit in all patients but 1. Eight of the 9 neonates survived. The wound was protected by silicone sheeting for 5.5 days on average. No wound infections developed, and no infant had evidence of mediastinitis.

The physiologic disorder in these infants is largely a result of water imbalance secondary to cardiorespiratory support during surgery. Persistent efforts to close the sternum prematurely can lead to the return of poor hemodynamics and pulmonary dysfunction. The use of silicone sheeting in place of sternal closure can provide the compliance critical to immediate cardiopulmonary function.

▶ The usefulness and safety of delayed sternal closure is well described in this short report. Delayed closure was used in 9 of 30 neonates, 8 of whom survived. The technique is well described. The absence of infection underlines the importance of the precise technique outlined.

A substantial period of time was required before the sternum could be closed, averaging more than 5 days; 2 patients recovered after the sternum was left open for 11 days and 12 days, respectively.—F.C. Spencer, M.D.

Symptomatic Visual Deficits After Open Heart Operations
Shahian DM, Speert PK (Lahey Clinic Med Ctr, Burlington, Mass; New England Deaconess Hosp, Boston)
Ann Thorac Surg 48:275–279, August 1989   17–17

Of 700 patients having open-heart surgery, 4 had symptomatic visual deficits. The causes included retinal embolism, occipital lobe infarction, and anterior ischemic optic neuropathy.

The incidence of neurologic dysfunction after open-heart surgery relates to how intensively it is sought. Retinal microembolism continues to occur despite improvement in arterial filtration and extracorporeal circulation. Ischemic infarction involving the central visual pathways can produce a homonymous hemianopia or, if bilateral, "cortical blindness." Anterior ischemic optic neuropathy is thought to result from interruption of blood flow to the optic nerve head. Neuropathy may occur immediately or after a period of weeks.

Visual complications can result from embolization of air or particulate debris, nonembolic hypoperfusion of the CNS, or optic nerve ischemia. Meticulous care in surgical technique can minimize embolization. Adequate perfusion flow and pressure must be maintained during cardiopulmonary bypass. Vasoconstrictors may dispose to ischemic neuropathy and should be used only if perfusion pressure and vascular resistance are reduced substantially. A hematocrit of less than 20% should be avoided. Prophylactic antiglaucoma drugs might help to prevent ocular complications of open-heart surgery.

▶ This short report calls attention to the occasional occurrence of significant visual defects after open-heart operations. This report describes 4 such patients following 700 operations, a frequency near 0.6%. Causes include retinal emboli, occipital lobe infarction, or anterior ischemic optic neuropathy. The latter condition is puzzling, as the evolution may be slow and not clearly understood. This article reviews the different concepts about this unusual condition. How these infrequent but serious disabilities can be avoided remains an unsolved problem.—F.C. Spencer, M.D.

Annular Destruction in Acute Bacterial Endocarditis: Surgical Techniques to Meet the Challenge

Ergin MA, Raissi S, Follis F, Lansman SL, Griepp RB (Mount Sinai Med Ctr, New York)
J Thorac Cardiovasc Surg 97:755–763, May 1989   17–18

Surgery with timely valve replacement is the established treatment for bacterial endocarditis. In some patients management of the condition is complicated by extension of the infectious process into the annular structures. Removal of the infected tissues and reconstruction of the annulus present a significant surgical challenge.

At 1 institution 15 of 82 patients who underwent surgical treatment for acute bacterial endocarditis during a 10-year period had extensive destruction of the annulus. Two of the 10 patients with prosthetic valves had each undergone 2 previous valve replacements. Diagnosis was obtained from clinical and bacteriologic findings confirmed by echocardiography. The most common organism cultured was *Staphylococcus aureus*.

Surgical treatment involved removal of the valve and all infected annular elements. Restoration of the annulus for anchoring of the prosthetic valve was accomplished by various means. The felt aortic root technique was used in 3 patients with native valve endocarditis; a valved composite graft replacement of the aortic root (the Bentall procedure) was used in 8 patients with prosthetic valve endocarditis. One patient with a mitral-aortic native valve underwent direct suture of the sewing skirts of the mitral and aortic prostheses, and 2 patients with mitral-aortic prosthetic valves were treated by composite patch reconstruction.

The surgical techniques described here proved safe and offered good long-term results. No intraoperative deaths occurred. One patient who was admitted in cardiogenic shock and renal shutdown died 45 days postoperatively of multiple organ failure. Heart block was the most common complication. At a mean follow-up of 23.7 months, 11 patients remained alive and well without complications. The 2 late deaths resulted from reinfection caused by continued intravenous drug abuse.

▶ Unusually complicated problems evolve when endocarditis extends into the perivalvular tissues with destruction of the annulus and adjacent structures. This report describes such problems in 15 patients, seen in a group of 82 patients treated for endocarditis over a period of 10 years.

A variety of ingenious reconstructive techniques were used, including Teflon felt patches, a valve composite graft replacement of the aortic root, and other types of reconstruction. The key principle was wide excision of all infected tissue, followed by restoration of anatomical continuity.

Remarkably enough, there was only 1 hospital death, with 2 subsequent deaths associated with continued intravenous drug use.—F.C. Spencer, M.D.

Myocardial Contusion: When Can the Diagnosis be Eliminated?
Miller FB, Shumate CR, Richardson JD (Univ of Louisville)
Arch Surg 124:805–808, July 1989   17–19

A 2-year study was conducted to evaluate the relative diagnostic value of ECGs, cardiac isoenzyme tests, and 2-dimensional echocardiograms in patients with myocardial contusion. Also, who needs to be monitored and for what length of time were determined.

Of 172 patients studied 28 had positive criteria for myocardial contusion. In 23 patients the injuries were caused by motor vehicle accidents; in 4 patients by motor vehicle or pedestrian automobile accidents; and in 1 patient, a fall. The diagnosis of myocardial contusion was based on ST-T changes observed on ECGs in 10 patients, cardiac rhythm in 8 electrical conduction in 6, increased creatine phosphokinase-MB in 15, 2-D echocardiograms in 5, and autopsy results in 3. Cardiac isoenzyme levels had negligible significance on outcome, and 2-D echocardiograms were not valuable as a screening technique. Myocardial contusion may have contributed to 1 of 3 deaths. All patients in whom myocardial contusion developed had ECG abnormalities, rhythm disturbances, or hemodynamic instability on admission or within the first 24 hours. No patients had late complications such as cardiac tamponade or myocardial infarction.

A protocol was developed based on these findings. Patients who have multiple injuries, hemodynamic instability, rhythm disturbance, or conduction abnormalities are admitted to an intensive care unit. After stabilization of these conditions for 24 hours, the patients are admitted to a telemetry unit for 24 hours; after this, if no instability of rhythm disturbances develop, they may be discharged from this unit and the hospital if they are well otherwise.

▶ The diagnosis of myocardial contusion was made in 28 of 172 patients seen after they had sustained blunt chest trauma. The value of 3 different diagnostic tests—determination of cardiac isoenzyme levels, ECG, and echocardiography—was analyzed. The significant finding emerged that virtually all abnormalities could be detected within 24 hours, after which time the likelihood of unexpected adverse changes was small. The ECG was the best indicator for cardiac monitoring. Cardiac enzymes and echocardiography were of minimal value.—F.C. Spencer, M.D.

Cardiac Contusion: The Effect on Operative Management of the Patient With Trauma Injuries
Ross P Jr, Degutis L, Baker CC (Yale Univ)
Arch Surg 124:506–507, April 1989   17–20

To evaluate the impact of cardiac contusion on subsequent management, data were reviewed on 64 patients with cardiac contusion substantiated by ECG and the creatine kinase MB (CK-MB) fraction assay after blunt chest injury. There were 45 male and 19 female patients aged 7–89 years. Most were injured in motor vehicle or motorcycle accidents; the remainder were injured in falls, industrial accidents, or as pedestrians. Additional chest injuries were present in 40 patients, and 18% were hypotensive.

Increased CK-MB levels were present in 58 patients; 35 of these had ECG abnormalities, including 25 with ST segment and T wave changes, 10 with premature ventricular contractions, 9 with right bundle-branch block, 3 with atrioventricular block, 3 with atrial fibrillation, and 2 with premature atrial contractions.

General anesthesia was used in 30 patients undergoing exploratory laparotomy, repair of complex lacerations, or open reduction and internal fixation of fractures. Perioperative complications occurred in 4 patients, including ventricular fibrillation, ventricular ectopy, nodal rhythm, and pulmonary edema. There were no deaths attributable to cardiac contusions. Complications appeared to be unrelated to older age, level of CK-MB, history of cardiac disease, or total number of systems injured.

Cardiac contusion is common in traumatically injured patients, but ECG manifestations of injury may be absent initially in up to 45%. Hemodynamic monitoring is suggested in patients with suspected cardiac contusion who require emergency surgery after trauma. Because preoperative factors do not identify patients at risk, preparations for early detection and treatment of arrhythmias should be made when patients undergo semielective surgery. Multiply-injured patients with cardiac contusions can undergo elective surgery with a low incidence of complications.

▶ The presence of cardiac contusion naturally evokes concern about the safety of semielective operative procedures in patients with multiple injuries. This important study assessed 64 patients with cardiac contusion, documented by ECG changes and a rise in the CK-MB fraction. Thirty of 64 patients subsequently underwent general anesthesia, with only 4 perioperative complications, primarily arrhythmias. There were no deaths attributable to cardiac contusion. These data indicate that such patients can be operated on safely if appropriate hemodynamic monitoring, including the detection of cardiac arrhythmias, is done.—F.C. Spencer, M.D.

Fracture of the Upper Ribs and Injury to the Great Vessels
Poole GV (Univ of Mississippi)
Surg Gynecol Obstet 169:275–282, September 1989   17–21

First rib fracture signifies severe trauma, and rupture of the thoracic aorta sometimes is an associated finding. Routine aortography for patients with fracture of the upper ribs is based on the assumption of an increased risk of disruption of the intrathoracic great vessels. This can occur without clinical manifestations and without x-ray evidence of mediastinal bleeding.

An association between fracture of the first or second rib and a high risk of injury of the thoracic aorta and its major branches has not been proved. Of 1,393 patients with blunt chest trauma whose first or second rib was the highest fractured, 6.2% had disruption of the thoracic aorta and 4.5% had injury of a great vessel. Fracture of the upper 2 ribs is found in about 25% to 30% of patients with disruption of the thoracic aorta. An association is most likely for injury to the ipsilateral subclavian artery.

Roentgenographic abnormalities are much more sensitive than are clinical signs of great vessel injury. A widened mediastinum is a frequent finding, but precise standards are lacking; possibly, too much importance has been placed on the singularity of this finding. An abnormal aortic outline is the other sensitive indicator of aortic rupture. The role of CT in making this diagnosis is uncertain, but experience to date suggests that arteriography may not be necessary when a blunt chest trauma victim has a normal thoracic CT scan.

▶ This collective review, with 60 references, well summarizes available data concerning traumatic injuries of the great vessels. Despite earlier impressions, there is no statistically increased risk of aortic injury with fracture of the first or second rib. The widened mediastinum is the most common radiologic abnormality, indicating that aortography should be done; what constitutes a "widened mediastinum" is somewhat subjective. Loss of definition of the aortic knob, or blurring of the contour of the aorta, is also a highly significant radiologic abnormality strongly indicating aortography. Scanning with CT, to date, has not been diagnostic.—F.C. Spencer, M.D.

Surgical Treatment of Aneurysms of the Transverse Aortic Arch
Kazui T, Inoue N, Komatsu S (Sapporo Med College, Sapporo, Japan)
J Cardiovasc Surg 30:402–406, May–June 1989   17–22

A total of 21 patients had surgery including aortic arch reconstruction for thoracic aortic aneurysms between 1983 and 1987; 16 patients had

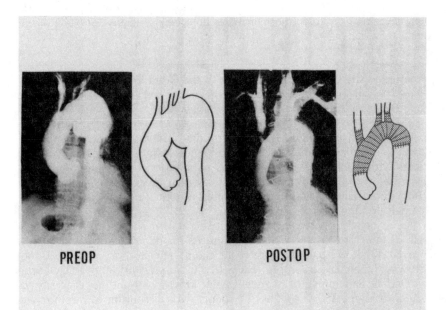

PREOP   POSTOP

Fig 17–2.—Preoperative and postoperative aortograms and line drawings showing the technique of operation in a patient with impending rupture of an aortic arch aneurysm. Resection and graft replacement of the ascending aortic arch and descending aorta with reconstruction of the arch vessels was performed with the aid of selective cerebral perfusion through a median sternotomy and left thoracotomy. (Courtesy of Kazui T, Inoue N, Komatsu S: *J Cardiovasc Surg* 30:402–406, May–June 1989.)

type A dissecting aneurysms of the aorta and 5 had atherosclerotic disease. Selective cerebral perfusion was used in 11 patients to prevent cerebral ischemia. Perfusion was at 25°C at a rate of 600 mL/min. The other 10 patients were managed by hypothermic circulatory arrest at 15°C. All patients but 1, who had patch angioplasty of the aortic arch, underwent resection of the aneurysm and Dacron graft replacement (Fig 17–2). Two patients had concomitant aortic valve replacement, and each had aortic cusp suspension and coronary bypass grafting.

The postoperative mortality rate was 14.3%; 2 patients who were treated with hypothermic arrest died of bleeding and renal failure at emergency surgery. No serious neurologic complications occurred. The average time of cerebral ischemia in the hypothermic arrest group was 35 minutes. The average cerebral perfusion time was 70 minutes. Fourteen patients were alive and well 4 months to 3 years after surgery.

The choice between selective cerebral perfusion and hypothermic circulatory arrest for patients undergoing aortic arch reconstruction depends on the site and type of the aneurysm, as well as the surgeon's preference and experience. The latter technique involves limited cerebral circulatory arrest time.

▶ This report, describing experiences with 21 patients having aortic arch reconstruction, indicates that selective cerebral perfusion may be employed effectively in selected patients. This approach was taken in 11 of the 21 patients, perfusing at a rate of 600 mL/min at 25°C into the innominate and left carotid arteries. Blood pressure, monitored through the right radial artery, ranged from 50 mm Hg to 70 mm.

Results were excellent. The unanswerable question is when selective cerebral perfusion should be used in preference simply to hypothermic circulatory arrest. The latter is preferable if the period of cerebral ischemia is not prolonged. The safe limit seems to be in the range of 45–60 minutes, but conclusive data are not available.—F.C. Spencer, M.D.

18 The Arteries, the Veins, and the Lymphatics

Alcohol Sclerotherapy of Nonparasitic Cysts of the Liver
Andersson R, Jeppsson B, Lunderquist A, Bengmark S (Lund Univ, Sweden)
Br J Surg 76:254–255, March 1989   18–1

Nonparasitic liver cysts are either congenital or acquired. Congenital cysts are more common and are considered to be embryologic malformations. Most congenital cysts remain asymptomatic and require no treatment. A high recurrence rate has been associated with conservative treatment of aspiration alone. A total of 9 patients had aspiration of nonparasitic liver cysts followed by instillation of a sclerosing agent.

The 9 patients (7 women, 2 men, aged 40–77 years) were treated between 1980 and 1987 and CT-guided percutaneous puncture and evacuation of the cyst contents followed by injection of absolute alcohol as a sclerosing agent. Multiple cysts were found in 6 patients and 3 had a single cyst. The largest cysts were between 5 cm and 20 cm in diameter.

After ethanol instillation some patients noted slight abdominal pain, and 1 woman had symptoms of moderate alcohol intoxication. A total of 29 punctures and injections were performed. A mean of 650 mL of cyst fluid was drained per procedure with a range from 50 mL to 3,100 mL. For 8–54 months, follow-up was performed with CT or ultrasonography. Results were considered to be good or excellent in 8 of the 9 patients; 2 were operated on because of residual or multiple cysts.

The procedure has not resulted in severe complications or signs of damage to liver tissue. Computed tomography-guided alcohol sclerotherapy appears to be a safe and effective initial therapy for nonparasitic liver cysts.

▶ The article presents encouraging results. It is certainly true that conservative treatment with aspiration of cyst fluid alone results in a high recurrence rate. The surgical management of these patients is relatively simple and involves merely unroofing the cyst widely. Some have advised using a sclerosing agent on the remaining cyst wall. It is somewhat surprising that sclerotherapy via CT-guided needle should be so effective; I would imagine that it would be difficult to expose all of the cyst wall to the sclerosing solution.—S.I. Schwartz, M.D.

Combining Clinical and Thallium Data Optimizes Preoperative Assessment of Cardiac Risk Before Major Vascular Surgery

Eagle KA, Coley CM, Newell JB, Brewster DC, Darling RC, Strauss HW, Guiney TE, Boucher CA (Massachusetts Gen Hosp, Boston)

Ann Intern Med 110:859–866, June 1, 1989   18–2

Preoperative cardiac evaluation of patients undergoing major vascular surgery is important to identify those at high risk in whom special monitoring or treatment may help to improve the outcome. Such evaluation is especially important in patients considered for major vascular surgery, in whom the prevalence of severe underlying coronary disease approaches 33% and in whom cardiac ischemic events account for more than 50% of postoperative deaths. The results of preoperative screening were reviewed and the ability of clinical features and dipyridamole-thallium imaging to predict postoperative ischemic events was compared in 200 patients undergoing nonemergent vascular surgery.

Thirty patients (15%) had 1 or more postoperative ischemic events. Six patients died of cardiac disease. Acute nonfatal myocardial infarction occurred in 4.5%. Of all patients with postoperative ischemic events, 83% had thallium redistribution on preoperative dipyridamole-thallium imaging. The univariate correlates of cardiac death or myocardial infarction included a history of angina, congestive heart failure, and diabetes mellitus. An S_3 gallop on evaluation and pathologic Q wave on ECG were correlated with postoperative ischemic outcomes. Two of 4 dipyridamole-thallium test variables correlated with ischemic events: ischemic ECG changes during dipyridamole infusion and thallium redistribution. Of the 64 patients with none of the 4 clinical variables—Q wave on ECG, age more than 70 years, history of angina, history of ventricular ectopic activity necessitating treatment, and diabetes mellitus requiring treatment—only 2 experienced postoperative cardiac ischemic events, and none died. Ten of 20 patients with 3 or more of these variables had postoperative ischemic events.

Preoperative dipyridamole-thallium imaging appears most useful in stratifying patients at intermediate risk according to clinical examination. Thallium redistribution correlates with a substantial change in probability of events in patients with 1 or 2 clinical predictors. However, for almost half of the patients, thallium imaging may be unnecessary because of very high or very low cardiac risk according to clinical assessment.

▶ Goldman has assessed the cardiac risks and complications of noncardiac surgery (1) and developed a multifactorial index score to estimate that risk. It is particularly pertinent to stratify vascular patients because of their high incidence of severe underlying coronary disease. The combination of pertinent clinical predictors and the salient imaging, when appropriate, appears to provide the most meaningful information.—S.I. Schwartz, M.D.

Reference

1. Goldman L: *Ann Surg* 198:780, 1983.

Limb Salvage Despite Extensive Tissue Loss: Free Tissue Transfer Combined With Distal Revascularization
Cronenwett JL, McDaniel MD, Zwolak RM, Walsh DB, Schneider JR, Reus WF, Colen LB (Dartmouth-Hitchcock Med Ctr, Hanover, NH; VA Med Ctr, White River Junction, Vt)
Arch Surg 124:609–615, May 1989   18–3

Extensive tissue loss may preclude limb salvage despite successful arterial reconstruction, particularly in diabetic patients with large hindfoot or ankle ulcers that expose tendon and bone with accompanying chronic infection. The combination of distal arterial reconstruction and microvascular free tissue transfer avoids limb loss in these patients. Fourteen patients, aged 33–74 years, with extensive tissue loss in 15 lower extremities exposing bone or tendon on the heel, ankle, lower part of the leg, or hindfoot, underwent distal arterial revascularization followed by free tissue transfer to achieve limb salvage. The mean ulcer size was 5 × 8 cm. Twelve patients had diabetes, and 4 had had previous contralateral below-knee amputations.

Femorotibial peroneal bypass was performed in 7 limbs, popliteal-distal bypass in 3, femoropopliteal bypass in 4, and tibial angioplasty in 1. Muscular or fascial free flaps combined with split-thickness skin graft or fasciocutaneous free flaps were used to obtain soft tissue coverage. Serratus anterior, scapular, latissimus dorsi, rectus abdominis, gracilis, ulnar, or temporalis free flaps were used. Both free flap and arterial reconstructive procedures were performed during the same operation in 2 patients. The mean interval between arterial reconstruction and free flap coverage was 13 days.

Limb salvage was achieved in 14 limbs (93%) during a mean follow-up of 24 months (range, 4–38 months). The single amputation occurred because of severe foot ischemia in a patient whose femorodistal bypass remained patent only to the viable free flap. Of the 13 patent bypass grafts, 1 required a subsequent vein patch angioplasty of the popliteal anastomosis to prevent thrombosis. Of the 17 free flaps, 12 healed primarily and 3 healed after minor surgical revision of the wound edges, for an 88% success rate. Of the 16 ulcers treated, 15 healed completely. Weight-bearing ambulation was achieved in 13 of 14 patients.

Lower-extremity revascularization combined with free tissue transfer may allow limb salvage in a subgroup of patients with severe ischemic tissue loss of a lower extremity. These patients usually have diabetes and have large, deep ulcers on the hindfoot or ankle that have developed in association with peripheral neuropathy.

▶ This exciting approach can be regarded as the ultimate refinement to achieve limb salvage. The first advance in achieving limb salvage was made by the vascular surgeon who effected successful arterial and, at times, venous reconstruction. The addition of microvascular free tissue transfer in ischemic limbs certainly addresses the issue of soft tissue defects that previously were not reconstructable. The authors are to be congratulated. The technique is applicable to trauma patients.—S.I. Schwartz, M.D.

Anaphylactoid Reactions to Protamine: An Often Lethal Complication in Insulin-Dependent Diabetic Patients Undergoing Vascular Surgery

Gupta SK, Veith FJ, Ascer E, Wengerter KR, Franco C, Amar D, El-Gaweet E-S, Gupta A (Montefiore Med Ctr-Albert Einstein College of Medicine, New York; New York Med College, Valhalla)
J Vasc Surg 9:342–350, February 1988   18–4

Protamine sulfate is used to reverse the anticoagulant effect of heparin in patients requiring short-term anticoagulation during cardiac catheterization, transluminal angioplasty, cardiac and vascular operations, and hemodialysis. Protamine is an extract isolated from the male gonads of salmon and other fish. Allergic reactions have been reported in patients with fish allergy, and a significant number of adverse reactions have been reported in diabetic patients treated with neutral protamine Hagedorn (NPH) insulin. It was postulated that the frequent small doses of NPH sensitize the patient. This is of special interest to the vascular surgeon because many patients requiring vascular surgery are diabetic.

Of 1,150 patients (table) 11 had major adverse reactions to protamine. After 10 minutes of protamine administration their blood pressures decreased to less than 60 mm Hg and major resuscitative efforts were required. Of the major reactions 9 occurred in 325 patients with insulin-dependent diabetes, an incidence of 3%. Only 2 reactions occurred in the 825 patients not receiving insulin, an incidence of 0.2%. The difference was significant. Of the 11 reactions, 10 occurred within 10 minutes of administration of 10 mg to 35 mg of protamine, and 1 reaction occurred immediately after a 5-mg test dose of protamine. Closed-chest message was necessary in 3. In 7 cases initial treatment was successful with epinephrine and steroids. Further resuscitation measures were needed in 4 patients; 1 had ventricular fibrillation and died. Including the 1 who died, 10 of the 11 patients had significant preexisting cardiac disease. Of the surviving 10, six had perioperative myocardial infarction and 3 died. The total mortality rate was 36%.

In diabetics, NPH insulin appears to produce an adverse reaction through immunologic presensitization. Protamine reactions can be lethal in older individuals with significant cardiac disease. Protamine therapy should be avoided in diabetic patients receiving insulin.

▶ The article brings into focus an uncommon but significant issue. The problem can be addressed by using smaller doses of heparin (30 mg/kg) but does not necessitate protamine reversal. In the discussion of this work, Wakefield reported the significant reduction in systemic arterial pressure associated with protamine reversal with heparin with drops as severe as 70

Information on 11 Patients With Major Adverse Reactions to Protamine

Patient No.	Age (yr)	Diabetes	Insulin	Cardiac history	Past history of protamine use	Total protamine dose (mg)	Time from dose to reaction (min)	Bronchospasm	Arrest	Postoperative MI	Death
1	75	No	None	AFIB	No	25	10	No	No	Yes	Yes
2	69	Yes	NPH	CABG	Yes	25	15	Yes	No	No	No
3	70	Yes	NPH	Angina	No	35	5	No	Yes*	Yes	Yes
4	46	Yes	NPH	MI	Yes	30	6	No	No	No	Yes†
5	75	Yes	NPH	MI	Yes	15	10	Yes	No	Yes	No
6	66	Yes	NPH	No	No	35	10	No	No	No	No
7	74	No	None	MI	Yes	25	10	No	Yes*	No	No
8	64	Yes	NPH	Angina	Yes	25	5	No	Yes*	Yes	Yes
9	57	Yes	NPH	MI	Yes	30	5	No	Yes	Yes	No
10	60	Yes	NPH	MI	No	25	10	No	No	No	No
11	72	Yes	NPH	MI	No	5	1	Yes	Yes	Yes	Yes

Abbreviations: MI, myocardial infarction; AFIB, atrial fibrillation; CABG, coronary artery bypass grafting.
*Required defibrillation.
†Died in the operating room.
(Courtesy of Gupta SK, Veith FJ, Ascer E, et al: *J Vasc Surg* 9:342–350, February 1988.)

mm Hg. Associated with the hypotension were changes in pulmonary artery pressure, bradycardia, thrombocytopenia, and leukopenia. It has also been demonstrated that protamine causes a decrease in systemic oxygen tension.—S.I. Schwartz, M.D.

Hypercoagulable States and Lower Limb Ischemia in Young Adults

Eldrup-Jorgensen J, Flanigan DP, Brace L, Sawchuk AP, Mulder SG, Anderson CP, Schuler JJ, Meyer JR, Durham JR, Schwarcz TH (Univ of Illinois College of Associated Health Professions, Chicago)
J Vasc Surg 9:334–341, February 1989   18–5

Deficiencies of natural anticoagulants, disorders of the fibrinolytic system, presence of lupus-like anticoagulants (LLA), or abnormalities of platelet function may cause hypercoagulable states. The latter may contribute to the progression of arterial occlusive disease and arterial thrombosis. Because young adults have a particularly severe and aggressive form of atherosclerosis, the relationship between hypercoagulability and arterial occlusive disease in young adults was evaluated in 20 patients younger than 51 years undergoing lower extremity revascularization for ischemia.

The patients, who ranged in age from 23 to 50, underwent operation for ischemia during a 20-month period. All had preoperative hypercoagulability followed by lower extremity revascularization. Of the patients 15 were male, 10 were black, 6 had hypertension, and 4 were diabetic. Rest pain or tissue necrosis in 18 patients and disabling claudication in 2 were indications for operation; 13 infrainguinal procedures and 7 aortoiliac procedures were performed. Of the patients, 9 had at least 1 abnormality of regulatory proteins or LLA: protein S deficiency in 4, protein C deficiency in 3, LLA in 3, and plasminogen deficiency in 2. Of 17 patients in whom platelet aggregation profiles were obtained, 8 had increased reactivity. Only 4 of 17 patients were normal when tested for all parameters. Within 30 days of operation arterial or graft thrombosis developed in 4 of 20 patients. In all 4 patients whose revascularization failed, hypercoagulability was found.

In patients younger than 51 years with lower limb ischemia requiring revascularization, a high incidence of hypercoagulable status was found. Hypercoagulability may have contributed to early postoperative thrombosis of the vascular procedure.

▶ There is a suggestion in the discussion that it may be appropriate to screen for hypercoagulable situations in young patients who have peripheral vascular disease. Towne has been unable to identify either protein C or protein S deficiency as a sole cause of arterial thrombosis. It is accepted that patients with antithrombin deficiencies should be treated with fresh-frozen plasma to replace the factor. Fresh-frozen plasma can also be used in treatment of protein C or protein S deficiency, or these patients can be managed with heparin and coumadin.—S.I. Schwartz, M.D.

Injuries to the Ascending Aorta, Aortic Arch and Great Vessels

Weaver FA, Suda RW, Stiles GM, Yellin AE (Los Angeles County/Univ of Southern California Med Ctr)
Surg Gynecol Obstet 169:27–31, July 1989   18–6

Fifty-one injuries to the ascending aorta, aortic arch, and great vessels were treated in 45 male and 1 female patient from 1977 to 1987. Forty-two patients had a single injury, most often to the subclavian or common carotid artery. Forty-two injuries (82%) were caused by penetrating trauma. Nine patients were hypotensive when admitted and 2 arrived in cardiopulmonary arrest. Sixteen patients (35%) required immediate operation. Lateral and end-to-end arterial repairs were done in 32 patients (62%). Prosthetic material was used in 11 of 12 patients who required an interposition graft.

All 49 arterial reconstructions remained patent after operation. One patient required reoperation for bleeding at the suture line. No extremity with concomitant venous injury had significant swelling whether the vein was repaired or ligated. Three patients with isolated injuries to the left subclavian artery died, 1 before repair was attempted.

Hemodynamically unstable patients with injury of the aorta or a great vessel require emergency exploration. Stable patients suspected of having arterial injury should have diagnostic angiography. A flexible surgical approach is best; left anterior thoracotomy and cervical exposure should be incorporated when indicated. Cardiopulmonary bypass should be available for repair of injuries to the ascending aorta.

► This is a relatively large series addressing an uncommon injury. Fortunately, management of these injuries has been refined to a degree that the mortality rate has been significantly reduced. The authors appropriately stress that emergency room thoracotomy for blunt injuries is uniformly fatal. A role should be reserved, however, for penetrating injuries, and it is interesting that one of their patients subjected to emergency room thoracotomy survived. In this area there is a little question that the liberal use of angiography is important and will define the presence of unsuspected injury.— S.I. Schwartz, M.D.

Aorta-Vena Cava Fistula

Alexander JJ, Imbembo AL (Case Western Reserve Univ)
Surgery 105:1–12, January 1989   18–7

Aortocaval fistulas can occur spontaneously or develop as a traumatic complication. Although early reports indicated that traumatic aortocaval fistulas were more common, spontaneous aortocaval fistulas are now seen more frequently and comprise 80% to 90% of all cases; traumatic injury accounts for the other 10% to 20%.

The spontaneous aortocaval fistula develops most often at, or immediately above, the venous bifurcation. About 90% of the spontaneous fistulas develop as a result of erosion or rupture of an atherosclerotic infrarenal aortic aneurysm into the vena cava. Rupture of an aneurysm caused by syphilis, bacterial infection, Marfan's syndrome, or Ehlers-Danlos syndrome is far less common in aortocaval fistula formation.

The traumatic aortocaval fistula may develop after blunt or penetrating injuries to the aorta and vena cava. A traumatic aortocaval fistula may also develop as a complication of lumbar disk surgery. Previous studies have reported that vascular injury complicates approximately 4% of all lumbar disk procedures, with arteriovenous fistula formation accounting for 10% to 45% of these vascular injuries.

The development of an aortocaval fistula results in extensive hemodynamic alteration as blood flow from the high-resistance arterial circuit is diverted into the lower-resistance, high-capacitance venous circuit. Such hemodynamic alterations cause cardiac hypertrophy, dilatation, and, eventually, intractable cardiac failure. The general clinical course of a patient with a spontaneous aortocaval fistula is characterized by progressive cardiac decompensation and death.

Treatment involves transaortic closure of the fistula and restoration of arterial continuity with a prosthetic graft. Surgical repair spontaneous aortocaval fistulas still has a reported early mortality rate of 22% to 51%. However, increasing experience has resulted in better understanding and improved surgical treatment of these large-vessel arteriovenous communications.

▶ This is an inclusive review of a rare disorder. As the authors point out, although the operative mortality is certainly significant, success can be achieved.— S.I. Schwartz, M.D.

Inflammatory Aneurysms of the Abdominal Aorta: Incidence, Pathologic, and Etiologic Considerations

Sterpetti AV, Hunter WJ, Feldhaus RJ, Chasan P, McNamara M, Cisternino S, Schultz RD (Creighton Univ, Omaha)
J Vasc Surg 9:643–650, May 1989   18–8

Inflammatory abdominal aortic aneurysm (AAA) is characterized by dense, fibrotic, perianeurysmal fibrosis. Although inflammatory AAA appears to be a distinct clinicopathologic entity, its cause, treatment and natural history are controversial. The records of 486 patients who underwent surgical repair of an AAA during a 12-year period were reviewed retrospectively.

Of the 486 patients, 30 had inflammatory AAA, based on the gross appearance of the lesion. Of these 30 patients, 27 had symptoms referable to their aneurysm, compared with 80 of the 456 patients with ordinary atherosclerotic AAA. Three patients with inflammatory AAA had significant weight loss, compared with 33 patients with atherosclerotic AAA. Six patients (20%) with inflammatory AAA had symptoms of obstructive uropathy, compared with 6 patients (1%) with atherosclerotic AAA.

A diagnosis of inflammatory aneurysm was suspected before operation in only 4 of the 30 patients, as diagnostic tests, including abdominal ultrasound and angiography, did not reveal the inflammatory nature of the aneurysm. At laparotomy the inflammatory aneurysm was seen to be encased in a thick, shiny, dense, whitish fibrotic process contiguous with the AAA and extending in all directions. All 21 surgical specimens of inflammatory AAA available for review had evidence of atherosclerotic disease of the aorta with intimal fibrosis and extensive mural thrombosis. On the other hand, 23 of 100 atherosclerotic AAA specimens had varying degrees of chronic inflammation.

Inflammatory AAAs are atherosclerotic aneurysms having an unusual accentuation of the chronic inflammatory process as compared with atherosclerotic aneurysms. As in patients with nonruptured atherosclerotic AAAs, excellent early and late results after operation can be expected in patients with inflammatory AAAs. Excessive dissection and lysis of the ureter and duodenum should be avoided.

▶ It is generally believed that if the diagnosis of an inflammatory aneurysm is suspected preoperatively, evaluation of the ureters should be performed. Many surgeons do not seem to need to dissect the ureters in these patients. Late ureteral obstruction is an uncommon circumstance. This would suggest that ureterolysis is not necessary. I've always wondered whether this inflammatory aneurysm is actually a misnomer, and that what we are considering is actually an atherosclerotic aneurysm that stimulated an inflammatory response in the surrounding tissue.—S.I. Schwartz, M.D.

Comparative Analysis of Retroperitoneal and Transperitoneal Aortic Replacement for Aneurysm
Leather RP, Shah DM, Kaufman JL, Fitzgerald KM, Chang BB, Feustel PJ (Albany Medical College, NY)
Surg Gynecol Obstet 168:387–393, May 1989   18–9

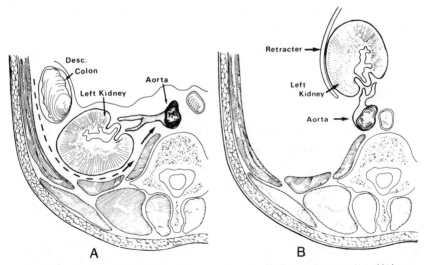

Fig 18–1.—**A**, plane of dissection into the retroperitoneal space. **B**, anterior retraction of kidney to expose the aorta. (Courtesy of Leather RP, Shah DM, Kaufman JL, et al: *Surg Gynecol Obstet* 168:387–393, May 1989.)

Retroperitoneal exposure with nonresective exclusion and inline aortic bypass is an effective approach to infrarenal aortic aneurysms. Morbidity may be less than with the conventional transperitoneal approach. The results of extended retroperitoneal surgery in 193 patients were compared with those of transabdominal operations in 106 patients. In most of the former patients the aneurysm was left intact after the infrarenal aorta was divided for end-to-end proximal anastomosis of an aortoaortic-to-iliac-to-femoral bypass. If a bifurcation graft was required, each graft limb was joined to the appropriate femoral or iliac vessel.

Operative mortality was 3.7%, with no difference between surgical groups. Perioperative morbidity also was comparable in the 2 groups. However, patients in the retroperitoneal group recovered more rapidly and resumed oral alimentation sooner. Blood loss was greater with transperitoneal surgery, and these patients required transfusions more frequently.

These findings support the routine use of retroperitoneal aortic exposure in elective operations for abdominal aortic aneurysm (Fig 18–1). The left extended retroperitoneal approach is recommended at present. Very short aneurysms are best managed by graft inclusion and larger ones by the exclusion technique.

▶ I was pleased to see this article reporting a large series, and the findings are in concert with my own observations. Rob (1) pointed out some of the intrinsic advantages of the extraperitoneal approach, and there is little question that it does represent an overall reduction in the physiologic disturbance of the patient. In the obese patient it offers a distinct advantage. Sicard et al. (2) compared the transabdominal and retroperitoneal approaches to reconstruction of the infrarenal abdominal aorta, and also concluded that the retroperitoneal approach was preferable. I have found that the same advantage can be applied to the distal splenorenal shunt in obese patients.—S.I. Schwartz, M.D.

References

1. Rob C: *Surgery* 53:87, 1963.
2. Sicard GA, et al: *J Vasc Surg* 5:19, 1987.

Ischemic Colitis Following Abdominal Aortic Reconstruction for Ruptured Aneurysm: A 10-Year Experience
Maupin GE, Rimar SD, Villalba M (William Beaumont Hosp, Royal Oak, Mich)
Am Surg 55:378–380, June 1989   18–10

Approximately half of all patients who reach the hospital alive with a ruptured abdominal aortic aneurysm (AAA) ultimately die of it. Survivors of emergency operation of an AAA are at increased risk for ischemic colitis. The frequency and severity of ischemic colitis in 103 patients who survived operation of a ruptured AAA were determined.

During a 10-year period, 88 men and 15 women aged 53–91 years

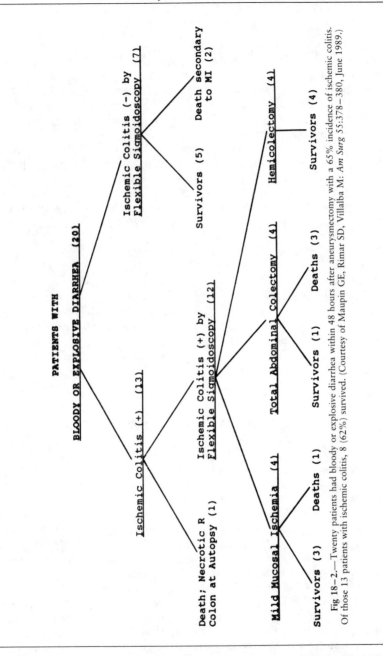

Fig 18-2.—Twenty patients had bloody or explosive diarrhea within 48 hours after aneurysmectomy with a 65% incidence of ischemic colitis. Of those 13 patients with ischemic colitis, 8 (62%) survived. (Courtesy of Maupin GE, Rimar SD, Villalba M: *Am Surg* 55:378–380, June 1989.)

(average, 73 years) underwent aneurysmectomy and aortic reconstruction of a ruptured AAA. Thirty-two of the 103 patients died during operation or by the first postoperative day; 39 patients died later from a variety of causes. The overall mortality was 69%. Ischemic colitis developed in 19 of the 71 patients who survived operation. This group included 16 men and 3 women aged 53–90 years (average, 72 years). Eleven of the 19 patients died and 8 survived, for a mortality rate of 58%.

Twenty patients had bloody or explosive diarrhea 24–48 hours after operation (Fig 18–2). One patient died of sepsis. The other 19 patients underwent flexible sigmoidoscopy. Seven of the 19 patients had no signs of ischemic colitis, 5 of whom survived; 2 died of myocardial infarction. Of the 12 patients with ischemic colitis, 8 survived and 4 died. Ischemic colitis was diagnosed between 9 and 20 days after operation in 6 additional patients. None of these 6 patients had diarrhea, but all had signs of increasing sepsis and all died of multiple organ failure related to ischemic colitis.

Because of the high incidence of ischemic colitis, routine flexible sigmoidoscopy within 48 hours of successful repair of a ruptured AAA is recommended, even in patients who have no diarrhea.

▶ Ischemic colitis represents one of the most major complications following abdominal aortic surgery. The proposal for the routine use of flexible sigmoidoscopy early in the postoperative period in all patients is an interesting one. Fiddian-Green et al. (1) proposed recording the intramural pH during aortic operations as a means of detecting sigmoid colon ischemia. They believe that reoperation may be wanted if the pH remains below normal after operation. It is appreciated that between 5% and 10% of patients having aortic surgery may have some type of bowel ischemia, but fewer than 1% progressed to infarction.—S.I. Schwartz, M.D.

Reference

1. Fiddian-Green RG, et al: *Arch Surg* 121:654, 1986.

Extraanatomical Bypass Procedures
Blaisdell FW (Univ of California, Davis, Sacramento)
World J Surg 12:798–804, December 1988   18–11

Femorofemoral, axillofemoral, and iliofemoral transobturator bypass procedures are used in the treatment of patients with vascular ischemic disease of the lower extremities considered at too high risk for conventional bypass procedures. Infection, which precludes graft placement in a conventional location in patients who require life- or limb-saving revascularization, is now an established absolute indication for extra-anatomical bypass. Associated disease and anticipated technical problems are deemed relative indications for extra-anatomical bypass. The use of an axillofemoral graft to bypass an aortic aneurysm remains a most controversial indication.

Axillofemoral bypass operations can be done with the use of local anesthesia but are preferably performed with light general anesthesia. The proximal one third of the axillary artery yields the best results in axillofemoral bypass procedures. Important technical requirements include

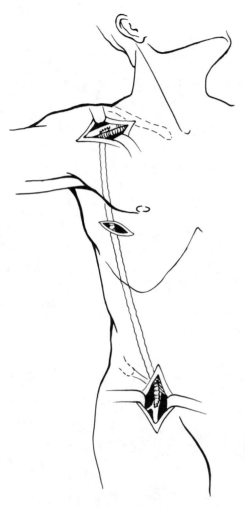

Fig 18–3.—Axillofemoral bypass. (Courtesy of Blaisdell FW: *World J Surg* 12:798–804, December 1988.)

the need to tunnel the graft well laterally so that it lies in the body's plane of flexion, and the use of a femorofemoral graft in conjunction with the axillofemoral graft to provide 2 outflow segments for the graft, 1 into the ipsilateral and 1 into the contralateral leg (Fig 18–3).

Technical requirements for the femorofemoral graft include the need to place the anastomoses in so as to avoid kinking and to place the graft in a subcutaneous or subfascial position, depending on the patient's degree of obesity or presence of existing scars. The technical aspects of the iliofemoral transobturator bypass vary, as they depend on the most accessible proximal vessel, usually the common iliac artery.

The literature reports wide variation in the results obtained with extra-anatomical bypass procedures (table). Reported 1-year patency rates for axillofemoral grafts have varied from 50% to 87%, with 5-year patency rates ranging from 25% to 76%. For the femorofemoral bypass, 1-year

Results of Axillofemoral Grafts

Year	N	Mortality (%) 30 day	Mortality (%) 5 yr	Patency (%) 1 yr	Patency (%) 5 yr	Graft Type	N	Patency (%) 1 yr	Patency (%) 5 yr	Comment
1977	130	8	23	77	70	AF*	64	64	37	No significant difference between PTFE and Dacron grafts.
						AFF	66	89	74	
1977	59	8	73	50	25	—	—	—	—	
1977	56	2	37	73	67	AFF	56	82	76	
1978	45	2	32			AF	25	60	51	
						AFF	20	90	90	
1979	84	3.7	32	84	72	AF	33	75	67	(96%)† 1 yr; (71%)† 5 yr AF
						AFF	21	90	77	(96%)† 1 yr; (77%)† 5 yr AFF
1982	220	3.6	24	87	66	—	—	—	—	
1985	56	5.3	57	75	47	AF	34	68	44	No significant difference between 8 and 10 mm Dacron grafts.
						AFF	22	84	50	
1986	88	2	47	(96)†	(75)†	AF	47	—	33	No significant difference between PTFE and Dacron patency.
						AFF	41	—	75	
1986	85	3.6	45	78	72	—	—	—	—	

*AF, axillounifemoral; AFF, axillobifemoral.
†Number in parentheses signifes patency with graft thrombectomy.
(Courtesy of Blaisdell FW: World J Surg 12:798–804, December 1988.)

patency rates varying between 82% and 93%, with 5-year patency rates varying from 56% to 86%, have been reported. The results of obturator bypass are not yet available.

▶ An article written by the individual who carried out one of the first extra-anatomical bypass procedures and was the major champion of the operation in the early 1960s is obviously significant. The author's use of external support for the graft is not endorsed by everyone. His emphasis on the principle of double outflow for the femoral anastomosis is appropriate. Johnson et al. (1) demonstrated that the axillo-bifemoral bypass graft is superior to the axillo-unilateral bypass graft.—S.I. Schwartz, M.D.

Reference

1. Johnson WC, et al: *Ann Surg* 186:123, 1977.

Vein Patch vs. Primary Closure for Carotid Endarterectomy: A Randomized Prospective Study in a Selected Group of Patients
Clagett GP, Patterson CB, Fisher DF Jr, Fry RE, Eidt JF, Humble TH, Fry WJ
(Univ of Texas, Dallas; Dallas VA Med Ctr)
J Vasc Surg 9:213–223, February 1989   18–12

To reduce complications, vein patch is often advocated for closure after carotid endarterectomy. However, vein patch closure is not without its own complications, and operating time is increased with this procedure. Because excellent results have also been reported with primary closure, many surgeons recommend selective, rather than routine, vein patch closure. During a 4-year period, 136 patients undergoing 152 carotid endarterectomies were randomized to receive either saphenous vein patch or primary closure of the arteriotomy.

Arterial dimensions and anatomy were carefully assessed at operation, before randomization. Patients with a small internal carotid artery (ICA) diameter or a twisted ICA, and those with longer arteriotomies, received an obligatory vein patch closure. The remaining patients were randomized. Patients were followed up every 3 months for 1 year and twice yearly thereafter by duplex scanning, ocular pneumoplethysmography, and neurologic evaluation.

Perioperative morbidity did not differ significantly between patients randomized for vein patch closure, those with primary closure, and those with obligatory vein patch closure. Operating time was significantly reduced in patients having primary closure. There were no deaths and no significant postoperative occlusions in any group. One patient in each group had a perioperative stroke. Recurrent disease was more common in patients with vein patch closure (12.9% vs. 1.7%), but recurrences were moderate stenoses not requiring additional surgery. In most recurrences there was evidence that thrombus layering in the dilated part of the saphenous vein patch reconstruction was responsible.

In men with carotid arteries of predetermined minimal dimensions who are undergoing carotid endarterectomy, results of saphenous vein patch closure are not superior to those with primary closure. The vein patch procedure is also associated with a higher incidence of early recurrence and longer operating time. The saphenous vein patch closure, however, is appropriate in selected patients.

▶ A similar randomized study, Eikelboom et al. (1) indicated that the rate of recurrent carotid stenosis after carotid endarterectomy was reduced more by patching than by primary closure, and that this was especially true in women. It has been suggested that hypercholesterolemia has a strong association with restenosis after carotid endarterectomy, and that it seems rational to perform a patch procedure in these patients. Stewart and associates (2) presented data to suggest that vein angioplasty has a positive effect.— S.I. Schwartz, M.D.

References

1. Eikelboom BC, et al: *J Vasc Surg* 7:240, 1988.
2. Stewart GW, et al: *Arch Surg* 122:364, 1987.

Recurrent Carotid Artery Stenosis: Resection With Autogenous Vein Replacement

Edwards WH Jr, Edwards WH Sr, Mulherin JL Jr, Martin RS III (St Thomas Hosp, Nashville; Vanderbilt Univ)
Ann Surg 209:662–668, June 1989   18–13

Recurrent carotid artery stenosis (RCAS) occurs in about 10% to 15% of patients after carotid endarterectomy (CEA). The RCAS may occur as early as 6 months after CEA and is estimated to become symptomatic in 3% to 5% of such patients. Although a second endarterectomy with patch graft is the most commonly used procedure in the treatment of RCAS, resection and vein graft interposition may offer a safe and effective alternative for restoring cerebral blood flow.

During a 14-year period, 3,711 CEAs were performed in 2,909 patients, 98 (3.5%) of whom required 106 reoperations. Most of the 98 had a second endarterectomy with patch grafting, but 9 men and 8 women (mean age, 66 years) underwent 20 resections of the common carotid artery and internal carotid artery with autogenous vein grafting. Of these 17 patients, 12 had undergone a previous CEA, 7 had 2 previous CEAs, and 1 had 3 previous CEAs. Indications for reoperation included hemispheric symptoms in 14 patients, asymptomatic tight stenosis of more than 80% in 3, and nonlateralizing symptoms and tight stenosis in 2. The interval between the last CEA and vein replacement ranged from 6 months to 10 years (average, 4.5 years).

No hospital deaths occurred. The patient who had undergone 3 previous CEAs had postoperative hypoglossal nerve palsy and hoarseness that

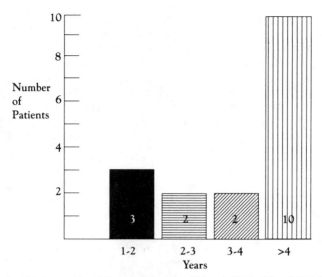

Fig 18–4.—Vein interposition (follow-up). (Courtesy of Edwards WH Jr, Edwards WH Sr, Mulherin JL Jr, et al: *Ann Surg* 209:662–668, June 1989.)

was slow to resolve. Another patient had contralateral hemiparesis 24 hours after operation; at emergency reoperation a thrombosed vein graft was found and replaced. Follow-up ranged from 6 months to more than 6 years, with a mean of almost 3 years (Fig 18–4). One patient had restenosis at the proximal suture line 4 months after vein grafting caused by a size mismatch between the common carotid artery and the vein graft. This patient died suddenly at home of myocardial infarction. The other 16 patients remained asymptomatic.

Resection of the common carotid artery and internal carotid artery with replacement by autogenous vein graft offers a safe and effective alternative to a second endarterectomy with patch grafting for restoring cerebral blood flow. This procedure also potentially prevents another recurrence of stenosis.

▶ This is a large experience directed at management of a difficult situation. It is particularly interesting in reference to the replacement by autogenous vein. In most instances, the stenosis has been managed by recurrent endarterectomy and angioplasty. The authors appropriately stressed the routine use of resection, and replacement of the vein is not justified.—S.I. Schwartz, M.D.

Intermittent Claudication—Surgical Reconstruction or Physical Training: A Prospective Randomized Trial of Treatment Efficiency
Lundgren F, Dahllöf A-G, Lundholm K, Scherstén T, Volkmann R (Univ of Göteborg, Sweden)
Ann Surg 209:346–355, March 1989   18–14

Previous studies found that patients with intermittent claudication who are treated conservatively are at low risk for limb loss and have a fairly good chance of spontaneous improvement of symptoms. The efficacy of conservative treatment in patients with arterial insufficiency, with respect to symptom relief, compared with that of arterial reconstruction was evaluated in 75 patients with moderate to severe intermittent claudication who were randomly assigned to reconstructive arterial surgery, physical training, or the combination of both. The mean age was 64 years, and 93% of the patients were smokers. There were no statistically signif-

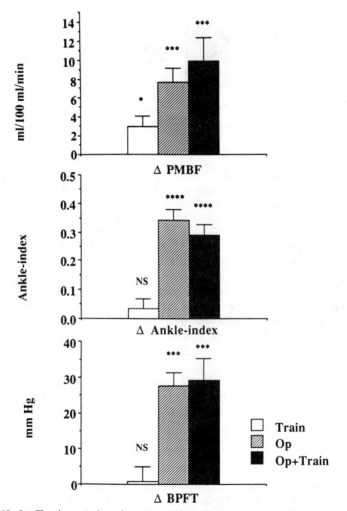

Fig 18–5.—The change in hemodynamic variables with treatment in the different groups. *MBF,* change in maximal calf blood flow measured with strain gauge plethysmography; *ankle-index,* change in ankle-arm blood pressure quotient; *BPFT,* change in blood pressure of the first toe. Data refer to the most symptomatic leg (Courtesy of Lundgren F, Dahllöf A-G, Lundholm K, et al: *Ann Surg* 209:346–355, March 1989.)

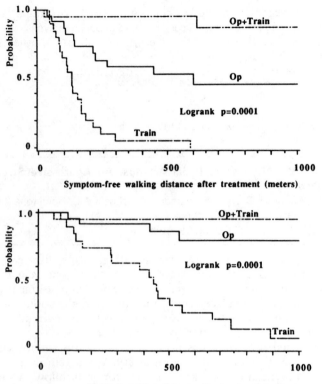

Fig 18–6.—Life-table representation of symptom-free and maximal walking performance after different treatments. Patients limited by symptoms other than intermittent claudication and those who walked farther than 1,000 m were right censored. (Courtesy of Lundgren F, Dahllöf A-G, Lundholm K, et al: *Ann Surg* 209:346–355, March 1989.)

icant differences between the 3 groups as to sex, age, presence of diabetes or associated atherosclerotic diseases, duration of arterial disease, ankle brachial blood pressure quotient, maximal plethysmographic calf blood flow, and walking performance before treatment.

After a mean 13-month follow-up, all 3 groups had significantly improved maximal plethysmographic calf blood flow (Fig 18–5) and symptom-free and maximal walking distance (Fig 18–6). However, patients who had physical training only showed no significant changes in ankle-index or blood pressure of the first toe.

Arterial reconstruction was clearly more effective than physical training alone. The addition of physical training to arterial reconstruction improved the symptom-free walking distance even further.

▶ A controversy remains regarding the advisability of femoral popliteal surgery in patients with intermittent claudication. After conservative treatment, particularly with physical training, the risk of limb loss is small. The durability of symptomatic relief related to training has not been defined, nor, on the other side, has the long-term patency and efficacy of femoral popliteal bypass in these patients. Wilson et al. (1) reported that the risk for limb loss in patients treated conservatively for intermittent claudication is smaller than 5% during a follow-up period extending to 8 years.—S.I. Schwartz, M.D.

Reference

1. Wilson SE, et al: *Am J Surg* 140:112, 1980.

Saphenous Vein Bypass to Pedal Arteries: An Aggressive Strategy for Foot Salvage

Harris HW, Rapp JH, Reilly LM, Orlando PA, Krupski WC, Goldstone J (VA Med Ctr, San Francisco; Univ of California, San Francisco)
Arch Surg 124:1232–1236, October 1989   18–15

Forefoot ischemia caused by advanced tibial artery disease presents a challenge to revascularization. Success with saphenous vein bypass to more proximal vessels led to a trial of this approach in 24 men with critical ischemia of a lower extremity that involved the foot. Two thirds were diabetic, half were hypertensive, and most were currently smoking. There were multiple tibial artery occlusions in all cases.

The preferred procedure has been to originate the in situ saphenous vein graft from the common femoral artery. When vein length is inadequate, the superficial femoral artery is used for graft inflow. A single vein sufficed in 23 cases. A modified Mills valvulotome was introduced through side branches of the vein to cut the valve leaflets. Heparin was given before occluding the arteries and low-molecular-weight dextran was infused.

Foot salvage was achieved in 83% of the patients during a mean follow-up of 14 months. Mean flow velocity in the bypass graft at the ankle was 60 cm/sec at discharge. Two grafts were treated successfully by percutaneous balloon angioplasty. Only 5 grafts failed, 3 of them within 2 months of surgery. Six major wound complications occurred.

Saphenous vein bypass to the pedal arteries provides salvage of extremities in patients who have severe infrapopliteal atherosclerosis and critical foot ischemia. Careful technique can reduce wound complications to an acceptable level.

▶ The salvage rate of 83% is certainly laudable. Other authors have indicated that the site of the distal anastomosis is usually the dorsalis pedis vessel, and it is rare that the posterior vessel is opened. Visualization of the vessels with arteriography is essential in planning the operative procedure. Most surgeons agree that the most sensitive technique for postoperative surveillance is duplex scanning, and the index for reintervention should be low.—S.I. Schwartz, M.D.

Monitoring Functional Patency of In Situ Saphenous Vein Bypasses: The Impact of a Surveillance Protocol and Elective Revision
Bandyk DF, Schmitt DD, Seabrook GR, Adams MB, Towne JB (Med College of Wisconsin, Milwaukee; VA Med Ctr, Milwaukee)
J Vasc Surg 9:286–296, February 1989   18–16

The steady decline of vascular graft patency with time mandates postoperative surveillance to identify grafts at risk for thrombosis. A postoperative surveillance protocol for monitoring in situ saphenous vein bypass patency was developed.

Between 1981 and 1988, 190 men and 41 women aged 42–92 years underwent 250 in situ saphenous vein bypass procedures because of occlusive or aneurysmal disease of a lower extremity. Of the 250 procedures, 163 were femorotibial bypasses, 83 were femoropopliteal, and 4 were isolated segment femoropopliteal. Indications for operation included critical limb ischemia in 232 (93%), popliteal aneurysm in 11 (4%), and disabling claudication in 7 (3%). All patients underwent preoperative and serial postoperative noninvasive hemodynamic testing at intervals of 1 and 7 days, 6 weeks, and 3 months after operation. Evaluation included arterial pressure measurements, continuous-wave Doppler spectral analysis, and duplex ultrasonography to assess patency and to detect and localize hemodynamic and anatomical changes indicative of graft stenosis.

Seventy (28%) of the 250 bypass grafts were identified as having correctable anatomical lesions, which required a total of 95 revisions. Ten bypass grafts were thrombosed at the time of graft revision. Correction of the vein conduit or anastomotic lesions was performed in 73 (77%) of the 95 revisions, correction of atherosclerotic lesions in the iliac accounted for 10%, and correction of infrapopliteal arteries accounted for 11%. The most commonly performed procedure was vein-patch angioplasty of a stenosis. Twenty-one graft lesions (10%) were corrected within 30 days of operation, 18 of which were identified by duplex scanning. The graft revision rate decreased to 7% per 6-month interval until 18 months after operation, and was 3% per year thereafter. The primary patency rate of grafts not identified as having a correctable lesion was 86% at 4 years, a level similar to the secondary patency of 81% for grafts requiring 1 or more revisions.

Surveillance by serial postoperative monitoring of functional patency of saphenous vein bypasses can identify grafts with correctable lesions before thrombosis occurs, thereby enabling timely elective revision of grafts at risk.

▶ There is little question that every attempt should be made to identify stenotic lesions before vein graft thrombosis occurs. Cohen et al. (1) reported on 29 patent grafts with stenoses identified by decreased ankle-brachial index. Patch angioplasty or percutaneous transluminal angioplasty resulted in a higher patency rate than thrombectomy did. Turnipseed and Acher also stressed the importance of preoperative surveillance as an effective means of detecting correctable lesions that threaten graft patency (2).—S.I. Schwartz, M.D.

References

1. Cohen JR, et al: *Arch Surg* 121:758, 1986.
2. Turnipseed WD, Acher CW: *Arch Surg* 123:324, 1985.

Initial Results of Laser Recanalization in Lower Extremity Arterial Reconstruction

Seeger JM, Abela GS, Silverman SH, Jablonski SK (Univ of Florida; VA Med Ctr, Gainesville, Fla)
J Vasc Surg 9:10–17, January 1989   18–17

Laser recanalization (LR) in the treatment of arteriosclerotic disease offers several advantages over more traditional techniques, particularly in elderly patients. However, the initial clinical results of trials in which LR was used to treat occluded superficial femoral or popliteal arteries have been somewhat disappointing. To identify those patients with peripheral arterial disease who would be most likely to benefit from treatment by LR, a 22-month study was undertaken in 195 patients with lower-extremity symptoms.

Of these 195 patients, 130 underwent angiographic examination to determine the site and degree of the occlusive disease; 110 were excluded because of inappropriate disease location. Another 39 patients were excluded because they had minimal symptoms, or the procedure was considered too risky. Only 46 patients (28%) were eventually considered suitable for LR treatment. Of these 46 patients, 19 had ischemic rest pain, 26 had claudication at less than 200 yd, and 1 had claudication at more than 200 yd.

Twenty-two of the 46 patients experienced relief of symptoms and had increased ankle brachial indexes after LR. The mean length of occlusion in these 22 patients was 8.8 cm, compared with 18.6 cm in patients in whom LR failed. However, 15 of the 22 patients in whom LR was successful subsequently required balloon dilatation because stenosis of more than 50% remained after LR. There were no complications in patients in whom LR was successful. Two patients experienced increased ischemia after LR failed, and 1 patient required emergency revascularization for ischemia after LR failed.

These results indicate that, at the present time and with the currently available instrumentation, LR has only limited usefulness in the treatment of peripheral vascular disease.

▶ Other recent articles have also addressed this issue. Wright et al. (1) assessed laser thermal angioplasty in 15 patients and concluded that, as it exists today, the technique has a limited role in the treatment of patients with limb-threatening ischemia. White and White, in an overview of the subject, find that recanalization of iliac-femoral and popliteal lesions can be accomplished in the majority of cases, with the chance of success being inversely proportional to the length of the occlusion. In tibial vessels results are also disappointing (2).— S.I. Schwartz, M.D.

References

1. Wright JG, et al: *J Vasc Surg* 10:29, 1989.
2. White RA, White GH: *J Vasc Surg* 9:598, 1989.

The Early Use of Operative Lumbar Sympathectomy in Peripheral Vascular Disease
Norman PE, House AK (Queen Elizabeth II Med Ctr, Nedlands, Western Australia; Univ of Western Australia, Nedlands)
J Cardiovasc Surg 29:717–722, November–December 1988   18–18

The present role of lumbar sympathectomy in the treatment of peripheral vascular disease is controversial. Since microsurgical vascular reconstruction has become available, lumbar sympathectomy has been reserved increasingly for the treatment of advanced vascular disease that is unsuitable for vascular reconstruction.

During a 13-year period 100 men and 53 women aged 38–91 years with intermittent claudication in 109 limbs and rest pain in 65 limbs underwent 174 standard L2–L5 operative lumbar sympathectomies as initial treatment. Twenty-one patients had bilateral symptoms. A below-the-groin vascular reconstructive procedure or amputation was performed thereafter only if symptoms were not alleviated by sympathectomy. All patients underwent arteriographic examinations, but the results did not affect patient selection for sympathectomy as long as the significant vascular occlusion was initially thought to be below the groin. Follow-up ranged from 4 to 13 years after sympathectomy.

After sympathectomy, the group with intermittent claudication had a postoperative mortality incidence of 0.9%, a 5-year survival of 60%, and a 10-year survival of 19%. The group with rest pain had a postoperative mortality of 4.6%, a 5-year survival of 32%, and a 10-year survival of 8%. The 5-year patient mortality from other manifestations of atherosclerosis was significantly greater than the sympathectomy failure rate after the first postoperative year. Limb survival contrasted with patient survival: 5 years after sympathectomy, 67% of the patients in the group with claudication and 54% of the patients in the group with rest pain had avoided further surgery. Limb survival in patients with diabetes did not differ significantly from that in patients who did not have diabetes.

Sympathectomy should be considered as first-line treatment in selected patients, as reconstructive surgery can still be performed if the procedure fails to produce adequate relief.

▶ The role of sympathectomy in arterial surgery remains controversial. Barnes et al. (1) have shown that when concomitant sympathectomy is performed during aortoiliac reconstruction there is no significant improvement in nutritional supply to the muscle, skin, or subcutaneous tissue. The limb survival data and the claudications have little meaning because one does not anticipate loss of limb in these patients. Few vascular surgeons would regard sympathectomy as a first-line procedure for patients with claudication or rest pain. The risks of reconstructive surgery are relatively low; it would be very difficult to select that group of patients in whom sympathectomy should be offered as the initial procedure.— S.I. Schwartz, M.D.

Reference

1. Barnes RW, et al: *Arch Surg* 112:1325, 1977.

Peripheral Arterial Embolectomy, Risks and Results
Takolander R, Lannerstad O, Bergqvist D (Univ of Lund, Gen Hosp, Malmö, Sweden)
Acta Chir Scand 154:567–572, October 1988   18–19

Risk factors for mortality associated with peripheral arterial embolectomy and the factors influencing limb salvage and long-term survival were analyzed retrospectively. The records of 221 patients (median age, 77) were reviewed. At the time of embolization 50% of the patients were already hospitalized for other reasons. The heart was the most probable source of embolus in 67% of cases. The mean follow-up time was 32 months (range, 1–128 months).

Of 263 embolectomies performed, 21% were done in the upper extremities. The amputation rate did not correlate with the interval from embolization to operation but was significantly lower in patients who received postoperative anticoagulant therapy. Operative mortality was 37%. Mortality was significantly higher among patients who were already in the hospital when embolization occurred, or in whom embolism was associated with myocardial infarction, as well as in those given oral anticoagulants postoperatively and those for whom the interval between embolization to operation was longer than 24 hours. The mortality rate increased directly with patient age. Multivariate analysis identified age, concomitant coronary artery disease, and oral anticoagulant treatment as independent predictors of operative mortality. The postoperative oral administration of anticoagulants was associated with significantly higher 5-year survival rates, as were operations performed by surgeons trained in vascular surgery vs. those operated on by other surgeons.

Data concerning amputation rate, perioperative mortality, and long-term survival in relation to oral anticoagulant treatment must be interpreted cautiously. Selective administration and the severely ill state of some patients when embolization occurred are factors to be considered. Certain factors may be deleterious in the outcome of arterial embolism. There is a need to define the treatment of patients with arterial embolism in terms of embolectomy, reconstructive procedures, or conservative management.

▶ The importance of anticoagulation in this group of patients is made apparent by the data presented. The fact that the amputation rate in this series was not related to the interval of time from embolization to operation is contrary to other reports. In the landmark article, Blaisdell and associates (1) emphasized that embolectomy could be avoided in some patients with acute lower extremity ischemia caused by embolism and thrombosis, and that the patients could be managed with anticoagulation instead. Green et al. (2) demonstrated that the lack of restoration of distal pulses after embolectomy does not preclude the outcome of a functional limb. They also strongly advised the use of heparin, initiating drug therapy immediately after the diagnosis is made, and continuing it postoperatively on a permanent basis.—S.I. Schwartz, M.D.

References

1. Blaisdell FW, et al: *Surgery* 84:882, 1978.
2. Green RM, et al: *Surgery* 77:24, 1975.

Chronic Compartment Syndrome: An Unusual Cause for Claudication
Turnipseed W, Detmer DE, Girdley F (Univ of Wisconsin Hosp and Clinics, Madison; Univ of Virginia Hosp, Charlottesville)
Ann Surg 210:557–563, October 1989   18–20

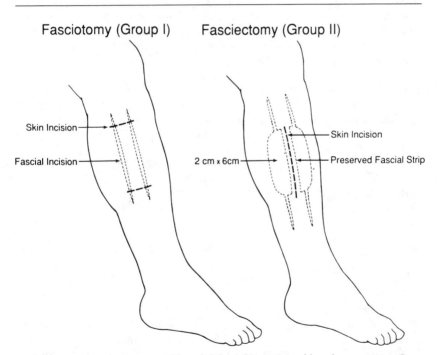

Fasciotomy (Group I)   Fasciectomy (Group II)

Skin Incision —
Fascial Incision —

2 cm x 6cm —
— Skin Incision
— Preserved Fascial Strip

Fig 18–7.—Surgical compartment release techniques for anterior and lateral compartments. Group I: subcutaneous fasciotomy is performed by using transverse skin incisions proximal and distal over symptomatic compartment. The compartment fascia is incised by passing scissors subcutaneously between skin incisions. Group II: open fasciectomy is performed by using a linear incision over the medial third of the anterior lateral surface of leg. Ellipse of the fascia approximately 6 cm long and 2 cm wide is removed from anterior and lateral compartments, leaving a strip of fascia over the intermuscular septum. This strip protects the superficial peroneal nerve from injury or scar adherence. Extended compartment release can be achieved by proximal and distal subcutaneous fasciotomy performed under direct vision. (Courtesy of Turnipseed W, Detmer DE, Girdley F: *Ann Surg* 210:557–563, October 1989.)

Chronic compartment syndrome (CCS) most often is related to overuse injury in athletes, but it also can occur in cases of blunt trauma, venous insufficiency, and tumor. The surgical treatment of 209 patients seen with CCS since 1976 was reviewed. Nearly 90% of the patients were athletes.

Claudication, tightness of muscle groups, and paresthesias were the most frequent symptoms. Compartment release involved subcutaneous fasciotomy in 100 patients and open fasciectomy in 109 others (Fig 18–7). In 59% of patients CCS was bilateral.

Complications occurred in 11% of the patients who had subcutaneous fasciotomy; the same proportion had recurrent symptoms. Most recurrences involved the anterolateral compartments and responded to open fasciectomy. Open fasciectomy combined with selective extended subcutaneous fasciotomy led to wound complications in 5.5% of the patients. Six patients had new symptoms of CCS in untreated compartments after surgery. In both groups the best results were achieved in patients with overuse injury. Patients were ambulatory within 48 hours of surgery and usually were jogging after 4 or 5 weeks.

Chronic compartment syndrome will not improve without surgery. Because open fasciectomy causes fewer complications than closed subcutaneous fasciotomy and recurrences are less frequent, open fasciectomy is the preferred surgical approach to CCS.

▶ As might be anticipated, this syndrome is usually reported in the sports medicine and orthopedic literature. As pointed out in the discussion, it is difficult to understand the etiology of the syndrome because the fascia should stretch if the abnormality is in the muscle per se. The authors indicate that in almost half of the patients there has been a mechanical explanation such as inflamed or traumatized fascia with myofascial scarring. The study does not truly confirm that an open fasciotomy is preferable to a semiclosed fasciotomy in management of this syndrome. It also would have been more meaningful if resting and postexercise compartmental pressures had been measured.—S.I. Schwartz, M.D.

Mesenteric Venous Thrombosis
Harward TRS, Green D, Bergan JJ, Rizzo RJ, Yao JST (Northwestern Univ)
J Vasc Surg 9:328–333, February 1989   18–21

Mesenteric venous thrombosis is a dangerous, rather uncommon abdominal event that has not been well reported in the literature. The records of all patients with documented mesenteric venous thrombosis treated during a 5-year period were reviewed retrospectively.

The study population consisted of 13 men and 3 women aged 22–76 years (average, 49.7 years). Twelve patients had progressive abdominal pain, 3 had mild to moderate gastrointestinal bleeding, and 1 complained only of general malaise. Associated symptoms included anorexia, nausea with or without vomiting, and diarrhea. Eleven patients with negative findings on routine gastrointestinal and hepatobiliary evaluation underwent contrast-enhanced CT. A correct diagnosis of mesenteric venous thrombosis was made in 10 of the 11 patients. Computed tomographic findings were confirmed by angiography in 6 patients, at operation in 2, and at autopsy in 2. Segmental intestinal necrosis was found in 3 patients with severe abdominal pain who required emergency laparotomy. Mesenteric venous thrombosis was confirmed in each of these patients, who had either protein C or protein S deficiency.

Three patients died in the hospital, but only 2 died of mesenteric venous thrombosis. The third patient died of biliary obstruction and sepsis secondary to pancreatic cancer. The other 13 patients survived to be discharged from the hospital. Nine patients had an identifiable coagulopathy, of whom 6 had a protein C deficiency, 2 had a protein S deficiency, and 1 had a factor IX deficiency. Seven patients had previously received treatment for deep vein thrombosis. None had congenital antithrombin III deficiency. Seven patients were treated for their coagulopathy with heparin or sodium warfarin.

Mesenteric venous thrombosis should be suspected in patients with a history of thrombotic events and known hypercoagulable states who have acute abdominal symptoms. Infusion CT is useful in the early diagnosis and treatment of this disorder.

▶ In our own experience (1), acute mesenteric ischemia in 10 of 49 patients was related to venous thrombosis. Three cases involved primary mesenteric venous occlusive disease; the others were secondary to sepsis, use of birth control pills, lymphoma, or thrombocytosis. Nine patients underwent segmental small bowel resection. Sixty-four percent of the patients survived, and this was the highest survival rate among any of the causes of the acute mesenteric ischemia. By contrast, none of the patients with arterial thrombosis survived, and only 35% of those with mesenteric ischemia to arterial embolization survived.—S.I. Schwartz, M.D.

Reference

1. Sachs SM, et al: *Surgery* 92:646, 1982.

19 The Esophagus

Current Results in Repair of Esophageal Atresia With Tracheoesophageal Fistula Using Physiologic Status as a Guide to Therapy
Randolph JG, Newman KD, Anderson KD (George Washington Univ; Children's Hosp Natl Med Ctr, Washington, DC)
Ann Surg 209:526–531, May 1989   19–1

From 1966 to 1982 the Waterston classification was the basis for the surgical management of infants with esophageal atresia (EA) and tracheoesophageal fistula (TEF). Since 1982, 26 infants with EA and TEF have been managed surgically, with selection of treatment based solely on physiologic status.

Infants who had stable cardiac and respiratory status were chosen for immediate repair. If an underlying irregularity was not life threatening or could be easily corrected, the infant was considered physiologically stable. Twenty-six of 39 infants met these criteria. Of these, only 9 would have been classified as Waterston A; 12 would have been classified as Waterston B, and 5 as Waterston C. The 26 infants underwent immediate primary repair via a right retropleural thoracotomy. In all cases a single-layer anastomosis was performed. Gastrostomy was avoided in all but 1 patient. On day 7, barium swallow was performed to assess esophageal function and the size and integrity of the anastomosis. Milk scan and pH probe were used to assess gastroesophageal reflux.

Thirteen patients had unstable physiologic status and did not undergo early repair. All of these patients would have been classified as Waterston C. All patients in this group had some form of staged repair. All infants with early primary repair survived. The survival rate was 77% in infants with staged repair.

Early surgical repair based solely on physiologic status has led to more and earlier primary repairs in infants with EA and TEF. Stable infants have had excellent survival rates. A staged approach is still suggested for some severely compromised infants.

▶ Several surgical approaches are possible in infants with TEF; these include immediate repair, delayed primary repair, and staged repair. Experiences with 118 patients are described. For the past 7 years at this medical center, physiologic status has been used as the sole basis for surgical management. Twenty-six children underwent immediate repair, with 100% survival. Thirteen with severe cardiopulmonary problems had a staged repair, with a 77% survival rate. The others received delayed primary repair with excellent results.—F.C. Spencer, M.D.

Primary Repair Without Routine Gastrostomy Is the Treatment of Choice for Neonates With Esophageal Atresia and Tracheoesophageal Fistula
Shaul DB, Schwartz MZ, Marr CC, Tyson KRT (Univ of California at Davis, Sacramento)
Arch Surg 124:1188–1191, October 1989   19–2

Staged repair with gastrostomy often is recommended for treating esophageal atresia with distal tracheoesophageal fistula (EA-TEF), especially in infants at high risk. In 42 consecutive infants treated between October 1980 and February 1988 routine staged repair was avoided. Fifteen infants were at high risk (Waterston class C). The fistula was divided via an extrapleural approach, and a primary single-layer end-to-end anastomosis was constructed. Four patients required proximal esophageal circular myotomy. Four early patients had a gastrostomy.

The 4 deaths were unrelated to EA-TEF. One anastomotic leak occurred and 4 patients required multiple dilatations for anastomotic stricture. Three patients with symptomatic reflux required fundoplication. The overall morbidity was 15% in this series. Waterston class C patients had a survival of 73% and an average hospital stay of 40 days. Only 1 patient in this group who had definitive repair died.

Primary repair without gastrostomy is suitable for most infants born with EA-TEF. The hospital period is shortened and the complications of gastrostomy placement are avoided. In high-risk infants with EA-TEF most deaths are caused by associated life-threatening anomalies.

▶ It is reasonable to categorize patients in such a fashion that gastrostomy does represent a useful adjunct in a limited number of cases. For full-term infants with no significant pneumonia, there is no question that primary repair without routine gastrostomy is a reasonable approach and, based on the findings of Spitz et al. (1), that a gastrostomy tube leads to an increase in gastrosophagy esophageal reflux, it does represent the preferred approach. As pointed out in the discussion of this paper, there is a role for gastrostomy if the infant has pneumonia or weighs less than 5 lb; the definitive operation must be deferred. The same applies to an infant with severe coexisting anomalies. The risk of reflux esophagitis associated with the gastrostomy has not been fully determined.—S.I. Schwartz, M.D.

Reference

1. Spitz L, et al: *Ann Surg* 206:69, 1987.

Spontaneous Rupture of the Esophagus: A 30-Year Experience
Pate JW, Walker WA, Cole FH Jr, Owen EW, Johnson WH (Univ of Tennessee, Memphis)
Ann Thorac Surg 47:689–692, May 1989   19–3

Boerhaave's syndrome, rupture of the esophagus, is a rare occurrence that is associated with a high mortality rate. Diagnosis is difficult because patients do not necessarily exhibit the classic symptoms: severe vomiting, epigastric or substernal pain, collapse, and shock. Data were reviewed retrospectively concerning 34 patients (median age, 53 years) with spontaneous rupture of the esophagus who were seen in a 30-year period. The condition was more common in men.

Rapid onset of pain (85%), vomiting (71%), or both, were the most frequent symptoms. The location of the pain was the abdomen in 16 patients, the thoracic area in 9, and the shoulder in 4. Physical examination yielded little specific information for diagnosis; the condition was correctly identified on admission in only 14 patients (41%). Routine chest roentgenographic examinations revealed nondiagnostic abnormalities in 24 patients. Pleural effusions were noted in 18 patients and mediastinal emphysema in 9.

Twenty-six patients underwent primary surgical repair, and pleural flaps were used to cover the suture line in 20 patients. Multiple antibiotics were given intravenously to all patients. Thoracotomy was performed in all except 4 patients. The rupture was most commonly located on the left wall of the distal esophagus.

The 14 patients who died included all 4 who did not have a thoracotomy. Delay in treatment (24 hours or more) did not significantly affect the mortality rate but caused a significant increase in complications. Surgical repair, even when delayed, offers the best chance of recovery. When an esophagogram was made the suspected diagnosis was confirmed in all but 1 patient. Undigested food found in pleural aspirates also strongly suggests esophageal rupture.

▶ This large series appropriately emphasizes that esophagography is indicated whenever the diagnosis is suspected. Although the authors indicate that a delay in diagnosis did not affect mortality rates in their series, many series report that a delay of more than 24 hours has a profound effect on mortality. A mortality rate of 41% bespeaks the serious nature of the lesion and is in keeping with other series. Although some, such as Cameron et al. (1) indicate that nonoperative conservative therapy can be used in patients with a perforation, this relates generally to iatrogenic perforations and not the true Boerhaave's syndrome.—S.I. Schwartz, M.D.

Reference

1. Cameron JL, et al: *Ann Thorac Surg* 27:404, 1979.

Diverticulopexy and Cricopharyngeal Myotomy: Treatment for the High-Risk Patient With a Pharyngoesophageal (Zenker's) Diverticulum
Konowitz PM, Biller HF (Mount Sinai Med Ctr, New York)
Otolaryngol Head Neck Surg 100:146–153, February 1989   19–4

Diverticulectomy is a successful procedure for treatment of Zenker's diverticulum; however, in the elderly the complications associated with this procedure may be devastating. Diverticulopexy is a good alternative in these patients because it avoids esophagotomy during diverticulectomy. From 1974 to 1987, 32 patients had dysphagia caused by a pharyngoesophageal diverticulum. Of the 32, 12 patients underwent diverticulopexy with cricopharyngeal myotomy. Others had 1-stage resection of the diverticulum with myotomy.

In both treatment groups complications occurred, but procedure-related morbidity was more common after diverticulectomy. Despite the low complication rate the patients who underwent diverticulopexy with myotomy were those who had risk factors that made them unsuitable for diverticulectomy. These risk factors included a debilitated state caused by the effects of the diverticulum, a history of postsurgical complications, multiple medical illnesses, advanced age with inability to ambulate, and insulin-dependent diabetes mellitus. After diverticulopexy, a nasogastric tube was not necessary, and this allowed for oral intake on the first postoperative day, immediate ambulation, and a shorter hospital stay.

Diverticulectomy has proved to be a relatively safe procedure. However, diverticuloplexy with cricopharyngeal myotomy is preferred for patients with a high risk of potential complications from the diverticulum excision or for whom prolonged hospitalization would be devastating.

▶ There is little advantage to this technique. Diverticulectomy alone is a procedure associated with a mortality of about 1% and a very low recurrence rate. The fistula rate is about 0.6%. Currently, with the use of nutritional support and excellent nursing care, the need for diverticulopexy should be extremely rare (1).—S.I. Schwartz, M.D.

Reference

1. Huang BW, et al: *Ann Thorac Surg* 37:189, 1984.

Myotomy for Reflux-Induced Cricopharyngeal Dysphagia: Five-Year Review

Henderson RD, Hanna WM, Henderson RF, Marryatt G (Univ of Toronto)
J Thorac Cardiovasc Surg 98:428–433, September 1989   19–5

Cricopharyngeal dysphagia is a prominent symptom in many patients with reflux. A total of 25 patients seen in a 5-year period had severe cricopharyngeal symptoms before surgery; 12 had reflux-induced dysphagia as the chief symptom and underwent cricopharyngeal myotomy. Six other patients did not have severe reflux symptoms but had failed to respond to intensive medical care. Cricopharyngeal myotomy also was carried out in these patients. Seven patients had myotomy after total fundoplication gastroplasty and esophageal dilation had failed to control cricopharyngeal dysphagia.

More than 90% of patients had manometric findings of cricopharyngeal incoordination. The myotomy was extended proximally to the pharynx and distally to the intrathoracic esophagus. All patients but 1 had excellent to satisfactory results. A wide range of myopathic degenerative changes was found in these patients.

These findings suggest an association between cricopharyngeal incoordination and responsiveness to cricopharyngeal myotomy. Aspiration no longer is a prominent problem. Cricopharyngeal myotomy is especially helpful to elderly patients with reflux.

▶ Experiences with 25 patients requiring cricopharyngeal myotomy are described, reported by the late Dr. Robert D. Henderson. Several important concepts are embodied in this report. These include the importance of radiologic diagnosis by manometry and a precise surgical technique with a long myotomy, extending into the pharynx superiorly and down into the intrathoracic esophagus inferiorly, a length of 6–7 cm. The condition is uncommon; Dr. Henderson performed only 25 such procedures in a series of more than 1,500 patients. The decision should be made carefully, because incompetence of the upper esophageal sphincter greatly increases the hazard of reflux and is often considered a contraindication to esophageal reconstruction by transplanting the colon or stomach into the neck.—F.C. Spencer, M.D.

The Treatment of Achalasia: A Current Perspective
Sauer L, Pellegrini CA, Way LW (VA Med Ctr, San Francisco; Univ of California, San Francisco)
Arch Surg 124:929–932, August 1989   19–6

Pneumatic dilatation has replaced the Heller myotomy as primary treatment for achalasia for more than a decade. Data were reviewed on the course of achalasia in 79 adults treated for this disorder from 1977 to 1988. Sixty-six patients had pneumatic dilatation as primary treatment. Eight patients had a modified Heller cardiomyotomy. Seven additional patients were seen after a Heller myotomy and other surgery elsewhere. Five ultimately underwent blunt esophagectomy with cervical esophagogastrostomy.

Fifty-three patients (80%) responded to primary dilatation, but 3 required immediate redilatation and 8 patients had esophageal perforation. Pulmonary aspiration occurred in 2 cases. Fifty percent of patients who had dilatation remained asymptomatic after 4 years. Thirty percent had symptoms of gastroesophageal reflux and 20% had persistent dysphagia.

Heller's myotomy gave excellent results in 7 of 8 patients, but 1 died in respiratory failure. All 7 patients originally operated on elsewhere recovered and were able to eat solid food.

Pneumatic dilatation is a reasonable initial approach to achalasia, but it may be less effective and less safe than hoped. Esophagomyotomy is more invasive, but it also is more reliable and is associated with low rates of mortality and morbidity. Unless the results of dilatation improve, surgery may well be used more often in the future.

▶ The results of pneumatic dilatation are similar to those reported by Donahue et al. (1) success was achieved in half of their patients. Esophagomyotomy alone led to definitive improvement in 12 of 19 patients in that series, whereas extended myotomy with an antireflux procedure was followed by relief in 12 or 13 patients. Little et al. (2) reported on 57 patients undergoing esophagomyotomy after previous pneumatic dilatation. Their approach was esophageal myotomy coupled with a Belsey repair. Assessing the results, I would agree with the authors' conclusions that pneumatic dilatation remains unperfected, and the need for surgical intervention should be reexpanded.—S.I. Schwartz, M.D.

References

1. Donahue PE, et al: *Ann Surg* 203:505, 1986.
2. Little AG, et al: *Ann Thorac Surg* 45:389, 1988.

Esophageal Resection for Achalasia: Indications and Results
Orringer MB, Stirling MC (Univ of Michigan)
Ann Thorac Surg 47:340–345, March 1989   19–7

The effectiveness of forceful dilation or esophagomyotomy in relieving esophageal obstruction in achalasia is well established. However, neither procedure is consistently reliable in the treatment of patients with either recurrent symptoms after a previous esophagomyotomy or a megaesophagus. Total thoracic esophagectomy was performed in 26 patients aged 15–84 years (average, 49) with achalasia. Eighteen patients had a history of a previous esophagomyotomy and 18 had a megaesophagus.

Twenty-four patients underwent a transhiatal esophagectomy without thoracotomy and 2 required a transthoracic esophagectomy because of periesophageal adhesions from previous operations. In all patients the stomach was positioned in the posterior mediastinum and a cervical anastomosis was performed.

The average intraoperative blood loss was 765 mL (range, 150–3,000 mL). Postoperative complications included mediastinal bleeding requiring thoracotomy in 2 patients, chylothorax in 2, an anastomotic leak in 1, transient laryngeal nerve paresis in 2, and a subdiaphragmatic abscess. There were no postoperative deaths. The average postoperative hospital stay was 10 days. Follow-up was complete for the 254 surviving patients and averaged 30 months (range, 3–91 months). Except for 1 patient with severe psychiatric disease, all other patients ate regular, unrestricted diets without postprandial regurgitation. Ten patients required early postoperative anastomotic dilation. The dumping syndrome occurred in 5 patients. None had pulmonary complications secondary to aspiration.

Total thoracic esophagectomy and a cervical esophagogastric anastomosis can be performed in patients with megaesophagus or a failed esophagomyotomy with far more reliable and favorable long-term functional results than esophagomyotomy, cardioplasty procedures, or limited esophageal resection.

▶ Esophagomyotomy represents the treatment of choice for achalasia. In the overwhelming majority of cases this has often been accompanied by a fundoplication. Pai et al. (1) indicated that in long-term follow-up, 94% of patients with esophagomyotomy alone had good results compared to 70% who had a concomitant antireflux procedure. The group of patients the present authors refer to is an interesting one, and in their hands the use of the transhiatal approach is reasonable. An increasing number of reports indicate that the stomach works well as a substitute esophagus, and it is being used more frequently than colon interposition.—S.I. Schwartz, M.D.

Reference

1. Pai GP, et al: *Ann Thorac Surg* 38:201, 1984.

Fifteen- to Twenty-Year Results After the Hill Antireflux Operation
Low DE, Anderson RP, Ilves R, Ricciardelli E, Hill LD (Virginia Mason Med Ctr, Seattle)
J Thorac Cardiovasc Surg 98:444–450, September 1989   19–8

Shorter-term studies have shown that the Hill antireflux procedure is an effective approach to resistant reflux, but long-term results are uncertain. A total of 441 patients who had the Hill repair for refractory esophageal reflux in 1968–1973 were evaluated. A late study group included 167 patients who were followed for an average of nearly 18 years. Of these, 15.6% had a previous antireflux operation.

The rate of subjectively good to excellent results was 82% after 5–10 years and 88% after 15–20 years. There were no serious late complications such as fistula formation, bleeding, or obstruction. Only 4 patients from the initial series required reoperation for recurrent symptoms during follow-up.

A properly performed standard antireflux operation in a correctly selected patient can be expected to give a highly favorable long-term outcome. Intraoperative manometry has made the Hill operation more precise; it has improved the short-term results and probably the long-term outcome as well. The lack of serious late complications contrasts with what is seen after the Nissen procedure.

▶ This report of follow-up studies in 441 patients, 167 of whom were followed for 15–20 years, describes what is probably the longest follow-up of patients treated with a standard operation. Good results were maintained in about 80% of the patients. An important point elaborated in the discussion of this report is recognition of an intractable stricture that should be treated by resection rather than by an antireflux operation.—F.C. Spencer, M.D.

Continued Assessment of the Combined Collis-Nissen Operation

Stirling MC, Orringer MB (Univ of Michigan)
Ann Thorac Surg 47:224–230, February 1989   19–9

In most patients requiring an antireflux procedure, the Collis-Nissen operation has been preferred at the University of Michigan. Previous experience at this institution and at others has shown that a complete fundoplication provides better reflux control than a partial gastric wrap, especially after construction of a Collis gastroplasty. The effectiveness of the Collis-Nissen operation in the long-term control of gastroesophageal reflux was evaluated. Between August 1976 and June 1988, 353 patients underwent the Collis-Nissen operation; 261 were followed for an average of 44 months.

Success was achieved in 75% of these patients. In the group experiencing complications (e.g., spasm, scleroderma, previous antireflux operation, stricture or paraesophageal hernia) patients were significantly less likely to have satisfactory results than those in the uncomplicated group, who had none of these features.

A recent modification in surgical technique has influenced results. A 54F dilator in women and 56F dilator in men have been used to construct both the gastroplasty and the fundoplication; the fundoplication has been limited to 3 cm in length and encircles only the distal gastroplasty tube. With this modification the overall clinical status has been enhanced and subjective reflux control has improved significantly. Postoperative dysphagia is also less. Obesity, advanced age (>70 years), and Barrett's epithelium have had no significant effects on clinical outcome.

Because of both recurrent or persistent reflux and dysphagia, especially in patients with complicated esophageal disease, surgical treatment of gastroesophageal reflux remains a challenge. Careful long-term follow-up and meticulous analysis of results of antireflux operations are necessary for future improvements.

▶ In the discussion of the presentation in this work, Pearson reported on his experience with 250 patients followed for more than 5 years and 100 patients followed for more than 10 years. There was a 93% incidence of satisfactory results. For repeat operations the good results diminished to 79%, and were most markedly decreased in the presence of an associated primary motor disorder, in which case the good results were only 50%. It is interesting that at the University of Michigan the Collis-Nissen procedure represented the procedure of choice for treatment of antireflux and the Nissen fundoplication, which is used in most centers, is done by the reporting group only in patients who are thin and without hiatal hernias, or with some hiatal hernias and minimal shortening without substantial esophagitis.—S.I. Schwartz, M.D.

Cervical Esophagogastric Anastomosis for Benign Disease: Functional Results

Orringer MB, Stirling MC (Univ of Michigan)
J Thorac Cardiovasc Surg 96:887–893, December 1988   19–10

The preferred organ with which to replace the esophagus in esophageal resection for benign disease has not yet been determined. Proponents of colonic interposition have said it is more physiologic to replace the esophagus with intestine and to leave the stomach in the abdominal cavity, preserving the gastric reservoir. The results of total thoracic esophagectomy and a cervical esophagogastric anastomosis were evaluated in 91 patients (average age, 49 years) requiring esophageal resection and reconstruction for benign disease. Follow-up was for 6–104 months.

Outpatient esophageal dilation was used liberally for any degree of postoperative cervical dysphagia. At their last follow-up visit, 43% of the patients could eat without dysphagia, 4% had mild dysphagia necessitating no treatment, 37% had undergone 1–3 dilations in the first 6–12 months after surgery for intermittent dysphagia, and 16% had more severe dysphagia necessitating regular anastomotic dilations. Mild regurgitation of gastric contents was experienced by 30%, especially when recumbent after eating. No patient had pulmonary complications from aspiration. Varying degrees of dumping syndrome occurred in 22%, but was generally transient and well controlled by medication; 2 needed an additional gastric drainage operation at 16 months and 82 months, respectively, after esophagectomy. Of the patients, 33% weighed 3–83 lb more than they weighed preoperatively, 38% weighed 5–40 lb less, and 29% had no change in weight.

The stomach functions well as a visceral esophageal substitute. As with the esophagus, it is more thick walled and resilient than colon. Significant

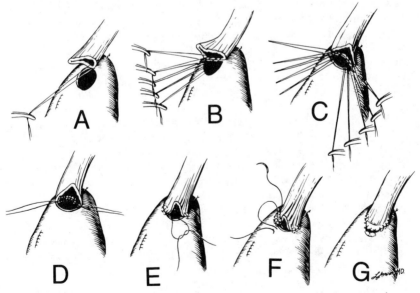

Fig 19–1.—A–D, completion of the posterior quadrants of the anastomosis by an interrupted suture technique with knots tied on the inside. E–G, anterior half of the anastomosis is completed with a 46F Maloney dilator (not shown) in the esophagus to insure an adequate, nonobstructed lumen. (Courtesy of Orringer MB, Stirling MC: *J Thorac Cardiovasc Surg* 96:887–893, December 1988.)

gastroesophageal reflux was uncommon after a properly performed cervical esophagogastric anastomosis. Postoperative dysphagia could be minimized by attention to technique in anastomosis construction (Fig 19−1). The stomach is the preferred organ for esophageal replacement for benign diseases as well as carcinoma.

▶ Spitz and associates (1), referring to their experience with a procedure in children, noted that it compared favorably with colon interposition. In adults, Curet-Scott et al. (2) reported that colon interposition for benign esophageal disease has a 30% complication rate and a 37% reoperation rate, but there was high ultimate patient satisfaction. Good results have also been achieved with jejunal interposition (3).—S.I. Schwartz, M.D.

References

1. Spitz L, et al: *Ann Surg* 206:69, 1987.
2. Curet-Scott MJ, et al: *Surgery* 102:568, 1987.
3. Wright C, Cuschieri A: *Ann Surg* 205:54, 1987.

The Results of Esophagogastrectomy Without Thoracotomy for Adenocarcinoma of the Esophagogastric Junction
Finley RJ, Inculet RI (Univ of Western Ontario, London)
Ann Surg 210:535−543, October 1989   19−11

Ninety-eight patients were seen with adenocarcinoma at the esophagogastric junction between 1980 and 1988. Eighty-two patients had resection of the celiac lymph nodes, the lesser curve and cardia of the stomach, and the thoracic esophagus via abdominal and neck incisions; thoracotomy was avoided. Eighty patients received a stomach tube and 2 received a colon tube.

The 2 hospital deaths were caused by pulmonary embolism. Survival was 55% at 1 year after resection and 31% at 2 years; the median survival was 16 months. Fifty percent of the patients with stage I−II disease were alive at 2 years. Patients with a columnar-lined esophagus did slightly better than the others.

The 2-year survival for patients with well-differentiated tumors was 73%. When only part of the esophageal wall was invaded, the 2-year survival was 46%, compared with 23% for patients with full-thickness invasion. Swallowing was maintained by resection in 75 patients.

Esophagogastrectomy without thoracotomy is an effective and relatively safe means of restoring swallowing in patients who have adenocarcinoma of the esophagogastric junction. Palliation has been better than with other techniques.

▶ In the discussion, Dr. Pearson reported on the Toronto experience, indicating that the results of a large series demonstrated as good, if not better, data related to mortality, morbidity, and survival in patients managed by this technique compared with those undergoing a more radical mediastinal dissection. The overall cure rate for lesions of the esophagogastric junction remains approximately 15% at 5 years. Orringer (1) reported essentially equivalent results for transhiatal esophagectomy. By contrast, Nishihira et al. (2), indicated that surgical excision using radical operation provided 5- and 10-year survival rates of 31% and 23%. The early results with combined modality therapy reported by Wolfe et al. (3) should encourage this multidisciplinary approach.— S.I. Schwartz, M.D.

References

1. Orringer MB: *Ann Surg* 200:282, 1984.
2. Nishihira T, et al: *World J Surg* 8:778, 1984.
3. Wolfe WG, et al: *Ann Surg* 205:563, 1987.

Surgical Treatment of Advanced Carcinoma of the Esophagus
Abe S, Tachibana M, Shimokawa T, Shiraishi M, Nakamura T (Shimane Med Univ, Izumo, Japan)
Surg Gynecol Obstet 168:115–120, February 1989   19–12

The role of surgery in the treatment of advanced epidermoid carcinoma of the esophagus was evaluated in 32 patients. All patients had histologically proved epidermoid carcinomas of the esophagus, representing stages III and IV of the tumor-node-metastasis classification. Esophagectomy, with or without reconstruction, was performed in 17 patients, bypass was performed in 6, and gastrostomy or esophagostomy or both, without esophagectomy in 4 (stoma group); the remaining 5 patients had no operation because of unresectability of the disease or complications.

The postoperative 1- and 2-year survival rates were 34.6% and 17.3%, respectively, in the esophagectomy group, whereas none of the patients in the bypass and stoma groups survived for 1 year. Median survival times after operation for the esophagectomy, bypass, and stoma groups were 199, 55, and 80 days, respectively. Thirty-day postoperative mortalities were 0%, 33.3%, and 25%, respectively. When grouped according to pattern of organ invasion, the postoperative survival time was significantly better in patients whose cancers spared the aorta or major respiratory tract. Complication-related mortality among the 27 patients who underwent surgery was 14.8%; this rate was 5.9% in the esophagectomy group and 50.0% in the bypass group. A total of 38 complications occurred in 17 patients in the esophagectomy group, and 9 in the 6 patients in the bypass group. Swallowing was improved in 58.8% of patients who had esophagectomy, but no patient had swallowing restored after bypass procedures.

Bypass procedures should not be the final resort after adjuvant therapy for patients with advanced esophageal carcinoma, considering the short postoperative survival time and frequent complications. Esophagectomy with reconstruction results in a longer survival time, but the procedure is accompanied by many complications and restoration of swallowing is not as satisfactory as expected. A randomized prospective study is recommended to compare resection with the newer nonsurgical therapy in patients with advanced carcinoma of the esophagus.

▶ Hankins et al. (1) compared the results of transhiatal vs. transthoracic resection in patients with carcinoma of the esophagus. The long-term survival was equivalent in each. Mannell et al. (2) reported 124 patients having bypass surgery for unresectable esophageal carcinoma; the operative mortality was 4% and the median length of survival was 5 months. Further, 89% of the survivors were able to eat an restricted diet on discharge. This poses an argument with those who suggest that esophagectomy is preferable. It may well be that in the article under review, the subsets of patients undergoing esophagectomy and bypass were different.—S.I. Schwartz, M.D.

References

1. Hankins JR, et al: *Ann Thorac Surg* 47:700, 1989.
2. Mannell A, et al: *Br J Surg* 75:283, 1988.

Surgical and Endoscopic Palliation of Esophageal Carcinoma
Segalin A, Little AG, Ruol A, Ferguson MK, Bardini R, Norberto L, Skinner DB, Peracchia A (Univ of Padua, Italy; Univ of Chicago)
Ann Thorac Surg 48:267–271, August 1989   19–13

To determine the effectiveness of palliative therapy for patients with advanced esophageal cancer, the data were reviewed on 732 patients with advanced disease, 156 of whom underwent palliative resection. Most of these patients had squamous cell carcinoma. Usually, the stomach was used for reconstruction.

Hospital mortality was 9.6% after resection. The median survival was about 8 months, and survival at 1 year was 29%. Excellent or good palliation was achieved in 78% of the patients who survived resection. Bypass procedures were done in 49 patients, and hospital mortality was 20%. Seventy-one percent of the survivors had excellent or good palliation. Another 254 patients had intubation of the tumor, with a 30-day mortality of 10% and a median survival of 4 months. None of these patients had excellent palliation.

Laser or photodynamic therapy provided excellent or good results in 83% of 50 patients, and there were no procedure-related deaths. None of these patients had a poor result.

Surgical palliation can be effective in patients with advanced esophageal cancer but at high cost, and resection is not recommended on a systematic basis for all patients. It should be done only when incurable disease is not confirmed until operation. Otherwise, comparable palliation can be achieved with less morbidity by such methods as intracavitary irradiation, radiation therapy, chemotherapy, and laser treatment. An esophageal bypass is used only if there is an esophagorespiratory fistula and no realistic alternative is at hand.

▶ This article addresses the state of the art, and the results achieved with laser or photodynamic therapy are most encouraging because they represent lesser procedures. The experience reported from South Africa by Mannell et al. (1) is truly extraordinary. In all, 124 patients underwent extrathoracic bypass operation for unresectable tumors. Of 110 survivors, 89% were able to eat an unrestricted diet on discharge. The stomach was used for bypass in the overwhelming majority of the patients. None had a thoracotomy.—S.I. Schwartz, M.D.

Reference

1. Mannell A, et al: *Br J Surg* 75:283, 1988.

20 The Stomach and the Duodenum

Changing Pattern of Admissions and Operations for Duodenal Ulcer
Bardhan KD, Cust G, Hinchliffe RFC, Williamson FM, Lyon C, Bose K (District
Gen Hosp, Rotherham; Trent Regional Health Authority, Sheffield, England)
Br J Surg 76:230–236, March 1989   20–1

Hospital admissions for duodenal ulcer, with or without complications, have been declining in the past 25 years. The increasing use of H_2-receptor antagonists (H_2RA) may affect admission rates of patients with duodenal ulcer.

Admission rates were expressed per 10^6 of the resident population. Use of H_2RA increased by 3.7-fold from 1978 to 1983. However, overall admission rates for perforation changed little: There were 99 between 1972 and 1976 before H_2RA, and 103 between 1977 and 1984 during H_2RA use. Admission rates for hemorrhage rose by 8%. The overall rates concealed large increases in admission rates for patients 65 and older of 33% for perforation and 28% for hemorrhage. Emergency admission rates for

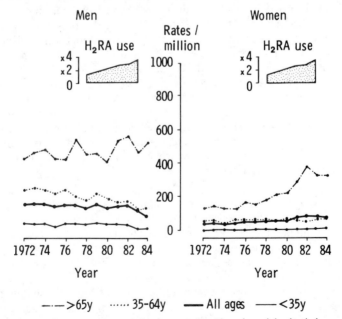

Fig 20–1.—Admission rates for men (a) and women (b) with perforated duodenal ulcer, subdivided by age. (Courtesy of Bardhan KD, Cust G, Hinchliffe RFC, et al: *Br J Surg* 76:230–236, March 1989.)

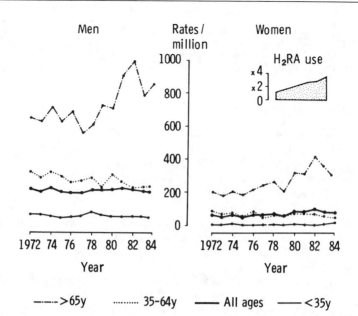

Fig 20–2.—Admission rates for men (a) and women (b) with uncomplicated duodenal ulcer, subdivided by age and operation rates. (Courtesy of Bardhan KD, Cust G, Hinchliffe RFC, et al: *Br J Surg* 76:230–236, March 1989.)

uncomplicated duodenal ulcer were unchanged, but the proportions operated on dropped by 58%. Waiting list admissions for uncomplicated duodenal ulcer dropped by 43%, from 187 in the pre-H$_2$RA period to 106 in the H$_2$RA period, and the proportions undergoing surgery fell from 162 to 76. The combined effect resulted in a decrease of 53% in the operation rates (Figs 20–1 and 20–2).

The use of H$_2$RA has not reduced emergency admissions in patients with duodenal ulcer but is associated with a reduction in waiting list admissions and in the number of patients undergoing surgery for uncomplicated duodenal ulcer. This reduction was even more pronounced when the drugs were used more intensively. Much of this decrease can be attributed to the changing natural history of the disease, but H$_2$RA has a significant additional effect.

▶ A decade ago we knew that hospital admissions for duodenal ulcer in the United States had decreased by 43% in the previous decade with no significant changes in the number of admissions for gastric ulcer (1). Six years ago, however, Peter Morris and colleagues in Oxford called attention to an increase in upper gastrointestinal hemorrhage in the previous decade, much of it caused by an increase in anti-inflammatory drug usage (2). The present study from Sheffield shows no significant changes in admissions for perforation or hemorrhage (admissions for older patients, in fact, rose significantly during the period). On the other hand, as noted by almost everyone else, intractable pain has plummeted in frequency as an indication for operation. The continued high incidence of life-threatening complications does, in fact, raise the question of whether or not the indications for operation in patients with long-standing ulcer disease, refractory to medical therapy, should not be liberalized in view of the low mortality risk and very low incidence of complications after selective proximal vagotomy (3, 4).—J.C. Thompson, M.D.

References

1. Elashoff JD, Grossman MI: *Gastroenterology* 78:280, 1980.
2. Morris P, et al: *J R Coll Surg Edinb* 29:134, 1984.
3. Thompson JC: *New Engl J Med* 307:550, 1982.
4. Jordan PH Jr, et al: *Ann Surg* 205:572, 1987.

Changes in Surgical Treatment of Peptic Ulcer Disease Within a Veterans Hospital in the 1970s and the 1980s
McConnell DB, Baba GC, Deveney CW (Oregon Health Sciences Univ, Portland)
Arch Surg 124:1164–1167, October 1989   20–2

Elective operations for chronic peptic ulcer have decreased but the incidence of complications remains constant. To learn whether the surgical experience at a Veterans Administration hospital is similar to that elsewhere, 104 patients having surgery between 1974 and 1977 and 61 having operations between 1984 and 1987 were compared.

In the 1970s group, 47% of ulcer operations were done for intractable symptoms, in contrast to only 18% of those in the 1980s group. The 2 groups overall were similar with regard to relative proportions of operations for bleeding, perforation, or obstruction, as well as in American Society of Anesthesiologists' physical status rating and fitness scores for assessing preoperative risk, both of which grant higher scores for higher risk. However, the 1980s patients with perforations were significantly older and their physical status and fitness scores were higher. No deaths occurred in patients with obstructions. The mortality for those with bleeding was 28%, a considerable decrease from the 1970s rates. For those with perforation, mortality in the 1980s series was 50%, a considerable increase from that in the 1970s series.

The safety of elective surgery for patients with chronic ulcer or obstruction was confirmed. However, the risk is high in patients with perforation or bleeding. The advancing age of the general United States population suggests that experience in private hospitals may begin to resemble that in VA hospitals.

▶ This paper is similar to the previous one (Abstract 20–1) in that there was a significant reduction (41%) in the overall number of procedures for peptic ulcer disease, whereas the number of patients operated on for complications of peptic ulcer remain unchanged. Again, the poor results obtained in the much older patients operated on for perforation raise the question of whether earlier treatment by selective proximal vagotomy might have improved the overall survival. I realize that, once invoked, the question is unanswerable, but it certainly deserves consideration.

In our experience, there is nothing wrong with H_2-receptor antagonist therapy as long as patients take their pills. When they leave the protective atmosphere of the hospital or clinic, go home, and then must buy the expensive medications on a weekly basis, often the cost of the drugs comes into competition with other expenditures in the family budget and the patient stops buying drugs. Because duodenal ulcer is a cyclic disease, they often meet with no symptoms when they stop treatment, so that they continue not taking their medication. After awhile, there is a cyclic recurrence of the ulcer diathesis and a life-threatening complication may ensue. The great advantage of operative achievement of acid reduction is that it removes the variable of patient cooperation from the therapeutic equation.—J.C. Thompson, M.D.

Costs of Medical and Surgical Treatment of Duodenal Ulcer
Sonnenberg A (VA Med Ctr, Milwaukee; Med College of Wisconsin, Milwaukee)
Gastroenterology 96:1445–1452, June 1989   20–3

Proximal gastric vagotomy (PGV) and intermittent and maintenance therapy with H_2-antagonists are all effective alternatives in the long-term treatment of duodenal ulcer. Assuming that inclusion of costs may narrow the overlap of success rates among these 3 interventions and thus allow a clear-cut choice favoring 1 over the other, the model Markov chain was used to compare their costs by a medical decision analysis. The expenditures were based on the American health care system.

With maintenance therapy the average costs per patient rose from $600 after 1 year to $7,600 after 15 years. Intermittent therapy cost as much as maintenance therapy, but the latter provided 8% and 4% more time spent free of ulcer relapse and pain, respectively. Although PGV was associated with less future costs of subsequent ulcer relapses, the high price of the initial procedure made PGV the most expensive therapy. In a sensitivity analysis, the order of the therapeutic options regarding their cost effectiveness remained robust to changes in the assumptions underlying the model. In the United States the initial gastric operation cost as much as two thirds of the gross average annual income, compared with only one seventh in European countries. Despite being expensive initially, PGV turned out to be the cheapest therapeutic strategy in European countries after 6 years.

In the United States, maintenance therapy provides the best long-term management of duodenal ulcer, whereas in Europe, gastric surgery may be a cost-effective therapeutic option for ulcer prevention.

▶ Economists at the Health Care Financing Administration (HCFA) must be pondering data like these and wondering over competing criteria for medical and surgical treatment of various illnesses (for example, just think of how they must be squirming in attempts to evaluate lithotripsy for gallstones). A few years ago, Dennis Jensen (1) suggested that maintenance drug therapy beyond 8 years may be more expensive than elective surgery for good candidates because of the high rate of ulcer recurrence after cessation of H_2-receptor blockade (up to 70% in some series). Also, if the HCFA rules in the future that cognition may take precedence over procedures in payment for physicians' services, the relative cost of the 2 procedures may require reevaluation. Again, the postoperative patient is far less likely to have an ulcer recurrence.—J.C. Thompson, M.D.

Reference

1. Jensen D: *Am J Med* 81:42, 1986.

A Multifactorial Analysis of Factors Related to Lethality After Treatment of Perforated Gastroduodenal Ulcer: 1935–1985
Svanes C, Salvesen H, Espehaug B, Søreide O, Svanes K (Haukeland Univ Hosp, Bergen, Norway; Univ of Bergen)
Ann Surg 209:418–423, April 1989   20–4

Mortality associated with perforated peptic ulcer remains high despite advances in surgical health care. The records of 1,128 patients treated for perforated gastric ulcer from 1935 to 1985 were studied retrospectively to identify factors that could influence posttreatment mortality. The data were analyzed by contingency tables and chi square testing; a stepwise logistic regression analysis was performed to identify interactions between variables and to describe the time trends in mortality rates. Most patients (97.7%) were treated surgically.

The total postperforation death rate was 7.4%. The death rate was 6.6% in patients treated surgically and 42.3% in those treated conservatively. Mortality decreased markedly with time but increased significantly with age of the patients. Logistic regression analysis showed that mortality was influenced significantly by year of admission, age of the patient, treatment delay, and localization of the ulcer. Treatment delay caused a significant but modest increase in mortality. Mortality was 3.6 times higher in patients with perforated gastric ulcer than in those with duodenal ulcer. Mortality did not differ between sexes, or between patients treated with simple suture or gastric resection.

Mortality after ulcer perforation has declined with time and is significantly influenced by the year of admission, patient's age, treatment delay, and localization of the ulcer.

▶ Multifactorial analysis allows dissection of what is important and what is not important in achieving an end. In this instance, the authors were looking at death, and they found that the age of the patient and delay in treatment were important, that gastric perforations are more dangerous than duodenal, and that mortality has diminished over the last half century. None of this is, perhaps, earth shaking, but when you look at the overall mortality rate here of 7% after perforation and compare it to 50% in old VA hospital patients in Mc-Connell's series (see Abstract 20–2), the factor takes on great significance. Whenever any of your medical colleagues suggest that a perforation might be treated nonoperatively, it is fortuitous to have this study at your fingertips, which shows that mortality was 7 times higher in those 2% of patients who were treated nonoperatively. Just as important in multifactorial analysis of those factors that are important are studies of those factors that have no bearing. A few years ago, a major study of mortality after coronary artery bypass demonstrated the surprising finding that the only factor that appeared related to death was anesthesia time.—J.C. Thompson, M.D.

Placebo-Controlled Trial With the Somatostatin Analogue SMS 201–995 in Peptic Ulcer Bleeding
Christiansen J, Ottenjann R, von Arx F, and the Study Group (Glostrup Hosp, Copenhagen; Krankenhaus München-Neuperlach, Munich)
Gastroenterology 97:568–574, September 1989   20–5

Previous studies have shown that natural somatostatin inhibits basal and stimulated gastric acid, pepsin, and gastrin secretion, and reduces splanchnic blood flow. A long-acting somatostatin analogue, SMS 201–995 (octreotide), acts similarly to natural somatostatin but has a longer half-life. To test its efficacy in the arrest of bleeding and prevention of rebleeding, a 5-day, double-blind, placebo-controlled trial was conducted in 23 centers; 273 patients were enrolled. Of these, 241 were assessable; 126 were given placebo and 115 were given octreotide. Only patients with severe and moderately active bleeding were included.

The efficacy rate for octreotide was 69.6% and for placebo, 70.6%. Patients in whom therapy failed were subdivided into 2 groups: those who did not stop bleeding—12.2% taking octreotide and 17.5% taking placebo; and those who stopped bleeding but rebled during the trial period—18.2% taking octreotide and 11.9% taking placebo. The surgery rate in the octreotide therapy group was 24.4%, and that in the placebo group, 23.0%. Ninety-nine of 115 patients given octreotide were transfused (mean, 2,392 mL of blood), as were 110 of 126 patients in given placebo (mean, 2,046 mL). In the octreotide group the 5-day mortality was 2.6%, and in the placebo group, 2.4%. Homogeneity was found in a retrospective subgroup analysis for age, sex, localization of the ulcers, severity of bleeding, and arterial spurting vs. oozing; no subgroup that would benefit from treatment with octreotide was identified. Both placebo and octreotide were well tolerated.

No statistically significant difference between octreotide and placebo was found with regard to the percentage of patients in whom bleeding stopped and no rebleeding occurred. In a well-defined subgroup of patients with upper gastrointestinal bleeding, natural somatostatin may have a beneficial effect, which could be addressed in a large prospective trial with strict protocol.

► Once a physiologic principle (in this incidence, reduction of splanchnic blood flow by somatostatin) is clearly established, the effort to put the idea into clinical practice is vastly seductive and apt to take on a life of its own, in spite of repeated negative trials. In reviewing a huge series of patients from Nottingham (1) in this section 5 years ago, I stated, "The results seem absolutely clear, and anyone who claims in the future that somatostatin is clinically useful in the treatment of upper gastrointestinal hemorrhage must plan on climbing, and refuting, this mountain of evidence." In this paper, Christiansen and colleagues have made the mountain 273 patients higher. The evidence against the clinical efficacy of somatostatin in the management of bleeding peptic ulcer seems irrefutable. Having said that, there are scattered case reports of success in the management of bleeding from a host of rare small bowel lesions (periarteritis, hemangiomas, parasitic infestation, *inter alia*).—J.C. Thompson, M.D.

Reference

1. Somerville KW, et al: *Lancet* 1:130, 1985.

A Simplified Technique for Rapid Truncal Vagotomy
Roberts JP, Debas HT (Univ of California, San Francisco)
Surg Gynecol Obstet 168:539–541, June 1989   20–6

A simplified technique of truncal vagotomy was developed that exploits the consistent anatomical relationships of the vagus.

Technique.—The constant presence and location of the hepatic branches of the anterior trunk of the vagus nerve and the celiac division of the posterior trunk of the vagus are used to identify the main nerve trunks. The peritoneum over the abdominal esophagus is incised horizontally and carried to the right onto the lesser omentum. The hepatic branches of the anterior trunk that are seen coursing toward the liver are held taut to bring the anterior vagal trunks into prominence. The nerve is then transected. Dissection is continued between the esophagus and the right crus of the diaphragm. The index finger is moved along the anterior surface of the aorta until the celiac artery and its left gastric artery are reached. With the left gastric artery held taut, the celiac division of the posterior trunk of the vagus becomes prominent, allowing identification of the posterior trunk. The nerve is sectioned.

This technique allows rapid identification of the vagal trunks without esophageal mobilization or extensive dissection. Vagotomy is performed under direct vision and with precision.

► The described technique is simple and effective. We do the operation frequently, and we do it quite differently, and we do it quickly. There are several ways to skin a cat, and this is one. Our cat skinning consists of using a Weinberg retractor to hold up the left lobe of the liver so you do not have to cut the triangular ligament. We palpate the nasogastric tube within the esophagus, lift the esophagus anteriorly, and break through the phrenoesophageal ligament that is posterior to it. We pass a Penrose drain behind the esophagus and pull inferiorly to exert traction so as to make the vagal fibers (which are less elastic than the esophageal muscle) stand out. It is then quite easy to palpate the relatively smaller anterior vagal trunk at about 1 o'clock (xiphoid is noon), and the much larger posterior vagal trunk at about 6:30 or 7 o'clock. It is important to dissect the vagal trunks up to the diaphragmatic hiatus because they often give off branches into the esophagus that must be divided. The vagi in the thorax decussate around the esophagus and may give branches into the esophageal muscle that run within the muscle down to the stomach. In some instances it is absolutely impossible to divide all vagal factors completely without dividing the esophagus. It is important to look for a branch of the vagus in the angle of His, a branch Grassi called the "criminal nerve." When we do a selective proximal vagotomy, we always identify the vagal trunks and put large sutures around them, so as to allow easy traction, which facilitates dissection and minimizes the chance of inadvertently dividing the vagal trunks as the dissection is carried up the lesser curvature toward the esophageal hiatus.—J.C. Thompson, M.D.

Decompression After Gastric Surgery: Gastrostomy Versus Nasogastric Tube
Pricolo VE, Vittimberga GM, Yellin SA, Burchard KW, Slotman GJ (Brown Univ; Rhode Island Hosp, Providence)
Ann Surg 55:413–416, July 1989   20–7

The relative efficacy, morbidity, and mortality of gastrostomy vs. nasogastric tube decompression were evaluated in 100 consecutive patients who underwent gastric surgery. Age, sex, and risk factors were equally distributed between the 2 groups. Perforated ulcers and emergency operations were more common and gastric resections less common in the group having gastrostomy.

Except for an increased incidence of atelectasis in the group having nasogastric tube decompression after elective procedures, postoperative morbidity was similar in both groups. Mortality was significantly increased in patients undergoing gastrostomy after emergency operations, and their hospital stay and hospital costs were significantly greater after emergency surgery compared with the other group. Furthermore, gastrostomy did not completely obviate the need for a nasogastric tube because, in addition to the gastrostomy, the latter patients required a nasogastric tube for an average of 2.9 days.

Gastrostomy offers no significant advantages over nasogastric tube decompression after gastric surgery. It should be limited to a select group of patients in whom gastric drainage is necessary and who would poorly tolerate a nasogastric tube.

▶ I am frequently surprised when visiting other clinics to find slavish adherence to the idea of postoperative gastrostomy for elective decompression.

First of all, we must realize that many surgeons over the world never (well, hardly ever) use gastric decompression postoperatively, and, secondly, that the putative bad effects of a nasogastric tube are difficult, if not impossible, to prove. The third thing to keep in mind is that patients die of leaking gastrostomies. I have never seen a patient die from a nasogastric tube (although I am sure that must have been reported), but I am personally familiar with 3 deaths caused by leaking gastrostomies that were in place simply for routine postoperative decompression. Why ever use a potentially lethal technique to accomplish a goal that is easily achieved otherwise?—J.C. Thompson, M.D.

Prospective Comparison of Gastric Secretory Function After Gastrectomy With Either Billroth II or Roux-en-Y Anastomosis
Rieu PNMA, Jansen JBMJ, Joosten HJM, Biemond I, Yap SH, Lamers CBHW (Canisius-Wilhelmina Hosp, Nijmegen; University Hosp, Leiden; St Radboud Hosp, Nijmegen, The Netherlands)
Surgery 105:331–336, March 1989   20–8

Erosive gastritis that may lead to atrophic changes may be caused by repeated exposure of the gastric mucosa to bile. The most pronounced changes, including mucosal atrophy, are noted within the first 2 years after gastric surgery. The effect of bile reflux on gastric secretory function after gastric surgery was determined in 22 patients with peptic ulcers before and 6 months after partial gastrectomy. The 2 groups of 11 patients each underwent either a Roux-en-Y diversion or a Billroth II anastomosis performed randomly. No significant differences in gastric secretory functions were observed preoperatively between the 2 groups.

In those patients having the Billroth II anastomosis, median fasting bile acids in the stomach increased from 0.35 to 16.10 μmol/hr postoperatively, but decreased significantly in the patients with Roux-en-Y anastomosis from 0.35 to 0.10 μmol/hr. A significant reduction of median values in basal acid output resulted from gastrectomy, with 4.6 vs. 0.6 mmol/hr for patients with the Billroth II anastomosis and 4.2 vs. 0.4 mmol/hr for patients with the Roux-en-Y anastomosis. Corresponding values for serum pepsinogen A were 121 vs. 86 μg/L and 92 vs. 45 μg/L, and for meal-stimulated serum gastrin secretion were 1,472 vs. 199 picomolars (pM)/60 min and 1,017 vs. 199 pM/60 min. Six months after surgery no significant differences in gastric secretory parameters were found between the 2 groups.

The secretory function of the gastric remnant after gastrectomy is not different in patients who have had either Billroth II or Roux-en-Y anastomosis. Both procedures resulted in marked improvement. Therefore, enterogastric reflux does not affect the secretory function of the gastric remnant within the first 6 months after surgery.

▶ As soon as someone (Drapanas?) advocated use of Roux-en-Y drainage of the stomach as a treatment for the nebulous condition of postoperative alkaline reflux gastritis, I knew that someone else would advocate Roux-Y drainage as a routine hook-up after gastrectomy for peptic ulcer disease. Sure enough, the present authors quote 3 articles recommending just such a course. The problem is, ultimately, that placing the defunctionalized jejunum at the unbuffered mercy of acid-peptic digestion (even after an acid-reducing procedure) increases the risk of marginal ulcer. We know that there is a finite risk of marginal ulcer with a Billroth I or II procedure, in both of which instances the small bowel mucosa is bathed by the benign influence of neutralizing bicarbonate from the pancreas and bile. When you create a Roux-Y limb, however, you expressly prevent such benign influences. I predict that in the next 10 years we will be taking down many of these Roux-Y hook-ups (we have already done 3 of these retrieval operations). I have been unremittingly skeptical about the whole significance of the diagnosis of bile reflux gastritis, and to have folks come along and advocate this physiologically dangerous (in my opinion) procedure on an elective basis seems wrong. The present authors have shown, moreover, that one of the putative justifications for the Roux-en-Y anastomosis, i.e., an increased secretory response to enterogastric reflux, does not exist.—J.C. Thompson, M.D.

The Need for Definitive Therapy in the Management of Perforated Gastric Ulcers: Review of 202 Cases

Hodnett RM, Gonzalez F, Lee WC, Nance FC, Deboisblanc R (Louisiana State Univ)
Ann Surg 109:36–39, January 1989   20–9

Frequently, perforation of a gastric ulcer is a fatal complication. Because these lesions are often grouped with the less lethal duodenal ulcer perforations, the mortality associated with the condition is underestimated. To identify those factors relevant to diagnosis and survival, a retrospective study was made of 202 patients who went to 3 Louisiana hospitals with perforated gastric ulcers. Only patients with gastric ulcers were included, not those with "channel ulcers" or peptic ulcers. Patients received surgical or medical treatment, or the diagnosis was made at autopsy. The median age was 55 years, with a range of 2 days to 99 years. Initial symptoms included abdominal pain in 93% of the patients, nausea and vomiting in 42%, and hematemesis in only 5%. Of 194 patients whose history was taken, 57% had no identifiable ulcer symptoms. Chest and abdominal x-ray examinations were the most helpful, showing pneumoperitoneum in 76% of those examined.

In 53 patients definitive surgery was performed; nondefinitive surgery was performed in the remaining 128 patients. Of 21 patients who did not undergo operation, 10 were treated medically, and in 11 the perforated ulcer was diagnosed at autopsy. In all, 20 deaths occurred in this group, accounting for a mortality of 95%. Overall mortality for the 202 patients was 26%. Mortality with operation was 18%; mortality without operation was 95%. There was a 29% mortality among the 128 patients treated with nondefinitive surgical procedures. Subsequent operative treatment was required in 25.7% of these cases. In the 53 patients treated with definitive procedures, the mortality was only 11.3%. The mortality was 52.8% among those who had a systolic blood pressure of 90 mm Hg or less. All 10 treated medically died. Of 26 patients treated operatively, the mortality was 35%. Forty percent of the patients survived operation without complication. The most common complication was atelectasis; sepsis and postoperative myocardial infarction were the most lethal events.

Immediate and aggressive surgical treatment is indicated by the high mortality among untreated and medically treated patients. The superiority of definitive operative procedures for patients with perforated gastric ulcer is shown by the higher mortality and need for reoperation in those who underwent nondefinitive operations. The Graham closure is inadequate for most patients with perforated gastric ulcer.

▶ First of all, "definitive" in this series means that some kind of acid-reducing procedure was performed in 53 patients (all but 3 had some form of distal gastric resection), whereas "nondefinitive" means simple closure of the perforation. The take-home message here is that there is a high mortality risk in patients with gastric perforations, and this and many other studies suggest that, whenever possible, a distal gastric resection should be performed if it encompasses the perforation. Many previous series (perhaps including this one) have a problem in interpretation of data in that the sickest patients were consigned to Graham closure of the perforation. It is important to operate on these patients early, and it appears also to be important to do a gastrectomy if the patient's condition and the anatomical situation appear to allow it.—J.C. Thompson, M.D.

Gastric Carcinoids

Aman S, Walia HS, Al Sayer H (Al Amiri Hosp, Kuwait)
J R Coll Surg Edinb 33:325–327, December 1988   20–10

Gastric carcinoid is a rare tumor, accounting for less than 3% of all carcinoids, and is not well understood. The average surgeon will encounter few cases. Three men and 1 woman with gastric carcinoid were seen from January 1982 to December 1986. All 4 were symptomatic on admission, with complaints of epigastric pain, upper gastrointestinal bleeding, and weight loss. The mean age at diagnosis was 40 years. Patient evaluation included hematologic investigations, a biochemical profile including SMAC-20, determination of serum gastrin levels and 5-hydroxytryptamine and 5-hydroxytryptophan concentrations, and 24-hour urinary estimation of 5-hydroxyindole acetic acid. A pentagastrin stimulation test was performed, as were chest x-ray examination, barium swallow, and ultrasound and CT scanning. All patients underwent endoscopic examination, and deep tissue biopsies were done.

Pathologic examination of the specimens showed a solitary carcinoid, ranging between 8 mm and 10 mm in diameter in 3 cases. In 1 case, there were multiple lesions, varying in size between 2 mm and 15 mm. All but

1 were broad-based polypoid lesions. On staining, all carcinoids were argyrophil positive but argentaffin negative with a predominantly trabeculated pattern.

Clinically, there were no distinguishing physical or radiologic features. One patient had an elevated 24-hour urinary 5-hydroxyindole acetic acid. All gastrin levels were normal, and no patient had pernicious anemia. The diagnosis was made and confirmed histologically in all patients before surgery.

Three patients underwent gastrectomy and in the fourth patient, who refused surgery, endoscopic resection was carried out in 2 stages. Follow-up included endoscopy of the remaining stomach, ultrasound, CT scan, and hormone assays every 3–6 months. All patients were alive at follow-up 3–6 years after surgery.

Conservative resection or simple endoscopic resection is adequate therapy for gastric carcinoids less than 1 cm in diameter.

▶ This paper, which is simply a case report of 4 patients, is included because gastric carcinoids may be caused by prolonged achlorhydria, and the tumors have been reported in rats treated for a long period with omeprazole. If omeprazole therapy becomes common, we will need to look for these tumors and familiarize ourselves with their life history. Some observers have predicted, in fact, that widespread adoption of omeprazole therapy for peptic ulcer patients will lead to the development of gastric carcinoid tumors as a complication in some of them. It is interesting that the 5-hydroxyindole acetic acid levels were elevated in 1 patient, and that the levels fell to normal on local resection. Because 5-hydroxytryptamine is metabolized on hepatic transit, I am not sure that I understand the elevated 5-hydroxyindole acetic acid level unless the tumor was producing massive amounts of 5-hydroxytryptamine.—J.C. Thompson, M.D.

Gastric Cancer After Peptic Ulcer Surgery: A Historic Prospective Cohort Investigation
Toftgaard C (Municipal Hosp, Aarhus, Denmark)
Ann Surg 210:159–164, August 1989   20–11

Studies on the relationship between gastric cancer and previous gastric surgery for benign peptic ulcer have yielded conflicting results. To examine the risk of the subsequent development of gastric cancer, 4,131 patients who had peptic ulcer surgery from 1955 through 1960 in 1 region were followed until cancer diagnosis or death, or to the end of the year 1982. Cancer incidence was compared with that in the total regional population in the same period.

The incidence of gastric cancer in the cohort was 46 observed vs. 47 expected. The incidence was less than expected until 15 years after surgery, but the risk increased by twofold to threefold after 20 years (Fig 20–3). The group having the highest risk comprised males with a Bill-

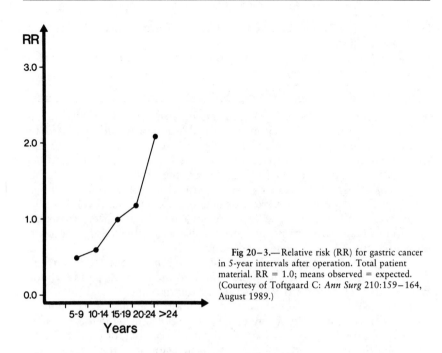

Fig 20–3.—Relative risk (RR) for gastric cancer in 5-year intervals after operation. Total patient material. RR = 1.0; means observed = expected. (Courtesy of Toftgaard C: *Ann Surg* 210:159–164, August 1989.)

roth II resection. The risk was similar for duodenal and gastric ulcers and whether symptoms were long lasting or were of shorter duration. There was no increased incidence of cancer in patients whose perforated ulcer had been treated by simple suture.

Peptic ulcer surgery may act as a precancerous agent. If a patient admitted because of stomach complaints has a history of peptic ulcer surgery more than 10 or 15 years previously, gastroscopy with multiple biopsies is recommended.

▶ Three years ago in this section I reviewed a study from England (see the 1987 YEAR BOOK OF SURGERY, pp 347–348) that summarized conflicting studies on the incidence of gastric carcinoma after gastric resection and concluded that one must follow patients for more than 20 years to demonstrate the phenomenon, which, I must say, appears to be real. Again, this paper from Denmark showed no great increase in risk until 20 years. It certainly does raise the question, however, of the possible carcinogenic effects of long-term acid suppression by highly effective drug therapy. If, as most physicians believe, there is an increased incidence of gastric cancer long after gastric resection, and if, as most also believe, that effect is caused by long-term suppression of acid secretion, we should expect to see the same thing in patients maintained by life-time suppression of acid secretion with H_2-receptor blockade or omeprazole. As far as I know, there has been no report of an increased incidence of gastric cancer after vagotomy without resection.—J.C. Thompson, M.D.

DNA Ploidy and Tumor Invasion in Human Gastric Cancer: Histopathologic Differentiation

Korenaga D, Haraguchi M, Okamura T, Baba H, Saito A, Sugimachi K (Kyushu Univ, Fukuoka, Japan)
Arch Surg 124:314–318, March 1989   20–12

That aneuploid tumors are usually associated with advanced disease and a poor prognosis has been confirmed for poorly differentiated tumors in carcinoma of the bladder, prostate, and breast, but not for gastric carcinoma. To assess the relationship between DNA ploidy and histopathologic features of gastric carcinoma, the DNA content of tumor specimens excised from 254 patients operated on for gastric carcinoma was measured. Specimens were classified as differentiated (DT) or undifferentiated (UT) tumors. The depth of invasion, tumor size, gross type, location, nodal involvement, and prognosis were reviewed in relation to individual tumor DNA ploidy and tumor type.

Of the 254 patients, 152 had low ploidy tumors and 102 had high ploidy tumors. Sixty-one low-ploidy tumors and 71 high-ploidy tumors were of the DT type, and 91 low-ploidy tumors and 31 high-ploidy tumors were of the UT type. Low-ploidy tumors confined to the mucosa were UT in histologic type, involved the middle third of the stomach, showed no lymph node metastasis, and were resectable for potential cure. High-ploidy tumors were associated with invasion into the serosal layer, were DT in histologic type, were located in the lower third of the stomach, showed no nodal involvement, and were not resectable for potential cure. For DT tumors, the rate of high ploidy was 42.9% at the mucosal stage and 68.4% at the serosal stage (Fig 20–4). Further, DNA ploidy was significantly correlated with prognosis, as the 5-year survival rate for patients with low-ploidy tumors was 90.6%, compared with 73.7% for patients with high-ploidy tumors. Thus aneuploidy is also a major prognostic factor for patients with gastric carcinomas.

▶ First of all, what is this ploidy business? Well, the normal DNA pattern of diploid chromosomes is 2c. The DNA distribution patterns can be divided into low and high groups according to the frequency of the aneuploid cell population, i.e., the frequency of high ploidy counts. A carcinoma with more than 10% of cells beyond the hexaploid (6c range) is designated as high ploidy (i.e., an aneuploid carcinoma); without such a proportion, the tumor is classified as low ploidy. Now there is general agreement that aneuploid tumors are usually related to advanced diseases, and this has been shown in carcinoma of the colon, esophagus, and prostate. The authors from Kyushu University have confirmed that some patients with gastric cancer have high ploidy tumors. When the authors went on to subject the prognostic data on their patients to multivariate analysis, they found that aneuploidy was a major independent factor for a poor prognosis.—J.C. Thompson, M.D.

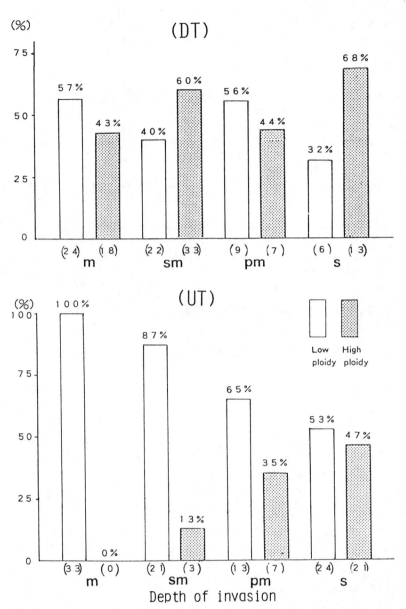

Fig 20–4.—Frequency of aneuploid carcinoma according to depth of invasion classified as differentiated *(at top)* or undifferentiated *(at bottom). Numbers in parentheses,* number of cases. *Asterisk,* significant difference compared with mucosa *(M) (P < .01)* and with submucosa *(SM) (P < .01). PM,* muscularis propria; *S,* subserosa and serosa; *shaded bars,* high ploidy; *open bars,* low ploidy. (Courtesy of Korenaga D, Haraguchi M, Okamura T, et al: *Arch Surg* 124:314–318, March 1989.)

Villous Tumors of the Duodenum

Chappuis CW, Divincenti FC, Cohn I Jr (Louisiana State Univ)
Ann Surg 209:593–599, May 1989   20–13

Villous tumors of the duodenum are relatively uncommon, but the incidence of malignancy in these lesions is high and the ampulla of Vater is frequently involved. Pancreaticoduodenectomy remains the procedure of choice for invasive cancer, but for those lesions that are benign or contain carcinoma in situ there is controversy about appropriate treatment.

Five patients had villous tumors of the duodenum involving the ampulla of Vater. Three patients were women, and average age of the 5 was 61 years. Before operation, all had endoscopic biopsies, and findings in specimens were interpreted as benign. The average size of the lesions was 3.3 cm, and all were sessile.

As an initial procedure 4 of the 5 patients had local excision; 1 had pancreaticoduodenectomy. Frozen sections prepared at the time of surgery in 4 patients were interpreted as benign. Subsequently, 2 were read as invasive carcinoma and 1 was read as carcinoma in situ, with foci of superficial microinvasion. One patient with a benign lesion had recurrence at 1 year, and the other had recurrence at 4 years. Both patients subsequently underwent pancreaticoduodenectomy and were alive and well 2 years and 5 years later. One of the 3 patients with carcinoma had a recurrence and died after 2 years. The other 2 are alive and well without evidence of recurrence at 2.5 years and 1.5 years.

Because of the risk of recurrence when local excision is used, and because of the difficulty in making an accurate preoperative diagnosis, pancreaticoduodenectomy should be strongly considered as the initial form of treatment of these lesions.

▶ The problem is that many of these tumors appear grossly benign. Endoscopists will look at them and take one of those minute fragmentary biopsy specimens that you get through an endoscope, and conclude that the tumor is benign and urge some kind of local resection. Local resections rarely work. This is just the lesion that the Whipple operation was designed for, and results will be uniformly good by using that great big operation for this relatively small tumor, which, if not completely removed, will recur and kill. In the Discussion of this paper, Kenneth Warren quotes Lord Smith in describing the pitfalls of local resection; he said, "You start out. It's a small tumor. It is a small cancer," and then goes on to tell about the need for wider, and wider, and wider resections, until the first thing you know is that you have taken the bile duct and the pancreatic duct or both apart from the duodenum. The best thing to do is to do a Whipple in the first place.—J.C. Thompson, M.D.

Endoscopic Laser Therapy for Duodenal Villous Adenoma

Paraf F, Naveau S, Zourabichvili O, Poynard T, Chaput JC (Hôp Antoine Béclère, Clamart, France)
Dig Dis Sci 34:1466–1467, September 1989   20–14

Villous adenomas of the duodenum occur rarely, but they present problems because of their propensity to become malignant, the difficulty in assessing the presence of malignancy, and controversy over the best way to treat them. Few descriptions of laser treatment have appeared.

Woman, 72, was seen because of melena. Endoscopy showed a sessile polyp 20 mm in diameter and 3 cm above the ampulla of Vater. Multiple biopsy samples revealed villoglandular adenoma with in situ focal carcinoma. The patient was considered inoperable because of a high-risk neurologic status, so therapy was carried out with the neodymium: yttrium/aluminum/garnet laser. Destruction of the entire adenoma required 6 laser sessions with a total of 24,217 J. Follow-up with endoscopic and histologic examinations for 30 months showed no recurrence.

Laser therapy should be considered for treatment of large, sessile duodenal villous adenomas in inoperable patients. Surveillance consisting of endoscopic examination repeated at 6-month intervals is suggested.

▶ Sure enough, you knew it would happen and here it is. There is no way in the world that you can tell whether the tumor is malignant if you zap it with a laser. This paper is included because it is, in my opinion, exactly what you do *not* want to do. You must excise the tumor so as to know whether it is malignant. It is extraordinarily difficult for a pathologist to know for sure even if he has the whole tumor available so that he can serially section it. If someone has vaporized it with a laser, you will not know until 7 or 10 or 12 years later when the tumor recurs in a malignant fashion.—J.C. Thompson, M.D.

True Clinical Entity of Vascular Compression of the Duodenum in Adolescence
Marchant EA, Alvear DT, Fagelman KM (Polyclinic Med Ctr, Harrisburg, Pa)
Surg Gynecol Obstet 168:381–386, May 1989   20–15

The superior mesenteric artery syndrome (SMAS) is defined as vascular compression of the superior mesenteric artery (SMA) at the root of the mesentery. Its existence remains a controversial subject because of the syndrome's nonspecific manifestations.

The signs and symptoms of SMAS were studied in 13 young patients, 9 females and 4 males aged 4–18 years. All except 1 complained of postprandial discomfort and early satiety. Acute vomiting and abdominal pain occurred in 12 patients, intractable bilious vomiting in 3, and severe dehydration in 2. In only 5 patients were significant differences noted between the age-related height and weight percentiles. The diagnosis was confirmed by roentgenographic studies of the upper gastrointestinal tract. All except 1 patient had duodenal obstruction without a systemic disorder or localized inflammation. Four patients were treated successfully with nasojejunal feedings alone. Nine underwent operative derotation; 6 of these patients had immediate relief of symptoms and only 1 required a gastrojejunostomy to bypass a persistent obstruction.

The SMAS is a distinct clinical entity that should be included in the differential diagnosis in any young patient with signs of obstruction of the upper gastrointestinal tract. Therapy is aimed specifically toward the problem of duodenal occlusion at the mesenteric root. All patients should initially be treated conservatively with nasojejunal feedings. Derotation proved to be the surgical procedure of choice.

▶ What is happening in Harrisburg? You would have a hard time getting together even 3 or 4 of these patients that you feel secure about—and their ages range all over the map—and here these folks find 13 adolescents in 1 hospital over a 12-year period. Most of them were found before Three-Mile Island, so we can't blame that. They do make a good case, however, and they provide good diagrammatic evidence of how compression of the duodenum comes about. They reiterate that diagnosis can be made by showing compression of the proximal third part of the duodenum, indentation of the superior mesenteric artery, and a to-and-fro motion of contrast media during fluoroscopy. In our experience, you can successfully treat the vast majority of these patients by getting them off their backs and having them lie on their stomachs (this is a marvelous indication for the circle electric bed) and putting some fat on them. I would certainly try to avoid operation, but if you must operate, I do not believe that gastrojejunostomy is the procedure of choice. Because the duodenum is obstructed, it should be decompressed and the jejunum should be anastomosed to the duodenum proximal to the compression. Best of all, get them off their backs and get them fat.—J.C. Thompson, M.D.

21 The Small Intestine

Surgical Implications of Jejunal Diverticula
Wilcox RD, Shatney CH (Univ of Florida, Jacksonville)
South Med J 81:1386–1391, November 1988   21–1

Because jejunal diverticulosis is uncommon, most physicians do not appreciate its potential clinical significance. To gain insight into the epidemiology, natural history, diagnosis, and management of jejunal diverticulosis, records from all teaching hospitals in the metropolitan area of Jacksonville were reviewed.

In 27 men and 59 women (mean age, 69.6 years) the diagnosis of jejunal diverticulosis was made ante mortem. In 71 patients the diagnosis of jejunal diverticulosis was made by upper gastrointestinal barium contrast study. Most of these patients had chronic abdominal pain or nonspecific gastrointestinal symptoms, such as nausea, diarrhea, or constipation. Mesenteric angiography or bleeding scan showed a jejunal source of massive rectal bleeding in 3 patients. Jejunal diverticulosis was discovered at laparotomy in the remaining 12 patients. In 6 of the 12 this was an incidental finding, and in the other 6 diverticular complications led to emergency operation.

Thirteen patients had complications of jejunal diverticulosis; 12 of these had multiple diverticula, of these, 4 had massive lower gastrointestinal bleeding, 3 had blind loop syndrome, 3 had small bowel obstruction, 2 had diverticular perforation, and 1 had chronic abdominal pain requiring jejunal resection. Another 12 patients had abdominal complaints consistent with jejunal diverticula, but none was operated on. Nine patients were treated successfully by resection and anastomosis for complications or symptoms of jejunal diverticula. Another 2 patients with jejunal diverticula were treated by diverticulectomy, but both died postoperatively.

When surgical intervention is indicated in patients with jejunal diverticulosis, resection and primary anastomosis is the operation of choice, even if only a solitary lesion is found. Local excision by diverticulectomy is not advisable. Of 11 patients operated on, the only deaths occurred in the 2 who had diverticulectomy. Breakdown of the diverticulectomy site and resulting intra-abdominal sepsis led to death in both patients.

▶ Diverticula of the small bowel are uncommon, and most of those that do occur are found in the duodenum (see a review of duodenal diverticula in the 1985 YEAR BOOK OF SURGERY, pp 374–376). This series of 86 jejunal diverticula occurring in 1 city during a 10-year period is remarkable, even if only 29% of the patients were symptomatic. The points to remember are these: not only Meckel's diverticula bleed, and any patient who is bleeding or has free intra-abdominal air may have a jejunal diverticulum as the etiology. All that I have seen have been incidental findings on small bowel series or operation, but I know of 2 that bled massively. There appears to be no justification for excising an asymptomatic jejunal diverticulum found incidentally at operation.—J.C. Thompson, M.D.

Gastrointestinal Tract Obstruction in the Fetus

Langer JC, Adzick NS, Filly RA, Golbus MS, deLorimier AA, Harrison MR (Univ of California, San Francisco)
Arch Surg 124:1183–1187, October 1989   21–2

The prenatal diagnosis of gastrointestinal tract obstruction is becoming more common. To help the consulting surgeon understand the natural course and prognosis, experience with 17 fetuses who underwent sonography in a 4-year-period was evaluated.

Complete proximal obstruction was found in 8 fetuses, 7 of whom survived after prompt neonatal surgery. Two had trisomy 18. Distal obstruction was diagnosed in 6 fetuses whose sonograms showed dilated bowel loops and increased peristaltic activity. Two of these died, 2 did well, and 2 had cystic fibrosis. Two had associated anomalies. All had polyhydramnios that appeared late and was not a sensitive or specific finding. Three fetuses had false positive sonograms, and all but 1 died of cytomegalovirus infection.

The prenatal diagnosis of gastrointestinal tract obstruction allows planned delivery and improved prognosis in most instances. In patients with proximal obstruction, karyotyping is recommended; in those with distal obstruction, the family history should be searched for cystic fibrosis. The development of ascites in the presence of documented bowel obstruction suggests perforation and should prompt early delivery. When the prenatal diagnosis is presented appropriately, the response of parents to a sick neonate is more positive.

▶ The first question is why in the world did these fetuses undergo sonographic examination in the first place? The authors state that all but 1 were studied because of a discrepancy between fetal size and date of gestation. Usually, that meant that polyhydramnios was suspected. Second, we should all realize that detection of intrauterine pathology may help us to meet difficult challenges; aggressive application of these techniques means that all pediatric surgeons will be waiting for a sick baby to come out (either by cesarean section or vaginal delivery). The third observation is that, compared with obstruction of the proximal small bowel, intrauterine obstruction of the *distal* small bowel has a much worse prognosis. Surgeons, pediatricians, radiologists, and colleagues in the fetal treatment program at The University of California at San Francisco are leaders in the study and treatment of sick fetuses and neonates. Prenatal diagnosis permits appropriate counseling of the parents, a carefully planned delivery, and prompt resuscitation and operation after birth.—J.C. Thompson, M.D.

The Role of Contrast Radiography in Presumed Bowel Obstruction

Riveron FA, Obeid FN, Horst HM, Sorensen VJ, Bivins BA (Henry Ford Hosp, Detroit)
Surgery 106:496–501, September 1989   21–3

Contrast radiography is used increasingly in the diagnosis of acute small bowel obstruction, but its value remains controversial. To assess its role in diagnosis, 229 patients whose final diagnosis was small bowel obstruction were studied. The observations from clinical examination and plain abdominal films were helpful enough to be the basis for diagnosis and management in 84 patients. Contrast studies—either upper gastrointestinal series, barium enema, or both—were used in 145 patients.

In the latter 145 patients there were 2 false positive results and 3 false negative results. Contrast radiography revealed no evidence of obstruction in 77 patients, low-grade or moderate obstruction in 21, Crohn's disease in 8, carcinoma or radiation changes in 16, and incarcerated ventral hernia in 1. In 22 patients contrast studies confirmed high-grade or complete obstruction that warranted early operation. No morbidity was directly attributable to the contrast studies. The mortality rate was 7.6% in those who had such studies and 6% in the others.

Contrast radiography is a safe and effective means of increasing diagnostic accuracy when the diagnosis of small bowel obstruction is equivocal. In such cases the studies should be performed early to differentiate between patients who need early operative intervention and those who can be managed conservatively.

▶ Can't these folks make a diagnosis of small bowel obstruction without a contrast radiographic study? Well, more than 63% of their patients had contrast studies, and even though I feel fairly enthusiastic about the study in appropriate cases (i.e., when I can't make up my mind) the high percentage seems excessive. The authors themselves state that the indications for the use of contrast radiography are (1) to assist when one cannot make the diagnosis otherwise, (2) to differentiate complete from partial obstruction, (3) to differentiate paralytic ileus from mechanical obstruction, and (4) to judge the relative safety of prolonged nonoperative management in high-risk patients. Even if you grant these assumptions, it seems unlikely that they would apply to nearly 2 of every 3 patients with small bowel obstruction. It is reassuring to see the authors state at the end of the article that the sun should never set on a bowel obstruction . . . as most such patients come in at night, we ought to say that the sun shouldn't rise on one either.—J.C. Thompson, M.D.

Enteroclysis in the Diagnosis of Intestinal Obstruction in the Early Postoperative Period

Dehn TCB, Nolan DJ (John Radcliffe Hosp, Oxford, England)
Gastrointest Radiol 14:15–21, Winter 1989   21–4

Intestinal obstruction after abdominal surgery is occasionally difficult to diagnose from clinical signs and plain abdominal radiographs. The enteroclysis technique—small bowel barium enema—is useful in demonstrating obstruction in the early postoperative period and in differentiating obstruction from ileus. Suspected intestinal obstruction was diagnosed successfully with enteroclysis in 14 patients (median age, 53 years).

Nine patients had undergone colonic or rectal resection, 3 had appendectomy, 1 had a laparotomy, and 1 had refashioning of an ileostomy. Symptoms included abdominal distention, failure of intestinal action, and persistent nasogastric output. Plain abdominal radiographs could not distinguish obstruction from ileus in 6 patients. The barium examination, performed at a median of 9 days after surgery, confirmed obstruction in all patients and identified the cause in 5. Laparotomy to relieve obstruction was necessary in 11 patients.

Small intestinal obstruction is associated with a high degree of morbidity and mortality. The complication is most common in abdominoperineal rectal and major colonic resections. In the early postoperative period the normal radiologic appearance of obstruction is obscured in some patients by fluid-filled intestinal loops. Although enteroclysis is not required in most patients when obstruction is difficult to determine, the use of barium is a safe and effective diagnostic tool.

▶ First, an enema is something you put through your rectum, and these patients were studied by means of injecting barium through a tube in the distal duodenum or proximal jejunum. We have been very pleased with enteroclysis in studying patients with early postoperative small bowel obstruction; in several instances, we believe that the instillation of contrast fluid has had a therapeutic effect, i.e., the patient had a more or less explosive episode of diarrhea afterward (our radiologists often use a liquid soluble iodine preparation with a high osmotic index). The study often shows complete bowel obstruction and serves as an impetus to early intervention.—J.C. Thompson, M.D.

Comparison of Five Methods of Assessment of Intestinal Viability
Brolin RE, Semmlow JL, Sehonanda A, Koch RA, Reddell MT, Mast BA, Mackenzie JW (UMDNF-Robert Wood Johnson Med School, New Brunswick, NJ)
Surg Gynecol Obstet 168:6–12, January 1989   21–5

A major unsolved problem in surgical treatment of the gastrointestinal tract is evaluation of the viability of ischemic small intestine. A strain gauge probe was designed that is capable of quantitative measurement of intestinal ischemic damage. This device, the electronic contractility meter, when clipped to the serosal surface of the small intestine, delivers a precisely controlled electrical stimulus that produces a well-defined smooth-muscle contraction over a 15-second response period. The minimum stimulus in milliamps necessary to produce a smooth-muscle contractile response is the threshold stimulus level (TSL). Resection and anastomosis in ischemic intestinal segments was carried out in 30 days to compare

TSL, intestinal color, peristalsis, Doppler ultrasound, and resection margin histology with survival.

Five fatal anastomotic leaks occurred, all resulting from intestinal necrosis. At 4 of the 5 anastomoses that leaked, there was no Doppler pulse in the marginal artery, whereas it was absent from only 8 of the 25 anastomoses that healed. The mean TSL at the resection site was 51 mA in nonsurvivors and 38 mA in survivors. In normal intestine the mean TSL was 22 mA. Both Doppler ultrasound and TSL correlated with resection margin histology. No correlation was found between presence of peristalsis and histologic grade or survival rate. Intestinal color correlated with resection margin histology but not with survival. The TSL measured by the contractility meter and marginal artery Doppler signal were the only 2 of the 5 methods of viability assessment that correlated with survival.

The results suggest that the quantitative electronic contractility meter measurements were more sensitive indices of viability than the presence of pulsatile arterial flow as measured by Doppler ultrasound.

▶ The problem with papers like this is that often they are set up as strawmen to prove the superiority of some arcane new device that the authors have invented, and they then proceed to show that their gadget is better than anything else. The present paper is true to form except that the authors also say that Doppler ultrasound, as well as myoelectric measurements by their electronic contractility meter, were both positively correlated with late viability. Three of the methods studied—intestinal color, presence of peristalsis, and histology of the resected margins—did not correlate with the intestinal survival rate in this experimental study in dogs. When I was 12, I went deer hunting with my father, and he eviscerated a deer he had killed early in the morning; when we came back around sunset, the mound of small bowel lying on the ground was still motile—so much for motility as an indicator of viability.—J.C. Thompson, M.D.

High-Output External Fistulae of the Small Bowel: Management With Continuous Enteral Nutrition

Lévy E, Frileux P, Cugnenc PH, Honiger J, Ollivier JM, Parc R (Hôp Saint Antoine, Paris; Hôp Laennec, Paris)

Br J Surg 76:676–679, July 1989   21–6

In the past 25 years modern principles have been formulated for the management of enterocutaneous fistulas. Total parenteral nutrition (TPN) has become the standard technique of provision of artificial nutrition to these patients, although most investigators believe that the usefulness of enteral nutrition with chemically defined diets is limited to low-output fistulas. The role of TPN was evaluated in 335 patients with high-output enterocutaneous fistulas arising from the small intestine.

The median fistula output was 1,350 mL/24 hr. In 165 patients (49%) the fistula opening was associated with abdominal wound dehiscence. In 75.5% of the patients at least 1 severity factor was present. Based on initial therapy, the patients were divided into 3 groups; 21 were referred in a moribund state and were not operated on (nonintervention); 80 were operated on as emergencies with the fistula either exteriorized or defunctional; and 234 (70%) received conservative management initially. In all cases appropriate local care and nutrition were provided. In 285 patients enteral nutrition was the exclusive nutritional support. Methods limiting fistula output or allowing reinfusion of chyme were required in 92 patients with proximal fistulas.

The overall mortality was 34%, but in the nonintervention group it was 100%. After emergency surgery mortality was 55%, and after conservative treatment, 19%. Eighty-eight of the 234 patients initially managed conservatively had spontaneous closure. In patients treated since 1980 the overall mortality was reduced to 19%.

In most high-output enterocutaneous fistulas, enteral nutrition with appropriate local care may be used, with an acceptable rate of spontaneous closure resulting. In the initial period treatment should be conservative. Emergency surgery carries a high risk of mortality and should be restricted to the treatment of hemorrhage or intra-abdominal abscesses associated with uncontrolled systemic sepsis.

▶ The interesting aspects of this study are the huge number of patients involved over 16 years, the high average fistula output (more than 1,300 mL/day), and the fact that 20 years age this group was using continuous enteral nutrition. The authors emphasize, as we all should, the importance of local control of fistula output so as to protect the skin from digestion.

I have problems understanding this study because the *British Journal of Surgery,* or these authors, give the caloric value of their enteral solution in kJ/mL (they aimed at a net intake of 209 kJ/kg/day), and I do not know how many calories equals a kiloJoule. They used parenteral nutrition only in the early days of resuscitation, and their excellent results appear to come from the enteral administration of nutrient fluids. The problem of when to operate on patients with fistula is of course not resolved and probably never will be. I am happy, when patients seem to start to get better, to then go ahead and operate. The mean duration of hospitalization was 72 days, with a mean stay in the intensive care unit of 43 days (I could not find the range of stay in the hospital). (You can't help but wonder where the diagnosis-related group business stands in France—the authors state that elective surgery should not be undertaken until at least 6 weeks after resolution of signs of intra-abdominal sepsis, and this often corresponds to 60–75 days after initial surgery.) Nonetheless, this is an extraordinary study and should energize us to the early use of enteral support. I wish they had told us how the fistula output responded to introduction of enteral feedings.—J.C. Thompson, M.D.

Extensive Short-Bowel Syndrome in Neonates: Outcome in the 1990s
Caniano DA, Starr J, Ginn-Pease ME (Ohio State Univ; Children's Hosp, Columbus, Ohio)
Surgery 105:119–124, February 1989

21–7

Data were reviewed concerning the clinical course, operative requirements, achievement of enteral alimentation, morbidity, and mortality of 14 infants with extensive short-bowel syndrome (SBS) treated from 1978 to 1987. Extensive SBS is defined as a residual jejunoileal length of 25% or less than the normal expected length for each infant's gestational age. Usually, SBS was caused by congenital abdominal well or midgut anomalies such as gastrochisis, jejunal atresia, midgut volvulus, and congenital SBS; in 2 patients SBS was caused by necrotizing enterocolitis.

The mean residual jejunoileal length was 32 cm (range, 15–53 cm), which represented an average 16% of normal expected jejunoileal length for gestational age. Problems related to total parenteral nutrition (TPN) accounted for the greatest morbidity and included catheter sepsis in 13 infants, cholestasis in 8, central venous thrombosis in 4, and cholelithiasis in 3. The survival rate was 86%; 2 infants died of end-stage liver disease. Eight of the 12 survivors achieved intestinal adaptation and discontinued TPN; 3 others are maintained with combined TPN-enteral feeding, and 1 receives TPN only. An intact ileocecal valve allowed intestinal adaptation and enteral alimentation in patients with shorter jejunoileal length. The mean cost of the initial hospitalization was $315,000, with an average stay of 450 days.

These data demonstrate that survival and eventual anteral alimentation can be anticipated in most neonates with extensive SBS. However, morbidity remains a problem, and methods to decrease the the morbidity of prolonged TPN and to enhance the adaptive process of the residual intestine must be developed. Home-based TPN and enteral feeding for infants with SBS may significantly lessen the economic impact of this condition.

▶ This extraordinary study forces us to face the issue of cost. How much is it worth to save a neonatal child? The authors tell us that the mean cost of initial hospitalization was $315,000 (range, $34,000 to $830,000) with an average initial hospitalization of 450 days (range, 68–1,151 days, or 3.15 years). Who has the right to judge how the resources of a society should be allocated? A Chinese female obstetrician who visited our institution, shocked by the presence of and outlook for some of the patients in our neonatal intensive care unit, suggested that we were interfering with Darwin. She asked if we were really so rich that we could afford this. I do not believe that anyone knows the answer to that now, but I believe that sooner or later we must face the question.

Nonetheless, consider that of the 12 surviving children, 3 had only 9% to 12% of their normal jejunoileal length yet eventually achieved complete enteral nutrition. It is truly a marvelous result, and the question of whether it is right or not will have to be answered by someone. I am not qualified.—J.C. Thompson, M.D.

Effect of Perioperative Blood Transfusion on Recurrence of Crohn's Disease
Williams JG, Hughes LE (Univ of Wales, Cardiff)
Lancet 2:131–132, July 15, 1989   21–8

Crohn's disease has a high rate of recurrence after surgical treatment. Because immunologic mechanisms may be involved in the etiology of this condition, the immunosuppressive effect of blood transfusion might influence the progression of Crohn's disease. The records of 60 consecutive patients were studied to determine the effect of transfusion on recurrence of the disease.

Twenty-eight patients undergoing a first resection of small-bowel Crohn's disease received a median of 3 units of whole blood or plasma-reduced heterologous blood perioperatively; 32 patients were not transfused. The groups were similar in age and duration of illness. Transfused patients, however, had longer lengths of affected bowel and midileal involvement, conditions usually associated with a greater incidence of recurrence.

At follow-up of approximately 5 years, those patients who received perioperative blood transfusions had a significantly lower recurrence rate (19%) than nontransfused patients (59%). Of 19 patients with a proven recurrence, 15 had not received transfusions (Fig 21–1). Blood transfusion may improve the outcome in Crohn's disease by its immunosuppressive effects, which include increases in suppressor T cells, in suppressor cell activity, and in numbers of immunoglobulin-secreting cells in the cir-

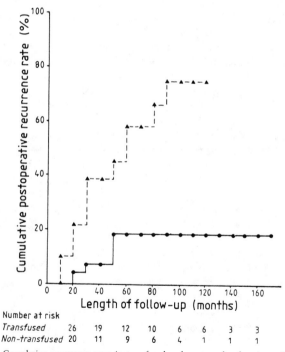

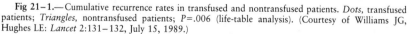

Fig 21–1.—Cumulative recurrence rates in transfused and nontransfused patients. *Dots,* transfused patients; *Triangles,* nontransfused patients; P=.006 (life-table analysis). (Courtesy of Williams JG, Hughes LE: *Lancet* 2:131–132, July 15, 1989.)

culation. In addition, natural killer cell activity and phagocytic cell activity are reduced.

▶ A glance at Figure 21 – 1 tells the story. The question is, can we assume that the protection conveyed by transfusion against recurrence of Crohn's disease can be ascribed to an immunologic mechanism? Well, just try to think of something else, as kidney transplant surgeons have for years, after learning that the survival of renal allografts is enhanced by previous transfusion.

Blood transfusions have been taking a drumming for their role in transmitting diseases; it is interesting to see that occasionally they may be helpful.—J.C. Thompson, M.D.

22 The Colon and the Rectum

The Consequences of Current Constraints on Surgical Treatment of Appendicitis
Cacioppo JC, Diettrich NA, Kaplan G, Nora PF (Columbus Hosp, Chicago)
Am J Surg 157:276–281, March 1989   22–1

During the past decade policies aimed at cost containment have altered many aspects of health care. Previous studies revealed that patients with cholelithiasis and inguinal hernias have not received adequate benefits, medically speaking, as a result of the constraints on elective surgical referral. Investigators chose a condition that does not offer options for medical or elective operative treatment—acute appendicitis—to determine whether similar trends are affecting these patients.

The records of patients undergoing appendectomy were reviewed for the years 1980 (76 patients), 1986 (61 patients), and 1987 (73 patients). Information was obtained concerning the stage of disease, delay in referral, morbidity and mortality, and length of hospitalization. Three stages of acute appendicitis were identified: uncomplicated (group A), complicated (group B), and advanced (group C).

The rate of negative appendectomy remained unchanged over the years. Most patients (82%) underwent surgery within 6 hours of evaluation. In no patient did perforation appear to have occurred between referral and surgery, and there were no deaths. But compared with 1980, significantly more patients progressed to advanced appendicitis with abscess (group C) in 1986 and 1987. A prolonged delay in hospitalization or surgical referral occurred in 37% of patients in 1986 and in 29% in 1987. As a consequence, over the course of the 1980s morbidity more than quadrupled, resulting in an extended hospital stay.

In patients whose condition requires urgent operative treatment, current policies result in deterioration in patient care and failure in cost containment. When acute appendicitis is suspected, immediate referral, hospitalization, and surgery, even though results may be negative, will actually lower costs.

▶ Almost any surgeon, I believe, would be willing to admit, in the abstract, that some control over rising costs of medical care is necessary, but so far we have not yet found the secret. Efforts at seeking second and third opinions, placing gatekeepers at the door of the hospital, requiring preadmission certification— all of these have doubtless changed the practice of surgery, but it would be difficult to document any savings because the cumbersome bureaucracy that maintains these hurdles is in itself expensive. Probably the most important change has been brought about by the diagnosis-related groups, which encourage both truncation of hospital stay and curtailment of extraneous studies. I do not know that we have experienced the delay in admission of patients with acute appendicitis that is detailed in this paper from Chicago, but the study does clearly point out the consequences that may accompany impediments to hospitalization, i.e., those who do get in may have complications that cost more money. Money, of course, is not the overwhelming factor here; our moral obligations to our patients are what is important, but we can measure money.—J.C. Thompson, M.D.

Incidence and Case Fatality Rates for Acute Appendicitis in California: A Population-Based Study of the Effects of Age

Luckmann R (Univ of California, Davis)
Am J Epidemiol 129:905–918, May 1989   22–2

The number of deaths from appendicitis has decreased substantially in the past 50 years in all but the older age groups. Perforation accounts for most deaths, and the proportion of cases with perforation is more than 50% in persons older than 60 years. Data from the California Health Facilities Commission were studied to determine the age- and sex-specific incidence and case fatality rates of appendectomy for acute appendicitis.

During 1984, there were 29,674 surgical procedures performed for acute appendicitis. Subclassifications were nonperforating, perforating,

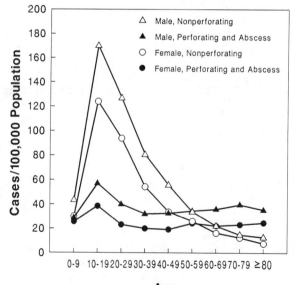

Age

Fig 22–1.—Incidence of appendectomy and drainage of abscess for appendicitis by age, sex, and type in California in 1984. Perforating appendicitis and appendiceal abscess are combined. (Courtesy of Luckmann R: *Am J Epidemiol* 129:905–918, May 1989.)

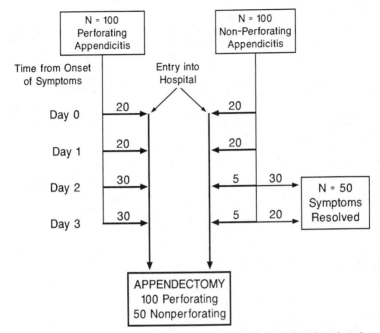

Fig 22–2.—Time course from onset of symptoms to hospital admission for 2 hypothetical types of appendicitis. *Numbers over arrows* indicate patients admitted to the hospital on the day after symptom onset shown on the same line. (Courtesy of Luckmann R: *Am J Epidemiol* 129:905–918, May 1989.)

and abscess. In males, nonperforating appendicitis peaked at 170 cases per 100,000 in the age groups 10–19 years. Females had a lower incidence in most age groups, although the rates grew closer after age 40 years and converged in those aged 80 years and older. Perforating cases were more equally divided between the sexes (Fig 22–1).

Patients older than 80 years were less likely than younger patients to have surgery on the day of hospital admission; most received timely surgery and tolerated it well. Age did not appear to affect the ability to tolerate uncomplicated surgery, but it did reduce a patient's ability to withstand infection. Older patients may not necessarily have a greater tendency to have perforation, but they have a decreased incidence of nonperforating appendicitis.

These findings suggest that nonperforating and perforating appendicitis may be 2 distinct entities, the former strongly related to age and the latter occurring at equal rates in all age groups. Obstruction appears to be involved in perforating appendicitis, whereas viral infection is linked to the nonperforating form of the disease. Symptoms tend to resolve in patients with nonperforating appendicitis, but they worsen when perforation occurs (Fig 22–2). If there are indeed these 2 types, early surgery would have little effect on mortality from nonperforating appendicitis.

▶ Surgical teaching for 50 years has been that appendicitis is most difficult to diagnose and most lethal in infancy and in very old age; this epidemiologic study confirms the latter teaching. Older patients tend to either tolerate or ignore minor signals from their belly, and a large number seek admission only after perforation occurs when they have ileus that is misdiagnosed as bowel obstruction. The suggestion that half of the patients with nonperforating appendicitis may experience spontaneous resolution of their symptoms is contrary to most teaching, but I am prepared to believe it (although I am not sure of the proper proportion). When I was in the Army taking care of young GIs who were often happy to be in the hospital, I saw an extraordinary number of very early cases of what appeared to be appendicitis in evolution, and in many instances the process resolved spontaneously. The authors suggest that there are 2 separate diseases—1 type that will perforate and another that will not. It is an interesting syllogism that, once invoked, is difficult to prove (or disprove).—J.C. Thompson, M.D.

Carcinoid Tumors of the Appendix in Children Younger Than 16 Years: A Retrospective Clinical and Pathologic Study
Jónsson T, Jóhannsson JH, Hallgrimsson JG (Icelandic Cancer Registry; Univ of Iceland, Reykjavik)
Acta Chir Scand 155:113–116, February 1989   22–3

Carcinoid tumors of the appendix are usually treated with standard appendectomy. However, there has been some support for more radical excision because of reports of metastasis. In view of the long life expectancy of children, the issue of more radical surgery has particular importance. The long-term outcome of standard appendectomy in the treatment of appendiceal carcinoid tumors in children was reviewed retrospectively.

During a 30-year period 14 girls and 4 boys aged 4–15 years underwent standard appendectomy in the treatment of carcinoid tumors of the appendix. Fifteen children had preoperative diagnoses of acute appendicitis. Histologic examination confirmed these diagnoses in 8 patients, 1 of whom had a perforated appendix. Two patients had only inflammation of the appendiceal serosa, suggesting inflammation elsewhere in the abdominal cavity. Carcinoid tumors were the only observed pathologic conditions in 5 patients. Tumor size ranged from 0.1 cm to 1.2 cm, with only 1 carcinoid measuring more than 1 cm. Carcinoid tumor was not suspected before operation in any of the patients.

Tumors were confined to the submucosa in 7 patients, had invaded the muscle layer in 1, the mesoappendix in 3, and the subserosal connective tissue in 7. None of the patients had metastasis at operation, and none underwent supplementary treatment.

After 2.2–29.3 years of follow-up after appendectomy, all 18 patients were alive without recurrence of carcinoid tumor. These findings support the view of other investigators that standard appendectomy is adequate treatment for carcinoid tumors of the appendix in children, regardless of invasion depth.

▶ Here is your chance to learn all about pediatric cases of appendiceal carcinoid in Iceland. The study was chosen for inclusion because of the long period of follow-up observation. There is nowhere to go (at least very far) in Iceland, so that follow-up studies are often models of completeness and differ greatly from those in the United States where half of our patients seem to be gypsies. I reviewed a study from the Mayo Clinic in this space last year that confirmed the general impression that metastatic disease is rare to absent in appendiceal carcinoids that are no larger than 2 cm (see the 1989 YEAR BOOK OF SURGERY, p 326). All of the tumors in this study from Reykjavik fall below that limit, so it is nor surprising to see good results.—J.C. Thompson, M.D.

The Efficacy of Oral Antimicrobials in Reducing Aerobic and Anaerobic Colonic Mucosal Flora
Groner JI, Edmiston CE Jr, Krepel CJ, Telford GL, Condon RE (Surgical Microbiology Research Lab, Milwaukee)
Arch Surg 124:281–284, March 1989   22–4

The impact of oral prophylaxis on the bacteriology of the colonic mucosal surface has not been examined. Intestinal antisepsis on the colonic mucosa-associated flora was investigated in 28 dogs. The animals were

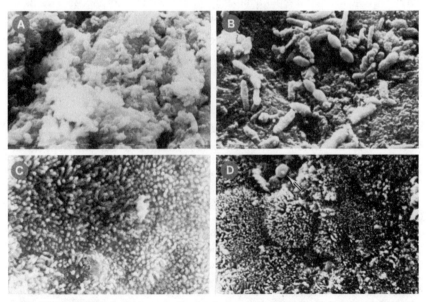

Fig 22–3.—**A,** SEM of colonic mucosal surface in group B dog (clear-liquid diet) demonstrating intact mucin sheath in which rods and cocci are embedded (original magnification, ×2,400). **B,** colonic mucosal surface in group C dog (mechanical preparation) demonstrates some mucus debris with heterogeneous mucosa-associated bacteria (original magnification, ×3,000). **C,** mucosal surface in group D (oral antibiotics) showing no microorganisms in proximal colonic biopsy specimen (original magnification; ×4,000). **D,** single cocci-like organism *(arrow)* residing on brush-border surface in another group D biopsy specimen (original magnification, ×3,200). (Courtesy of Groner JI, Edmiston CE Jr, Krepel CJ, et al: *Arch Surg* 124:281–284, March 1989.)

assigned randomly to 4 groups. Group A received no bowel preparation; group B, a 3-day clear-liquid diet; group C, mechanical cleansing of the bowel; and group D, mechanical cleansing followed by oral neomycin and erythromycin. Mucosal biopsy specimens were taken for bacteriologic and scanning electron microscope (SEM) examination.

There was no significant difference in recovery of mucosal bacteria between groups A and B. A significant reduction in recovery of aerobes was noted in group C, and a significant reduction in both aerobes and anaerobes was noted in group D compared with group A. Enterobacteriaceae and *Bacteroides fragilis* were eliminated or greatly diminished. Scanning electron microscope analyses revealed a marked decrease in mucosa-associated microflora in group D compared with groups B and C (Fig 22–3).

Oral treatment with neomycin and erythromycin produced a significant quantitative decrease in the colonic mucosa-associated bacterial population in dogs, including the potentially pathogenic *Escherichia coli* and *B. fragilis* isolates. These mucosa-associated bacteria are a likely source of abdominal cavity and wound contamination at the time of colon surgery.

▶ This paper substantiates Edgar Poth's suggestion (1) nearly 40 years ago that bowel flora are best reduced by mechanical cleansing plus administration of neomycin and some other antibiotic. Dr. Condon and colleagues have been leaders in studies on bowel preparation, and this represents another strong contribution in which they actually studied the diminution in mucosal surface bacteria by scanning electron microscopy.—J.C. Thompson, M.D.

Reference

1. Poth E: *JAMA* 153:1516, 1953.

Volvulus of the Colon: A Review of 93 Cases and Current Aspects of Treatment

Påhlman L, Enblad P, Rudberg C, Krog M (Univ Hosp, Uppsala, Sweden; County Hosp, Västerås, Sweden)
Acta Chir Scand 155:53–56, January 1989   22–5

Volvulus of the colon is a fairly common condition, occurring most often among elderly patients. A number of treatment strategies are available, although no consensus exists on the optimal management of this condition. Different therapies were compared retrospectively in emergency and elective cases.

During a 15-year period, 93 patients were treated at 2 Swedish hospitals. Volvulus of the sigmoid colon was more common among men (46 of 53 patients). Women had a greater incidence of cecal volvulus (26 of 40 patients) (Fig 22–4). Volvulus of the sigmoid colon was treated with immediate decompression in 17 patients, emergency surgery in 28, and elec-

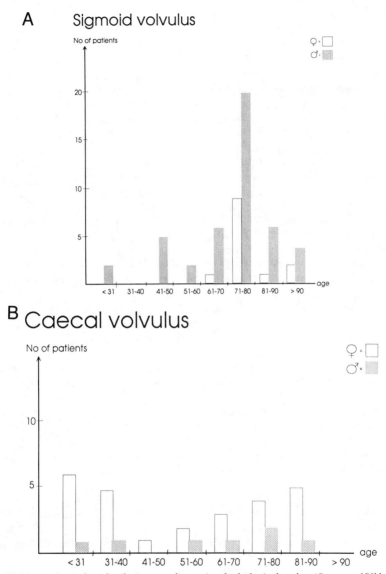

A   Sigmoid volvulus

B Caecal volvulus

Fig 22–4.—Age and sex distribution according to site of volvulus in the colon. (Courtesy of Påhlman L, Enblad P, Rudberg C, et al: *Acta Chir Scand* 155:53–56, January 1989.)

tive surgery in 13. Two patients were untreated. Thirty-one of the 33 patients with cecal volvulus underwent emergency laparotomy.

Nine patients with sigmoid volvulus and 8 with cecal volvulus died. Two patients had volvulus of both the cecum and sigmoid, a rarely reported occurrence. Most deaths were among those treated on an emergency basis, indicating the danger of this approach. Cecal volvulus, however, almost always requires emergency surgery; it is difficult to diagnose preoperatively and cannot be decompressed easily by colonic intubation.

Sigmoid volvulus without signs of gangrene can be managed by tube decompression followed within 2–3 days by sigmoid resection. When accompanied by peritonitis, emergency laparotomy and resection are necessary. The optimal treatment for cecal volvulus may be immediate colonoscopic decompression followed by a semiemergent surgical procedure.

▶ The mortality for sigmoid volvulus in most series is higher than that for cecal volvulus. Mortality rates are the same in this Swedish paper, which is surprising because the patients with sigmoid volvulus were older. Attempts should certainly be made to decompress sigmoid volvulus by insertion of a tube or by colonoscopy, bearing in mind Ben Eiseman's apocryphal suggestion that after such a maneuver it is often easier to get a new proctoscopist than it is to clean off the old one. The important thing to remember is that endoscopic decompression of sigmoid volvulus should be followed in 2 or 3 days by operation, and that the best operation to perform is sigmoid resection, getting rid of all the redundant colon. I would not agree with the authors' suggestion here that patients with cecal volvulus should first have colonoscopic decompression. That would be applicable, in my opinion, only when the world's slickest colonoscopist was on 24-hour call. Otherwise, the resultant delay in getting the patient with a cecal volvulus to the operating room would lead to an increased mortality risk.

The sexual predilection of these conditions is puzzling: I never will understand sex, and I certainly do not understand sex as it influences choice of disease. Why are 87% of the patients with sigmoid volvulus men, whereas 65% of those with cecal volvulus are women? In the paper from Iceland previously reviewed in this section (Abstract 22–3), why were 78% of children with carcinoid tumors of the appendix girls? This is a major conundrum. If we could solve it we could make, I am sure, an absolutely vital observation. As yet, we do not even know how to begin to attack the problem.—J.C. Thompson, M.D.

Primary Repair of Colon Wounds: A Prospective Trial in Nonselected Patients

George SM Jr, Fabian TC, Voeller GR, Kudsk KA, Mangiante EC, Britt LG (Univ of Tennessee, Memphis)

Ann Surg 209:728–734, June 1989   22–6

Surgical practice in dealing with wounds of the colon has been based on trauma surgery protocols developed during wartime. The most frequently used approach, exteriorization of the wounded colon as a colostomy, however, may not be necessary in most civilian wounds. Primary repair may be possible in all patients without any anastomotic failure. In a prospective study penetrating wounds to the intraperitoneal colon were treated on the assumption that primary repair would be possible in most nonselected patients.

Of 102 consecutive patients, 92 were male and 10 were female; the mean age was 30 years. Injuries resulted from gunshot (67%), stab (24%), and shotgun (9%) wounds. Of 175 associated injuries, 47 occurred in the small bowel. Most patients (66%) had mild contamination; about a third required 4 or more units of blood. Treatment consisted of primary repair of the colon wound in 81%, resection and primary anastomosis in 12%, and resection with end colostomy in 7%.

Septic complications occurred in 33% of the patients but was unrelated to primary repair. Development of an intra-abdominal abscess was related to significant contamination, more than 2 associated injuries, and transfusion with 4 or more units of blood. None of the 3 deaths was directly related to the colon wound. In the 93% of patients in this trial who were treated with primary repair or anastomosis, only 1 failure occurred.

Such treatment has a number of advantages over colostomy closure, including lower cost and decreased morbidity. Colostomy can be reserved for patients with a prolonged delay to surgery, or for those with severe blood loss that requires packing for coagulopathy.

▶ This study corroborates the ongoing experience from Baylor (1), but goes even further in concluding that " . . . nearly all penetrating colon wounds can be repaired primarily or with resection and anastomosis, regardless of risk factors." One of the first things that happens in any war that this country gets into is that an edict appears from the Surgeon General's office that colon wounds will be managed by colostomy. Now that many inner city hospitals are working in a de facto combat zone, now that many civilian injuries are caused by rifles with high-muzzle velocities, and now that there is great experience in the primary management of colon injury (direct suture of small wounds and resection and anastomosis with devascularizing injuries), you cannot help but wonder whether combat casualties could now now be safely managed in a primary fashion. We all pray that we do not have to find out.—J.C. Thompson, M.D.

Reference

1. Burch JM, et al: *Ann Surg* 203:701, 1986.

Evaluation of Right Hemicolectomy for Unexpected Cecal Mass
Riseman JA, Wichterman K (Southern Illinois Univ, Springfield)
Arch Surg 124:1043–1044, September 1989   22–7

Finding an unexpected ileocecal mass at laparotomy for presumed appendicitis presents a therapeutic dilemma to the surgeon because the diagnosis is not always clear. Whereas the differential diagnosis of neoplasm, diverticular disease, inflammatory bowel disease, or severe appendicitis involving the ileocecal region may usually be obvious, in some cases it can be confirmed only with the pathology report.

During a 5-year period an unexpected ileocecal mass was found in 13 of 1,445 patients who underwent operation for presumed appendicitis.

Preoperatively, all patients had reported pain and tenderness in the right lower quadrant, and all had leukocytosis with low-grade fever. Seven patients (average age, 58 years) had an appendiceal phlegmon and underwent right hemicolectomy for appendicitis. Five of these patients had correct preoperative diagnoses of appendicitis; 1 was operated on for presumed cecal carcinoma that proved to be an appendiceal mass. Hepatic dysfunction resulting from an antibiotic drug reaction developed in 1 of these patients. Inflammatory bowel disease or tumor was eventually diagnosed in 6 patients (average age, 47 years), but only 1 of these 6 had a correct diagnosis before operation. One patient in this group died secondary to steroid-dependent chronic obstructive pulmonary disease 45 days after operation.

For patients in whom an unexpected mass is found at operation for presumed appendicitis, right hemicolectomy as an emergency procedure in an unprepared bowel is reasonably safe, allowing resolution of the immediate problem with acceptable morbidity.

▶ There is no way to distinguish safely between a paracecal or a para-right-colonic phlegmon that is caused by a ruptured appendix, a perforated cecal diverticulum, or a perforated cecal carcinoma. It has been, I believe, standard surgical practice for some time to treat all of these by excision of the right colon. In doing so, we take no more than 4 or 5 cm of the terminal ileum (unless inflammation dictates), and we try to leave in as much of the right colon as possible. There is nothing magical about taking out the hepatic flexure. Whether or not to do a primary anastomosis, or whether to do a diverting ileostomy, depends on whether the patient is in good condition generally and whether there is free local pus. If there is abundant local pus, and if the bowel is inflamed and edematous, temporary exteriorization of the ileum and colon often prevents leakage from an ileocolostomy. It took me a long time to learn that, but sitting at our weekly Morbidity and Mortality Conference for years has confirmed the wisdom of that approach.—J.C. Thompson, M.D.

Obstructing Carcinomas of the Colon
Serpell JW, McDermott FT, Katrivessis H, Hughes ESR (Monash Univ; Alfred Hosp, Victoria, Australia)
Br J Surg 76:965–969, September 1989   22–8

From 7% to 29% of all patients with colorectal cancer have obstruction of the large bowel. These patients have significantly poorer prognoses than patients with colon cancer without obstruction. To explain this finding, the clinicopathologic and survival data of 908 patients with colon cancer were analyzed. Of these, 148 had complete bowel obstruction at first examination, 280 had partial obstruction, and 480 had no evidence of bowel obstruction. All underwent standard resections appropriate to the tumor site and presence of obstruction.

Tumor staging revealed that only 7.4% of the patients with complete obstruction had Dukes' stage A tumors, compared with 17.9% of the patients without obstruction. Any difference in the distribution of Dukes' B and Dukes' C tumors was not significant. However, only 24.8% of the patients without obstruction had Dukes' D tumors, compared with 39.2% of those with complete bowel obstruction.

The overall rate of cancer recurrence in patients without obstruction

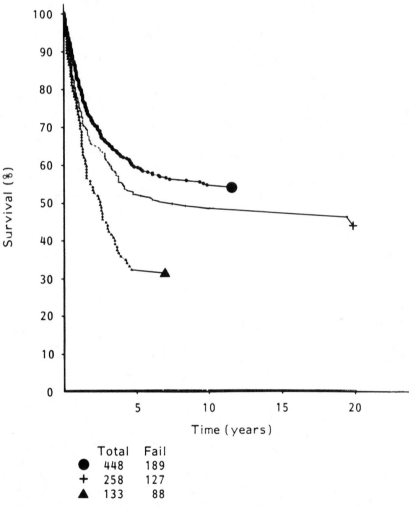

	Total	Fail
●	448	189
+	258	127
▲	133	88

Fig 22–5.—Cancer-specific survival rates in relation to no obstruction *(circles)*, partial obstruction *(plus sign)*, or complete obstruction *(triangle)* for the total series. Patients dying of complications within 90 days were excluded *Fail* signifies death from cancer of the colon; each mark on the survival curve represents an individual patient's death from recurrence. The heavier markings during the earlier postoperative years are consequent to an increased frequency of deaths during this period. Each survival curve attains a plateau after the last mark, which represents the time of death of the patient who to date has survived the longest before dying of colon cancer. The no-obstruction and complete obstruction groups have been followed for a period comparable to that for patients with partial obstruction (P<.04) and comparing complete with no obstruction (P<.001). (Courtesy of Serpell JW, McDermott FT, Katrivessis H, et al: *Br J Surg* 76:965–969, September 1989.)

was 25.4%, compared with 41.3% in patients with obstruction. The overall 5-year cancer-specific survival rate for patients without obstruction was 59.1%, compared with 31.8% for those with complete bowel obstruction (Fig 22–5). The 5-year cancer-specific survival rate after curative resection was 54.1% for patients with obstruction, compared with 78.9% for those without obstruction.

The data suggest that colonic cancer completely obstructing the bowel is more aggressive than other types of colon cancers. Whether the obstruction process itself affects the relationship between the tumor and host resistance has not yet been determined.

▶ As this experience suggests, a partial explanation for the poor prognosis in patients with obstructed colon cancer lies in Dukes' observation that survival is related to the depth of cancer penetration. Patients with obstructed cancers usually have full-thickness involvement. Also, they may have intraperitoneal seeding. In this series, obstruction cut the survival rate almost in half, which is slightly higher than figures usually quoted in the United States, although the overall survival rate of nearly 60% is 10% or 15% better than usually reported for all comers in this country.

An incidental curiosity is that 7% of patients with obstruction had Dukes' A tumors—that is fairly mysterious in itself.—J.C. Thompson, M.D.

Surgical Treatment of Recurrent Colorectal Cancer: Five-Year Follow-Up
Mäkelä J, Haukipuro K, Laitinen S, Kairaluoma MI (Oulu Univ Central Hosp, Finland)
Arch Surg 124:1029–1032, September 1989   22–9

The recurrence of colorectal cancer after primary resection for cure should be detected early to improve the chances of survival; otherwise, surgical treatment can be only palliative. To determine whether the latent interval and diagnostic delay differ among local, regional, and distant recurrences, records of 173 patients who underwent operation for primary colorectal cancer with curative intent during a 10-year period were studied.

Of 81 recurrences during a minimum follow-up of 5 years, all 6 local recurrences, 25 of 31 regional recurrences, and 31 of 44 distant recurrences developed within 2 years. Forty-seven of the 81 patients underwent reoperation, and 34 had conservative treatment. Thirty-five patients in the surgical group and 24 in the conservatively managed group had specific symptoms at the time of detection.

The mean delay in diagnosis of a recurrence was 3 months for both treatment groups. Thirty-one of the 47 surgically treated patients underwent resection, 8 of which were radical procedures. Six patients had abdominal exploration only, and 10 underwent palliative procedures. Six of the 47 patients died after operation. The overall postoperative morbidity was 45%; intra-abdominal hemorrhage was the most common complication. The median durations of survival were 24 months after resective

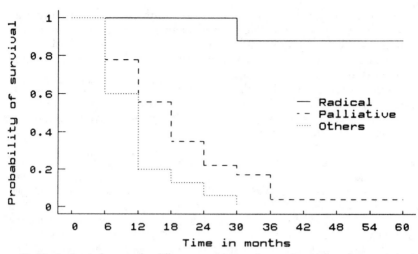

Fig 22–6.—Survival curves after different operative procedures performed for recurrent colorectal cancer. Spread of cancer is not equal among the treatment groups. (Courtesy of Mäkelä J, Haukipuro K, Laitinen S, et al: *Arch Surg* 124:1029–1032, September 1989.)

surgery and 8 months after nonresective surgery. Twenty-six (55%) surgically treated patients and 18 (53%) conservatively treated patients survived for more than 1 year. The overall 5-year cumulative survival was 18% in the surgical treatment group and 3% in the conservative treatment group (Figs 22–6 and 22–7).

The mean duration of symptom relief after surgical treatment was 13 months for patients with local recurrences, 3 months for those with regional recurrences, and 4 months for those with distant recurrences. Twenty (65%) of 31 resected patients had good relief of symptoms for

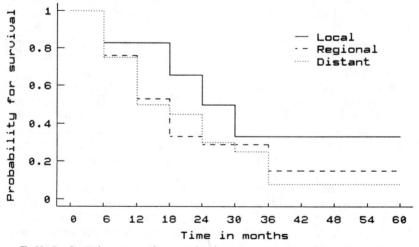

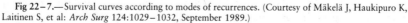

Fig 22–7.—Survival curves according to modes of recurrences. (Courtesy of Mäkelä J, Haukipuro K, Laitinen S, et al: *Arch Surg* 124:1029–1032, September 1989.)

more than 3 months; 17 for more than 6 months; and 12 for more than 1 year. Seven of 16 nonresected patients had good relief for more than 3 months, as did 3 for more than 6 months and 1 for more than 1 year. The median relief of cancer symptoms was 8 months after resection and 2 months after nonresective surgery.

Radical re-resection after the detection of recurrent colon cancer is clearly associated with a longer survival period than palliative and non-resective procedures. However, survival after nonresective procedures is not longer than that after conservative treatment.

▶ The authors make the obvious but memorable statement that recurrent cancer is caused by failure to remove the original tumor. Seventy-seven percent of recurrences in their series appeared within 2 years. How aggressive should we be in caring for these patients? The 5-year survival of nearly 1 of every 5 gives impetus to adoption of an aggressive attitude. Interpretation of the 2 figures obviously requires some experience. In Figure 22–6, radical surgery is far and away the better pick. If you think about how you would handle these patients, you would realize that the findings are, in fact, self-evident. You do radical operations on patients who have a chance of cure. In Figure 22–7 we see that local recurrence is better than distant spread. The message is this: If we know a patient has distant spread, operation is futile. Survival was no better than with nonoperative treatment.—J.C. Thompson, M.D.

Death From Unsuspected Colorectal Cancer
Armstrong CP, Whitelaw SJ (Derriford Hosp, Plymouth, Devon, England)
Ann R Coll Surg Engl 71:20–22, January 1989   22–10

Colorectal cancer is a common malignancy and a major health problem in the Western world. During the past 2 decades the outcome for patients with colorectal cancer has remained unchanged, probably because so many tumors are detected only at an advanced stage. Newer screening techniques should result in earlier diagnosis, although a significant number of patients are not routinely examined and die of unsuspected colorectal cancer.

In 1 health district in England 61 patients with 62 tumors died of undiagnosed colorectal cancer between 1977 and 1986. These patients accounted for 4.1% of all cases of the malignancy in this area. Because autopsies were not performed in most cases, death caused by unsuspected colorectal cancer may occur with even greater frequency than is believed. Based on the findings in this health district, 800 cases may occur each year in the United Kingdom.

Flexible sigmoidoscopy might have detected 41 of the 62 tumors, and curative resection would have been possible in 34 patients. A simple rectal examination would have found 10 tumors. Large bowel cancer was the cause of death in 57 of these patients. Screening of asymptomatic persons older than age 50 years would detect colorectal cancer at an early stage—before metastases occur and when curative surgery is still possible.

▶ Not only a digital rectal examination but also sigmoidoscopy is indicated in any patient with a lower abdominal complaint or with guaiac-positive stools. Yet, in the Plymouth Health District in England, an average of 1 patient every 2 months for 10 years died of unsuspected colorectal cancer, and in nearly all the cases the cancer was the primary cause of death. The problem is that none of these patients had sought help for any symptom related to the large bowel. Not until there is a safe, effective, and low-cost method developed for mass screening will we get ahead of this problem. What will it be? A dye in the drinking the water? A labeled monoclonal antibody introduced into wheat flour? Get cracking! This problem is solvable.—J.C. Thompson, M.D.

Neuroendocrine Carcinomas of the Colon and Rectum: A Clinicopathologic Evaluation
Staren ED, Gould VE, Warren WH, Wool NL, Bines S, Baker J, Bonomi P, Roseman DL, Economou SG (Rush-Presbyterian-St Luke's Med Ctr, Chicago)
Surgery 104:1080–1089, December 1988   22–11

Between 1980 and 1987, colon cancers were removed from 683 patients. Thirteen of these had neuroendocrine carcinomas. The 7 men and 6 women had a median age of 72 years. Six patients had a significant elevation of serum carcinoembryonic antigen, and 7 had elevated alkaline phosphatase values. Of 12 evaluable lesions, 10 were Dukes' stage C2 or D. Eight patients had regional node and 6 had liver or bone metastases.

Ten patients underwent definitive surgical resection, whereas 3 had biopsy only. All of the tumors were large, fungating, focally ulcerated masses. Small cell lesions were most frequent. Eight tumors had foci of glandular or squamous differentiation. All tumors immunostained for at least 1 panneuroendocrine marker—neuropeptide or serotonin. Eight patients died within a year of diagnosis; the median survival was 7 months.

Neuroendocrine tumors of the gastrointestinal tract are more frequent than generally realized. Intermediate cell and small cell carcinomas of the colon and rectum tend to be advanced at diagnosis and to behave aggressively.

▶ What these folks are talking about would be called malignant carcinoids by most everyone else, but they think that the term carcinoid is indistinct and reserve it for benign or low-grade malignant variants of these neuroendocrine tumors. The major problem in trying to learn about these tumors is their rarity— the 13 tumors reported here constitute a large series, yet we would surely be laughed out of town if we tried to make generalizations regarding the treatment of cholecystitis by reporting 13 patients. The observation that well-differentiated tumors do best is expected and the lack of incitement of any recognizable endocrine syndrome by these tumors (even though they consist of cell types that have great secretory capabilities) is also expected. Most large experience with malignant carcinoids of the colon report a preponderance of rectal cancers, which this series does not. The median survival of 7 months suggest great lethality but, again, this and all previous series are so small as to make any kind of generalization tricky.—J.C. Thompson, M.D.

Hypoplasia of Defunctioned Rectum

Appleton GVN, Williamson RCN (Bristol Royal Infirmary; Hammersmith Hosp, London)
Br J Surg 76:787–789, August 1989   22–12

It is common practice to defunction temporarily the large bowel in patients with inflammatory bowel disease by proximal colostomy or ileostomy to rest the inflamed intestine. Although studies of rats have demonstrated progressive hypoplasia after surgical defunction of the colon, little is known about the cytokinetic changes in the human defunctioned large bowel. A close association between rates of colonic cell turnover and susceptibility to neoplasia has previously been demonstrated. Adaptation in the human defunctioned rectum was assessed by measuring crypt size and crypt cell production rate (CCPR) in 11 patients (mean age, 59.7 years) who had undergone surgical colorectal defunctioning and in 14 patients (mean age, 61.2 years) who had no known colorectal disease. Indications for surgical defunctioning of the bowel included diverticular disease in 5 patients and colon cancer in 3. Three patients had other indications. Mucosal biopsy specimens taken from the upper rectum 2 months to 5 years after surgical defunctioning of the bowel were established in organ culture, and the CCPR was determined 16 hours later.

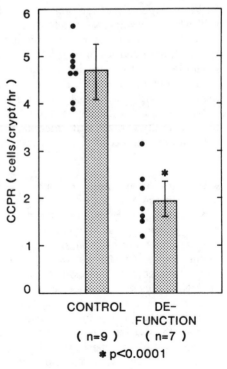

Fig 22–8.—Mean cell birth rates in rectal mucosa from controls *(left column)* and patients with colorectal defunction *(right column)*; CCPR, crypt cell production rate. The values for individual patients *(circles)* and the standard deviations are shown. (Courtesy of Appleton GVN, Williamson RCN: *Br J Surg* 76:787–789, August 1989)

For technical reasons the CCPRs for 5 of the 14 control cultures and 4 of the 11 patient cultures could not be measured. The mean CCPRs for the 7 remaining patients with a defunctioned rectum was 1.96, compared with 4.65 for the remaining 9 controls (Fig 22–8). There was no correlation between CCPR and either the patient's age or length of time since surgical defunction was performed. Similarly, crypt length in patients with defunctioned rectums was 24% less than that in controls, and crypt width was 38% less. Thus surgical rectal defunctioning causes profound and persistent hypoplasia in man.

▶ This proves what you always knew, i.e., when you defunctionalize the rectum it becomes hypoplastic. When you defunctionalize the left colon it turns into a narrow pipe without haustra and the rectum gets smaller, but this is the first demonstration I know of that provides direct evidence of atrophic or hypoplastic changes. Robin Williamson and colleagues have developed a test for measuring rates of crypt cell production that provides a clear index of the frequency of cell turnover (he calls it "mean cell birth rate"). Their other studies show that the defunctionalized rectum is truly shorter and narrower, just as you would expect. It would be important to repeat these studies after the defunctionalized rectum has been reconnected to the enteric tube and see how long it takes for the a return to the normal cell birth rate in the rectum (the authors state that the process takes up to 3 months after colostomy closure in animals).—J.C. Thompson, M.D.

Evaluation and Management of Massive Lower Gastrointestinal Hemorrhage
Leitman IM, Paull DE, Shires GT III (New York Hosp—Cornell Med Ctr, New York)
Ann Surg 209:175–180, February 1989   22–13

Most patients with lower gastrointestinal (GI) hemorrhage stop bleeding during resuscitation. In patients who continue to bleed, the use of early nuclear bleeding scans and arteriography may result in localization of the bleeding site. When the site is localized, patients with continued hemorrhage may have segmental bowel resection rather than subtotal colectomy. The clinical course of patients with massive lower GI bleeding was examined to determine the appropriate assessment and treatment in this group.

A total of 68 patients with massive lower GI bleeding underwent emergency arteriography. Patients required transfusion of an average of 6 units of packed red blood cells within 24 hours of admission. The source of bleeding was localized by arteriography in 40% of the patients, with a sensitivity of 65% among those requiring emergency resection. However, 12 patients (29%) with a negative arteriogram still required emergency intestinal resection for continued hemorrhage. Radionuclide bleeding scans had a sensitivity of 86%.

The most common site of bleeding, identified in 35% of the patients,

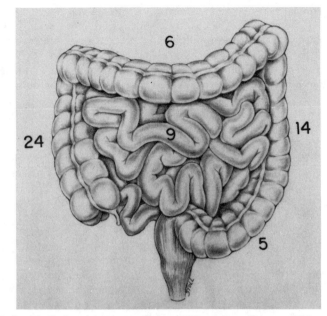

Fig 22–9.—Distribution of sites for massive lower GI hemorrhage. (Courtesy of Leitman IM, Paull DE, Shires GT III: *Ann Surg* 209:175–180, February 1989.)

was the right colon (Fig 22–9). The most common causes were diverticulosis and arteriovenous malformation. Selective intra-arterial infusion of vasopressin and embolization were successful in 36% of the patients in whom it was used, but the procedure contributed to the deaths of 2. Segmental resection was done in 23 patients, and 7 required subtotal colectomy for multiple bleeding sites or negative studies in the face of continued bleeding. Intraoperative infusion of methylene blue through angiographic catheters permitted successful localization and resection of bleeding small bowel segments in 3 patients.

Overall, 21% of the patients died. The mortality for those without a malignancy, with a positive preoperative arteriogram, and who had emergency segmental resection was 13%. Patients in whom transcatheter treatment failed had a 38% death rate.

▶ All in all, the picture is fairly bleak, and you cannot help wondering whether adoption of a routine policy to perform total abdominal colectomy with ileal-rectostomy in all patients with massive colonic hemorrhage might not be the best solution, except for the fact that anything you do is a choice among rotten apples. What we all pray for is that the patient stops bleeding spontaneously. The preoperative diagnosis is beset with practical problems. Angiography should be the answer but rarely is, because the act of sending a patient to the radiology suite magically halts bleeding, and arteriographic demonstration depends on continued intraluminal leakage at exactly the time the dye is injected. Radionuclide scans should be better and are, fractionally, but even the best are not very good. If the patient is to be operated on and if you are not satisfied that you have detected the point of hemorrhage, a total colectomy will usually prevent the need for reoperation and will probably give the best survival rate. Zealots are always writing about some new test that fills the bill, but practical application of any of them has been disappointing.—J.C. Thompson, M.D.

Bleeding Stomal Varices Treated by Sclerotherapy
Mosquera DA, Walker SJ, McFarland JB (Royal Liverpool Hosp, England)
J R Coll Surg Edinb 33:337, December 1988   22–14

Minor stomal bleeding is common and responds to local care. Recurrent severe bleeding, which is uncommon, may be related to stomal varices with underlying portal hypertension. Injection sclerotherapy may be a safe and simple technique in these patients.

Woman, 65, had recurrent severe stomal bleeding 12 months after a Hartmann's procedure for sigmoid colon carcinoma with multiple hepatic metastases. The source of bleeding was not identified until discrete bleeding points at the mucocutaneous junction were noted. Bleeding was poorly controlled with silk sutures. Her condition had the appearance of classic peristomal varices secondary to portal hypertension. Subcutaneous injection sclerotherapy was done on 3 occasions. Lidocaine, 1%, was infiltrated subcutaneously into the peristomal area, and 4 mL to 8 mL of ethanolamine oleate was distributed to the varices around the stoma at the 4 compass points. Injection was painless. The only complication was tissue necrosis localized to a small area around 1 of the injection sites at which 2 mL was injected. In the next 7 weeks the patient had only 1 further episode of stomal bleeding. Her hemoglobin level was maintained, and the patient remained relatively well until she died of disseminated carcinoma.

Peristomal sclerotherapy merits more widespread consideration. It is a safe, simple, effective local treatment for control of recurrent stomal bleeding.

▶ This paper was included because it describes what appears to be a simple and effective way of handling an extremely rare problem that, when it does occur, can often be maddening to both patient and surgeon. Any patient with portal hypertension who has an enteric stoma is at risk of bleeding varices developing at the site, and local sclerotherapy appears to be a useful method of management.—J.C. Thompson, M.D.

23 The Liver and the Spleen

Diagnostic and Therapeutic Approaches to Pyogenic Abscess of the Liver
Klatchko BA, Schwartz SI (Univ of Rochester)
Surg Gynecol Obstet 168:332–336, April 1989

Data were reviewed on 33 patients with a mean age of 51 years who were treated in the past 7 years for pyogenic abscess of the liver. Biliary causes were identified in 12 patients and infection by the portal venous route was identified in another 12. Four patients had traumatic abscesses, 4 had infection by the hepatic artery route, and 3 had cryptogenic abscesses. The median time from onset of symptoms to diagnosis was 2 weeks. Findings were positive on ultrasonograms and CT scans in most of the patients studied, but findings on radionuclide studies were less consistently positive.

Ten abscesses that developed from a biliary route required surgical drainage. Five of the 12 patients with portal abscesses were effectively managed roentgenologically. Two of 5 patients died after primary surgical drainage. The other patients were all successfully drained surgically. Three patients who had diffuse or multiple abscesses were managed successfully by primary hepatic resection.

Surgical drainage remains the standard management of pyogenic abscess of the liver, although roentgenologically controlled drainage may be effective in some cases. Drainage generally is done via a transperitoneal route so that causative factors can be corrected.

▶ The use of hepatic resection in 3 patients represents a unique departure from the conventional therapeutic approach. The message of the article is that both radiographically directed drainage and surgical drainage play roles that should be regarded as complementary rather than competitive. The proposal that medical treatment alone would be sufficient in the case of an established abscess violates most surgical principles.—S.I. Schwartz, M.D.

Intraoperative Ultrasound of the Liver Affects Operative Decision Making
Parker GA, Lawrence W Jr, Horsley JS III, Neifeld JP, Cook D, Walsh J, Brewer W, Koretz MJ (Virginia Commonwealth Univ)
Ann Surg 209:569–577, May 1989

Surgeons must determine the feasibility of resection of primary and secondary liver neoplasms and the appropriate magnitude of resection re-

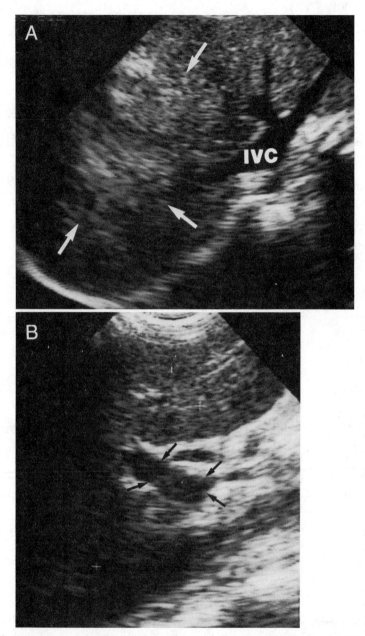

Fig 23–1.—A, transverse IOU through the inferior vena cava and confluence of hepatic veins shows a large solitary metastasis *(arrows)* in the right lobe. **B,** oblique IOU through the liver hilum shows an unsuspected tumor thrombus *(arrows)* in the main portal view. (Courtesy of Parker GA, Lawrence W Jr, Horsley JS III, et al: *Ann Surg* 209:569–577, May 1989.)

quired. To ascertain which tests best aid the surgeon in making these decisions, preoperative CT of the liver and intraoperative ultrasound (IOU) were compared in 42 patients with liver tumors undergoing 45 exploratory operations. Primary disease included colorectal cancer metastases in 27 patients, hepatoma in 11, and metastatic cancers of other origins in 4.

The malignancy of 89 identified hepatic lesions was confirmed by resection, biopsy, or continued growth on follow-up CT. The sensitivity for detecting these lesions was 77% on CT and 98% on IOU (Fig 23–1). In 13 patients resection was not possible. Five had extrahepatic disease; in 4, more nodules were discovered by IOU; in 3, tumor involvement in all 3 hepatic veins was found by IOU. One patient had portal vein invasion. In 4 patients, tumors identified by CT as involving all 3 hepatic veins were free of at least 1 hepatic vein, permitting resection. In a patient who had previous surgery, a tumor thought to involve the remaining right hepatic vein was free of the vein, also allowing resection. Intraoperative ultrasound was helpful in determining the extent of resection. Lesser procedures than anticipated were possible in 7 patients with the use of IOU. In 2 patients, IOU indicated that a more extensive resection was necessary. Operative treatment was influenced by IOU in 22 (49%) of the 45 operations.

For evaluating the feasibility and extent of resection needed for primary and secondary hepatic cancers IOU is superior to preoperative CT and surgical exploration. It appears that IOU is the most sensitive indicator of number of lesions in the liver. Its ability to determine hepatic venous anatomy is a useful adjunct in determining tumor resectability.

▶ It is now generally agreed that intraoperative ultrasound is the most sensitive indicator of the number of lesions present in the liver, and it also plays a distinct role in defining the intraparenchymal vascular anatomy, thus facilitating resection. Traynor et al. (1) conducted a retrospective review of case reports of 672 patients and noted that supplementary information was obtained by the use of paraoperative ultrasonic examination in 155. It is true that preoperative ultrasound of the liver is useful in detecting small tumors, but it is important to recognize that many of these small tumors may not represent malignancy; rather, they are benign lesions such as hemangiomas, thus the very demonstration of an unexpected lesion may not preclude resection.—S.I. Schwartz, M.D.

Reference

1. Traynor O, et al: *Br J Surg* 75:197, 1988.

Infantile Hepatic Hemangiomas: Clinical Features, Radiologic Investigations, and Treatment of 20 Patients
Stanley P, Geer GD, Miller JH, Gilsanz V, Landing BH, Boechat IM (Childrens Hosp of Los Angeles; Univ of Southern California; Univ of California, Los Angeles)
Cancer 64:936–949, Aug 15, 1989   23–3

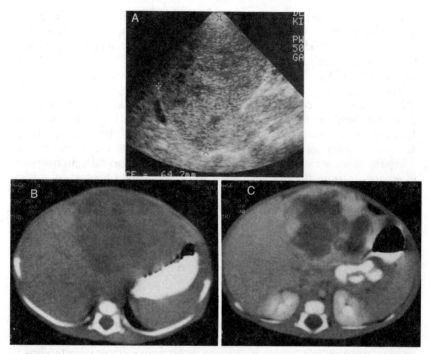

Fig 23–2.—A, ultrasound shows moderately well-defined heterogeneous mass of increased echogenicity within left lobe of liver. **B,** precontrast CT scan demonstrates mass of low attentuation within left lobe of liver. **C,** after bolus injection of contrast medium there is peripheral enhancement of mass with frond-like centripetal extension. (Courtesy of Stanley P, Geer GD, Miller JH, et al: *Cancer* 64:936–949, Aug 15, 1989.)

Twenty infants were seen with hepatic hemangioma between January 1974 and September 1988. The mean age of the 10 female and 10 male infants at presentation was 8 weeks, but 8 infants were seen in the first week of life. Eighteen had a palpable abdominal mass and 11 had high-output cardiac failure. Nine had a consumptive coagulopathy and 5 had microangiopathic anemia. Seven infants had other hemangiomas, most often in the skin.

Angiography consistently demonstrated a large feeding artery to the tumor and diminution in size of the aorta distal to the origin of the celiac axis. Findings on CT scans before and after injection of contrast medium and findings at ultrasonography are shown in Figure 23–2. Hypervascularity and prolonged pooling of contrast fluid or a persistent stain were consistent findings.

Four patients had primary operative treatment and 14 were initially managed medically, most often by steroids. Seven patients received radiation therapy. Two of 5 patients initially treated with steroids alone had a good response. Seventeen of the patients were well 6 months to 13 years after diagnosis.

If an hemangioma is found as an asymptomatic mass, only serial imaging studies are required. Steroids are the first line of medical management. If the lesion fails to respond, therapeutic embolization may be considered in place of radiation therapy. Severe heart failure is treated with steroids, digitalis, and diuretics. Other options for resistant hemangiomas include cyclophosphamide and surgical excision. Surgery is recommended for solitary, large hemangiomas and for lesions that have ruptured. Resolution is best monitored by serial ultrasonography.

▶ The clinical manifestations of hemangioma in infants are significantly different from those in adults. Consumptive coagulopathy and heart failure with hepatic rupture are rare complications of the adult hemangioma. Of the fewer than 10 spontaneous ruptures associated with hemangiomas reported in the world, half occurred in neonates. Management of the newborn infant with hemangioma and cardiac failure has proponents for both conservative and aggressive surgical approaches. Nguyen et al. (1) managed 5 children conservatively during the first year of life without steroids or radiotherapy. Ligation of the hepatic artery alone has successfully reversed cardiac failure. Linderkamp's review suggests that in infants with giant solitary hemangioma, excision of the tumors is the treatment of choice, because there was only 1 death among 22 surgically treated patients with symptoms during the first year life, whereas 15 of the conservatively treated patients died (2).—S.I. Schwartz, M.D.

References

1. Nguyen L, et al: *J Pediatr Surg* 17:576, 1982.
2. Linderkamp O, et al: *Eur J Pediatr* 124:23, 1977.

Liver Cell Adenomas: A 12-Year Surgical Experience From a Specialist Hepato-Biliary Unit
Leese T, Farges O, Bismuth H (Hôp Paul Brousse, Villejuif, France)
Ann Surg 208:558–564, November 1988   23–4

The incidence of liver cell adenomas has increased since the introduction of oral contraceptives. These tumors are usually benign and are seen primarily in women during the reproductive years. Treatment remains controversial. To define a logical approach to the indications and technique of surgical resection of these tumors, data were reviewed on 24 patients with a definite diagnosis of liver adenoma seen between 1976 and 1987. The patients ranged in age between 4 and 45 years. The diagnosis was made on the basis of histology of the resected specimen in 21 patients or from biopsy performed at laparotomy in 3. Differentiation was made between these lesions and focal nodular hyperplasia or well-differentiated hepatocellular carcinoma.

Of the 24 patients 6 had multiple adenomas, associated in 4 with glycogen storage disease. Two of these 6 had polyadenomatosis; liver transplantation was successful in 1 of the 2 after malignant transformation to hepatocellular carcinoma. Of the 24 patients 18 had either a solitary adenoma or 2 adenomas; there were 15 women and 3 men. Eleven of the

15 women had taken oral contraceptives and 2 had taken other hormone preparations. Half of the patients experienced sudden upper abdominal pain after hemorrhage into an adenoma. In 17 patients complete resection of 1 or both adenomas was achieved; 8 had tumorectomy, 5 had right hepatectomy, 3 had left lobectomy, and 1 had trisegmentectomy; 1 patient received treatment to reduce tumor size before surgery. The median amount of blood transfused was 3 units, and the median postoperative stay was 12 days. On follow-up, all patients were alive and well.

Surgical excision of liver adenomas is advocated when it can be done without mortality or severe morbidity. Excision eliminates the patient's symptoms and also removes the complications of hemorrhage and malignant transformation.

▶ This is an impressive series. I agree that resection is indicated for liver cell adenoma based on the risk of hemorrhage and malignant transformation. Our own experience is that most patients who have had hemorrhage have bled either within the tumor or have presented with a subcapsular hematoma. We have seen 1 patient with a 1-cm lesion that caused a significant subcapsular hematoma. If you consider the patients with hepatic cell adenoma who present with intratumoral, subcapsular, or intraperitoneal bleeding, nearly 90% are women who have been using contraceptive medication. The issue of multiple liver cell adenomas associated with type I or III glycogen storage disease is a difficult one. Although hepatic transplantation has been proposed, I would anticipate that the donor liver would eventually develop adenomas.—S.I. Schwartz, M.D.

Results of Treatment of Patients With Hepatocellular Carcinoma With Severe Cirrhosis of the Liver
Fujio N, Sakai K, Kinoshita H, Hirohashi K, Kubo S, Iwasa R, Lee KC (Osaka City Univ, Japan)
World J Surg 13:211–218, March–April 1989   23–5

More than 70% of patients in Japan with hepatocellular carcinoma (HCC) also have liver cirrhosis. A cohort of 201 patients treated for HCC in a 6-year period were retrospectively classified by the results of tests of 15-minute indocyanine green retention ($ICGR_{15}$) done at the time of admission.

Of the 201 patients, 36 had $ICGR_{15}$ values of less than 10% (group 1), 81 had $ICGR_{15}$ values of 10.1% to 20% (group 2), and 84 had values of 20.1% or more (group 3). Overall, 72% of the patients had liver resection, including 78% in group 1, 80% in group 2, and 62% in group 3. The cirrhosis of patients in group 3 was considered severe. Fifty-two of these patients underwent liver resection, with approximately half receiving preoperative transcatheter arterial embolization. Another 9 received both transcatheter arterial embolization and portal vein embolization before surgery. At 2 and 3 years, the survival rate was significantly higher when transcatheter arterial embolization was used preoperatively than when resection alone was done (Fig 23–3).

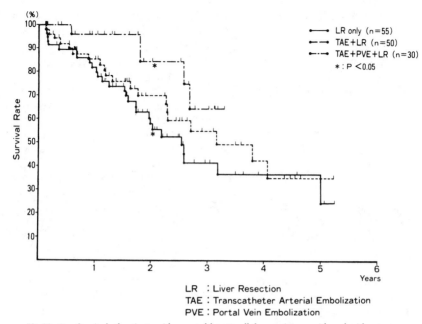

LR : Liver Resection
TAE : Transcatheter Arterial Embolization
PVE : Portal Vein Embolization

Fig 23–3.—Survival of patients with resected hepatocellular carcinoma with and without preoperative therapy. (Courtesy of Fujio N, Sakai K, Kinoshita H, et al: *World J Surg* 13:211–218, March–April 1989.)

Liver resection is the most effective therapy for patients with HCC and severe cirrhosis of the liver. However, cirrhosis prevents liver resection in some patients. Preoperative transcatheter arterial embolization and portal vein embolization appear to improve the survival rate of patients undergoing liver resection.

▶ Others have previously tried preoperative embolization before hepatic resection and could find no significant difference in long-term prognosis between treated and untreated patients. Transcatheter arterial embolization is also associated with operative difficulties such as cholecystitis and perivasculitis. The results of the present article are impressive but need confirmation.—S.I. Schwartz, M.D.

Long-Term Survivors After Resection for Primary Liver Cancer: Clinical Analysis of 19 Patients Surviving More than Ten Years
Zhou X-D, Tang Z-Y, Yu Y-Q, Yang B-H, Lin Z-Y, Lu J-Z, Ma Z-C, Tang C-L (Shanghai Med Univ)
Cancer 63:2201–2206, June 1, 1989   23–6

Primary liver cancer (PLC), rare in the Western world, is one of the most common fatal tumors in Asia and Africa. Surgical resection is the only effective treatment, but long-term survival rarely results. From 1958 to 1978, 333 patients with pathologically proved PLC were admitted to a university hospital in Shanghai; of these, 132 underwent resection. Nineteen patients survived for more than 10 years.

All 19 patients had radical resection, including right hemihepatectomy in 2 patients, left hemihepatectomy in 10, left lateral segmentectomy in 3, and local resection in 4. The patients were alive without disease for 10–26 years after the procedure, with a mean follow-up of 15 years. The patient with the longest survival had a tumor measuring 10 cm × 8 cm × 6 cm and underwent local resection. Two patients with intraperitoneal ruptured tumors have survived for 19 years and almost 17 years, respectively, after surgery and have returned to work.

Early and radical resection is the main factor influencing long-term survival. Reoperation for subclinical recurrence and solitary metastasis remains an important strategy for prolonging survival further. Intraperitoneal rupture of PLC does not exclude the possibility of cure. New surgical techniques, including cryosurgery and bloodless hepatectomy, were effective in some patients.

▶ The rate of 14% survival for more than 10 years is in keeping with other series. Lin et al. (1) reported a 5-year survival of 18%. Kinami et al. (2) reported on hepatocellular carcinoma associated with cirrhosis. The 5-year survival for large tumors was 0.—S.I. Schwartz, M.D.

References

1. Lin TY, et al: *Br J Surg* 74:839, 1987.
2. Kinami Y, et al: *World J Surg* 10:294, 1986.

Lack of Intrahepatic Recurrence of Hepatocellular Carcinoma by Temporary Portal Venous Embolization With Starch Microspheres
Matsumata T, Kanematsu T, Takenaka K, Sugimachi K (Kyushu Univ, Fukuoka, Japan)
Surgery 105:188–191, February 1989   23–7

Immediate recurrence in the hepatic remnant sometimes develops after curative resection for hepatocellular carcinoma (HCC). A possible cause is multiple dissemination of tumor cells through the portal vein in the remnant liver as a result of operative manipulations. In an attempt to prevent such recurrences, ultrasonically guided, intraoperative portal embolization with starch microspheres was done in 1 woman and 7 men (average age, 58 years) with HCC.

Technique.—An ultrasonic probe is applied to the surface of the liver. The portal venous branch supplying the tumor-bearing subsegment is punctured under ultrasonic guidance with a 23-gauge needle. Starch microspheres are then injected into the portal branch (Fig 23–4). Microsphere doses are determined with reference to those used for hepatic arterial administration. The right lobe is mobilized, and subsegmental hepatic resection without hilar dissection is done.

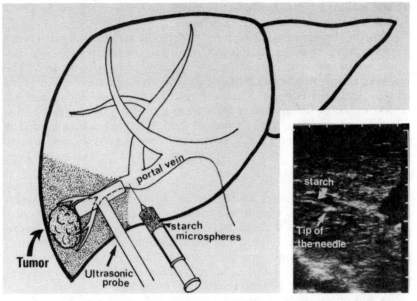

Fig 23-4.—Tip of the needle and injected starch microspheres are recognized ultrasonically. (Courtesy of Matsumata T, Kanematsu T, Takenaka K, et al: *Surgery* 105:188-191, February 1989.)

The starch microspheres lodge only temporarily in the microvasculature and do not produce adverse effects such as a rise in portal pressure or postoperative liver dysfunction. None of the 8 patients has had a recurrence to date.

▶ This is an addendum to the technique of resection. It does not seem logical to conclude that embolization precludes spread during dissection. Yoshida et al. (1) addressed the issue of surgical margin and resection in patients with hepatocellular carcinoma to determine whether 1 cm beyond the gross tumor was sufficient. The data suggest that in patients with tumors less than 4 cm in diameter, recurrence is not linked to the extent of margin. However, in larger tumors, 1 cm of margin appears to be inadequate.—S.I. Schwartz, M.D.

Reference

1. Yoshida Y, et al: *Ann Surg* 209:297, 1989.

Major Hepatic Resection Under Total Vascular Exclusion
Bismuth H, Castaing D, Garden OJ (Hôp Paul Brousse, Villejuif, France)
Ann Surg 210:13-19, July 1989   23-8

Blood loss is a major problem in liver resection, especially when the lesion is located close to or involves the hepatic veins and the inferior vena cava. Total vascular exclusion is one method of establishing control of the major vascular structures. This technique was evaluated in 51 resections performed over a 9-year period.

Most of the patients (62%) were undergoing treatment for liver metastases. After a vascular clamp was applied to the hepatic pedicle to occlude inflow, the vena cava was clamped below and above the liver. The mean operating time was 5.8 hours, and the average time of vascular exclusion was 46.5 minutes. Patients received 4.5 units of blood and 8.2 units of plasma, usually before the start of total vascular exclusion. During the exclusion procedure crystalloid fluid, 2,631 mL was infused. The mean systolic blood pressure, mean central venous pressure, and urinary output all fell temporarily but returned at least to pre-exclusion values after declamping.

There were 8 complications (16%), including respiratory infection and biliary fistula. One patient died of sepsis and multiorgan failure postoperatively on day 45. This low mortality rate indicates that total vascular exclusion is a safe and useful technique in resection of hepatic lesions that involve the hepatic veins. The technique may not be well tolerated, however, in hypovolemic patients because it results in a significant reduction in venous return to the heart. Preoperative ultrasonography is essential in evaluating the hepatic lesion and tumor invasion of the hepatic veins and portal venous branches.

▶ In most instances, as the authors point out, inflow occlusion is all that is required, but the demonstration that total vascular exclusion can be accomplished safely is an important one in a small group of patients. It is essential to expand the blood volume with crystalloid before clamping. Ryan and Faulkner (1) have shown that vascular isolation before parenchymal division significantly decreases the need for transfusion. In a group of 58 hepatic resections, including 13 right lobectomies, 3 extended right lobectomies, and 4 left lobectomies, there was no need for transfusion in a significant number of patients. This is a most laudatory accomplishment.—S.I. Schwartz, M.D.

Reference

1. Ryan JA, Faulkner DJ: *Am J Surg* 157:472, 1989.

Intra-Abdominal Sepsis After Hepatic Resection

Pace RF, Blenkharn JI, Edwards WJ, Orloff M, Blumgart LH, Benjamin IS (Royal Postgrad Med School, London; Queens Univ, Kingston, Ont)
Ann Surg 209:302–306, March 1989   23–9

Postoperative intra-abdominal sepsis is a well-documented complication of hepatic resection. Postoperative subphrenic or perihepatic abscess traditionally has been treated by reoperation. Modern imaging and percutaneous radiologic methods currently offer a noninvasive alternative to this approach. A series of 130 patients who underwent hepatic resections in an 8-year period was reviewed to identify risk factors associated with posthepatectomy intra-abdominal infection and to assess changing trends in management.

In 36 of 126 patients surviving for more than 24 hours postoperatively, culture-positive intra-abdominal collections developed. The diagnoses of trauma or cholangiocarcinoma and the need for reoperation to control bleeding during the postoperative period were significantly independently associated with intra-abdominal sepsis. Over the years, operative drainage in the treatment of infected fluid collections was largely replaced by percutaneous methods, which have proved effective in most patients.

▶ Our own experience parallels that of the authors; we have had a 20% incidence of subphrenic abscess or infected fluid collections in patients after major hepatic resection. In the past 8 years we have not had to reexplore any of these patients, and they have been managed successfully with radiographically directed percutaneous insertion of catheters.—S.I. Schwartz, M.D.

Endoscopic Sclerotherapy in the Management of Esophageal Varices in 61 Children With Biliary Atresia
Stringer MD, Howard ER, Mowat AP (King's College Hosp, London)
J Pediatr Surg 24:438–442, May 1989   23–10

The number of long-term survivors after surgery for biliary atresia has grown, producing an increasing cohort of children with portal hypertension prone to variceal bleeding. Only a few patients with this condition have been treated with endoscopic sclerotherapy. Success has been variable over follow-up periods rarely exceeding 1–2 years.

Sixty-one children surviving for more than 2.5 years after corrective surgery for biliary atresia were followed prospectively with endoscopy for up to 6 years. Esophageal varices were found in 41 children, 17 of whom had had episodes of variceal hemorrhage. Variceal bleeding was controlled with endoscopic injection sclerotherapy in all except 1 child, who died of hemorrhage before treatment could be completed. Treatment complications included bleeding episodes before variceal obliteration, esophageal ulceration, and stricture. Conservative therapy resolved these complications without long-term effects. During a mean 2.8 years of follow-up after variceal obliteration, rebleeding from recurrent esophageal varices occurred in 1 child, who responded to further sclerotherapy.

Endoscopic sclerotherapy is associated with low mortality from variceal bleeding and a rebleeding rate from recurrent varices of 7%. Because results are superior to those of surgical procedures for portal hypertension in biliary atresia, endoscopic sclerotherapy is the recommended treatment.

▶ These are very encouraging figures. Endoscopic sclerotherapy represents the preferred approach to these patients because it will not compromise liver transplantation in those patients for whom that becomes appropriate therapy.

Okamoto et al. (1) reported that esophageal transection and devascular procedures do not yield superior results.— S.I. Schwartz, M.D.

Reference

1. Okamoto E, et al: *Exerpta Medica* 283, 1983.

A Comparison of Sclerotherapy With Staple Transection of the Esophagus for the Emergency Control of Bleeding From Esophageal Varices
Burroughs AK, Hamilton G, Phillips A, Mezzanotte G, McIntyre N, Hobbs KEF
(Royal Free Hosp and School of Medicine, London; Univ of Milan, Italy)
N Engl J Med 321:857–862, Sept 28, 1989   23–11

Emergency sclerotherapy in the treatment of acute esophageal variceal bleeding, with or without earlier balloon tamponade, is more effective than balloon tamponade alone. Sclerotherapy is now the treatment of choice in many centers, with operation a second-line treatment. Emergency esophageal transection with a staple gun has effectively controlled esophageal variceal bleeding in many patients, and mortality has been similar to that associated with emergency sclerotherapy.

In a prospective, randomized study endoscopic sclerotherapy was compared with staple transection of the esophagus in the emergency treatment of esophageal variceal bleeding in 101 patients with cirrhosis of the liver and bleeding esophageal varices. Four of 50 patients assigned to sclerotherapy and 12 of 51 assigned to staple transection did not actually undergo those procedures, but all statistical analyses were made on an intention-to-treat basis.

Sclerotherapy controlled the variceal bleeding in 41 patients (82%) and transection controlled the bleeding in 49 (96%). Twenty-two patients in the sclerotherapy group (44%) and 18 in the transection group (35%) died within 6 weeks of treatment. The difference was not statistically significant. However, blood and plasma requirements during the procedures and the first 5 days thereafter were substantially lower in the group having transection. The incidence of rebleeding after treatment was also lower in the transection group: A 5-day interval without bleeding was achieved after a single injection in 88% of the transection group but in only 62% of the sclerotherapy group.

Staple transection of the esophagus as an emergency treatment for variceal bleeding in patients with cirrhosis of the liver is as safe as sclerotherapy and is more effective than a single sclerotherapy procedure.

▶ This is a most provocative article indicating that surgery should play a greater role in the management of the patient with acutely bleeding varices. Cello et al. (1) concluded that, although endoscopic sclerotherapy was as good as surgical shunting in the acute management of massively bleeding varices in the poor-risk patient, elective surgery should be considered in those in whom the varices are not obliterated. As is the case with sclerotherapy, esophageal transection represents a temporizing procedure. We certainly agree with the conclusion of the authors that staple transection, based on their data, has a role as a first-line treatment in the emergency management of bleeding esophageal varices.—S.I. Schwartz, M.D.

Reference

1. Cello JP, et al: *N Engl J Med* 316:11, 1987.

Endoscopic Elastic Band Ligation for Active Variceal Hemorrhage

Stiegmann GV, Goff JS, Sun JH, Wilborn S (Univ of Colorado; Denver VA Hosp)
Am Surg 55:124–128, February 1989   23–12

Endoscopic variceal ligation (EVL) is a new means of controlling active esophageal variceal hemorrhage. Small elastic "O" rings are used to strangulate and thrombose the varices mechanically. During a 16-month period, 68 consecutive patients with actively bleeding esophageal varices underwent EVL performed with a flexible gastroscope.

Endoscopic variceal ligation successfully controlled the bleeding in 23 patients (34%). Eleven of the 23 patients had no previous therapy; the other 12 had received EVL, sclerotherapy, or operation for variceal hemorrhage previously. All patients, who ranged in age from 10 to 71 years (mean, 40 years), were treated within 8 hours of hospital admission; most were treated between 2 and 4 hours after admission. Repeat EVL was performed as needed for bleeding and at 2-week intervals thereafter until varices were grade I or eradicated.

Endoscopic variceal ligation initially controlled active variceal bleeding in 22 of the 23 patients, of whom 16 required 1 EVL treatment and 6 required 2 treatments. Initial bleeding control could not be attained by EVL in the remaining patient who died of exsanguination after a technically successful portacaval shunt. In all, 9 patients (39%) died during the course of the study, 5 of hepatic failure with no recurrence of bleeding and 4 as a direct consequence of recurrent bleeding. All deaths occurred within 3 to 24 days of initial EVL treatment. During a mean follow-up of 9 months, 6 of the 14 survivors experienced 7 episodes of recurrent variceal bleeding. Twelve had variceal eradication or a reduction in variceal size to grade I or less after a mean of 5.5 repeat EVL sessions. Excluding rebleeding, there were no treatment-related complications in 80 EVL sessions.

Endoscopic variceal ligation is effective in the initial and long-term control of variceal hemorrhage and appears to be associated with a low incidence of nonbleeding complications. The procedure is technically not more difficult to perform during active variceal hemorrhage than endoscopic sclerotherapy.

▶ This represents a unique approach to local management of bleeding esophagogastric varices. It could be used in lieu of sclerotherapy. It offers certain advantages over sclerotherapy related to esophageal stricture and perforation. If there is confirmation that it is as effective as endoscopic sclerotherapy in eradicating varices and diminishing the risk of recurrent bleeding, it will represent a significant addition to our therapeutic armamentarium.—S.I. Schwartz, M.D.

H-Type Shunt With an Autologous Venous Graft for Treatment of Portal Hypertension in Children

Gauthier F, De Dreuzy O, Valayer J, Montupet Ph (Hôp de Bicêtre, Le Kremlin Bicêtre, France)
J Pediatr Surg 24:1041–1043, October 1989   23–13

An H-type shunt in which an autologous vein is used has replaced the interposition shunt in the routine treatment of extrahepatic portal hypertension (EHPO) in children at Bicêtre Hospital. Between 1980 and 1988 a total of 86 consecutive children aged 16 months to 16 years (mean age, 6.6 years) had this operation. The usual indication for operation was portal hypertension with gastrointestinal bleeding, but 11 children had not bled. The etiology of hypertension was EHPO in 59 patients and idiopathic in 37.

Portal pressure declined by a third or more of the preanastomotic value in 58 cases. Early abdominal ultrasonography showed signs of patency in 48 of the 79 patients studied, but it was inconclusive in the others. In 29 of 33 patients who had early esophagoscopy the varices appeared less tense, and in 9 cases they were no longer visible. Four children had recurrent gastrointestinal bleeding, including 1 whose shunt was patent. No patient had encephalopathy. Two of 6 children with shunt failure had a successful reoperation.

With an approximate success rate of 95% the H-type shunt with venous graft is recommended for use in treating young children who have portal hypertension of extrahepatic origin. The operation usually is less demanding than traditional portosystemic shunt procedures.

▶ This is a most impressive series with outstanding results. Boles et al. (1) pointed out that splenorenal or mesocaval shunting is consistently effective in children who have had extrahepatic portal hypertension, but makeshift shunts fail. This series is particularly significant because no case of encephalopathy was reported. This has paralleled our experience (2).—S.I. Schwartz, M.D.

References

1. Boles ET Jr, et al: *Am J Surg* 151:734, 1986.
2. Graver SE, Schwartz SI: *Ann Surg* 189:566, 1979.

Distal Splenorenal Shunt With Splenopancreatic Disconnection: A 4-Year Assessment

Henderson JM, Warren WD, Millikan WJ, Galloway JR, Kawasaki S, Kutner MH (Emory Univ)
Ann Surg 210:332–341, September 1989   23–14

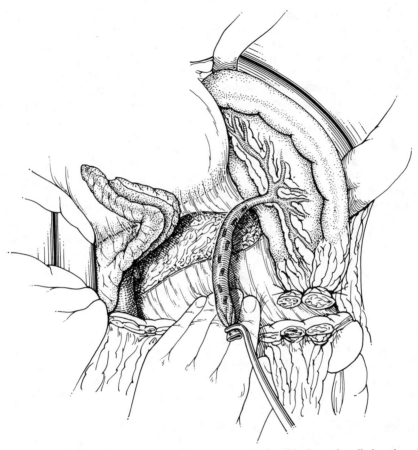

Fig 23–5.—Schematic of concept of DSRS-SPD. Splenic vein should be dissected totally free of pancreas before anastomosis to left renal vein. Pancreas cannot always be "swung up" as indicated, but the vein may be passed freely from inferior to superior to pancreas. (Courtesy of Henderson JM, Warren WD, Millikan WJ, et al: *Ann Surg* 210:332–341, September 1989.)

Complete disconnection of the splenic vein from the pancreas (SPD) was introduced as a modification of the distal splenorenal shunt (DSRS) to maintain portal flow and prevent the siphoning of hepatotrophic factors from the pancreas. Interruption of all pancreatic tributaries to the splenic vein (Fig 23–5) prevents the development of pancreatic collateral vessels. The splenic vein is brought down to the left renal vein and anastomosed.

In 1983 through 1987 DSRS-SPD was done in 78 patients; 35 had alcoholic cirrhosis. Thirty-two patients were in Child's class A, 25 were in Child's class B, and 21 were in Child's class C. All but 1 patient had a patent shunt in the early postoperative phase. Eleven patients (14%) had recurrent upper gastrointestinal bleeding. After 4 years portal perfusion was maintained in 84% of the alcoholic patients and in 90% of the others. Liver function was maintained in both groups. The operative mortality was 6.4% and overall mortality was 30%; rates were similar in the alcoholic and nonalcoholic groups.

This experience validates the use of DSRS-SPD in patients with alcoholic cirrhosis who require a selective shunt to control variceal bleeding. In other patients the advantage over standard DSRS is not proved, but interruption of the pancreatic siphon also should benefit these patients.

Prograde portal venous perfusion is nearly always maintained after disconnection. Langer has cautioned that the modified procedure is technically difficult, is not required to prevent encephalopathy, and is associated with an increased rate of bleeding.

► As pointed out by Dr. Langer in the discussion, the controlled trials did not show any progressive increase in the instance of encephalopathy even though portal perfusion was lost. The pertinent question is this: As the operation is more difficult and does not appear necessary to protect against encephalopathy, how widely should it be recommended? Paquet reported improved results with distal splenorenal shunt in a selected patient population (1). Operating on only Child's A and B patients, no development of rebleeding encephalopathy or shunt thrombosis was recorded.—S.I. Schwartz, M.D.

Reference

1. Paquet KJ: *Ann Surg* 210:184, 1989.

Appraisal of Distal Splenorenal Shunt in the Treatment of Esophageal Varices: An Analysis of Prophylactic, Emergency, and Elective Shunts
Nagasue N, Kohno H, Ogawa Y, Yukaya H, Tamada R, Sasaki Y, Chang Y-C, Nakamura T (Shimane Med Univ, Izumo; Hiroshima Red Cross and Atomic Bomb Hosp, Japan)
World J Surg 13:92–99, January–February   23–15

The distal splenorenal shunt is widely used in the treatment of esophagogastric varices. All patients who underwent elective, emergency, or prophylactic distal splenorenal shunts between 1969 and 1987 were reviewed retrospectively.

The study population consisted of 52 males aged 32–71 years and 26 females aged 16–76 years with portal hypertension and esophagogastric varices. Thirty-seven patients were chronic alcoholics. Hepatitis B surface antigen was positive in only 11 patients (15.5%). Of the 78 patients, 67 had cirrhosis of the liver, 5 had chronic hepatitis, 4 had idiopathic portal hypertension, 1 had primary biliary cirrhosis, and 1 had fatty liver. Fifty-two patients were in Child's class A, 18 in Child's class B, and 8 in Child's class C. The operations were urgent in 9 patients, elective in 40, and prophylactic in 29. Prophylactic operations were performed on Child's class A and class B patients only. Forty-two patients had the original Warren shunt; 36 patients had a modified distal splenorenal shunt with expanded polytetrafluoroethylene interposition.

The operative mortalities were 11.1% in the emergency group, 2.5% in the elective group, and 3.4% in the prophylactic group. The overall operative mortality was 3.8%; the overall in-hospital mortality was 7.7%. Three patients with an original Warren shunt had occlusion of the shunt, yielding a patency rate of 94.1%. The incidence of rebleeding in esophageal varices was 3.8%.

Fifteen patients died after discharge; at the time of the report, 57 patients were still alive. The 1-, 2-, and 3-year survival rates of patients in the emergency surgery group were all 77.8%. The 1-, 2-, 3-, 5-, and 10-year survival rates in the elective surgery group ranged from 86.9% to 29.4%. The 5-, 10-, and 15-year survival rates in the prophylactic surgery group were all 85.5%. The long-term prognosis was poorest for chronic alcoholics and patients in Child's class C.

The distal splenorenal shunt is a reliable technique in the treatment of esophagogastric varices associated with portal hypertension, and it can be used safely in emergency, elective, and prophylactic situations.

▶ This is another confirmatory article related to the efficacy of the distal splenorenal shunt. The operative mortality of 11% in the group having emergency surgery is certainly most unusual. Most series have reported more than 40% mortality in this group. The significance of this article is that it defines the course of patients followed for longer than 10 years. I would agree with the discussion by Dr. Millikan questioning the use of an interposition H-graft of Gore-Tex because interposition shunts certainly have a tendency to occlude over time in the venous circulation. Also, complete separation of the splenic vein from the pancreas leads to improved preservation of postoperative portal perfusion.—S.I. Schwartz, M.D.

Long Term Results of Treatment of Budd-Chiari Syndrome by Side to Side Portacaval Shunt

Orloff MJ, Girard B (Univ of California, San Diego, La Jolla)
Surg Gynecol Obstet 168:33–41, January 1989   23–16

Budd-Chiari syndrome caused by hepatic vein occlusion is characterized by rapid progression of liver damage, ineffectiveness of medical treatment, and a very high mortality rate, mainly among young adults who were often in good health before onset of symptoms. Side-to-side portacaval shunt may be effective in the treatment of hepatic vein occlusion. The procedure decompresses the liver by creating a new outflow tract.

The patient population included 7 men and 6 women aged 19–45 years who were seriously ill with Budd-Chiari syndrome caused by hepatic vein occlusion. Symptoms included abdominal pain, marked ascites, hepatosplenomegaly, wasting, and disturbed liver function. The presumed etiology was the use of oral contraceptives in 3 patients, polycythemia rubra vera in 2, and Behçet's disease in 1; the cause was unknown in 7 patients. Side-to-side portacaval shunt operations were performed from 4 to 78 weeks after onset of symptoms. In all patients the elevated wedged hepatic vein pressure was much higher than the inferior vena caval pressure. Liver biopsy showed centrilobular congestion and necrosis.

Side-to-side portacaval shunt effectively decompressed the liver, reducing the mean corrected portal pressure from 240 mm of saline solution before operation to 7 mm of saline solution afterward. Of the 13 patients, 12 (92%) survived to hospital discharge; 1 patient died 6 days after operation of a recurrent thrombosis. The patient with Behçet's disease died 2 years after operation of symptoms not attributable to Budd-Chiari syndrome. The remaining 11 patients were alive 3 to 16 years after operation, for a long-term survival rate of 85%. All survivors were free of ascites without diuretic therapy. Hepatic function returned to normal, and hepatosplenomegaly disappeared in all but 2 patients, who already had cirrhosis at presentation. None of the patients had portosystemic encephalopathy. Serial liver biopsy specimens showed a much-improved liver architecture, disappearance of necrosis, and a decrease in centrilobular congestion. In all patients a patent portocaval shunt was observed on serial angiography.

The side-to-side portacaval shunt appears to be extremely effective in the treatment of Budd-Chiari syndrome and should be done early in the course of the disease.

▶ The excellent long-term results reported in this series should lay to rest the use of the LeVeen shunt as therapy for ascites associated with the Budd-Chiari syndrome. As has been pointed out on many occasions, the use of a peritoneal venous shunt does not address the basic pathologic issue. Ahn et al. (1) reported on the simultaneous retrohepatic inferior vena cavaplasty and side-to-side portacaval shunt for recurrent thrombosed mesoatrial shunt in the Budd-Chiari syndrome. Cameron et al. (2) reviewed an experience with 12 patients with a mesenteric systemic shunt; in 5 of these a mesocaval shunt was performed and in 7 a mesoatrial shunt. Shunt thrombosis occurred in many of these patients.—S.I. Schwartz, M.D.

References

1. Ahn SS, et al: *Surgery* 101:165, 1987.
2. Cameron JL, et al: *Ann Surg* 198:335, 1983.

Mesoatrial Shunt: A Surgical Option in the Management of the Budd-Chiari Syndrome
Stringer MD, Howard ER, Green DW, Karani J, Gimson AS, Williams R (King's College Hosp, London)
Br J Surg 76:474–478, May 1989   23–17

Patients with Budd-Chiari syndrome have enlargement of the liver, ascites, and abdominal pain as a result of hepatic venous outflow obstruction. The condition is often complicated by inferior vena caval occlusion.

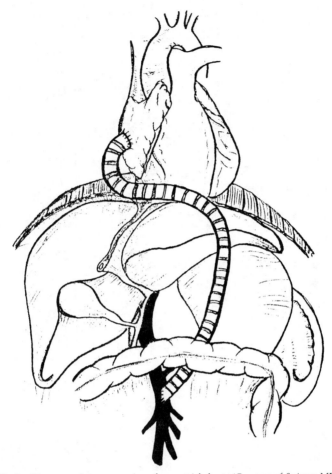

Fig 23–6.—Diagrammatic representation of mesoatrial shunt. (Courtesy of Stringer MD, Howard ER, Green DW, et al: *Br J Surg* 76:474–478, May 1989.)

In some patients an acute onset is followed rapidly by death; others have a more chronic course, but only 50% of these survive for 2 years. Various surgical treatments have been proposed, most of which have involved portosystemic shunting. A modification of the mesoatrial shunt, first reported in 1978, was constructed in 5 patients aged 14–54 years with Budd-Chiari syndrome. Four had an underlying myeloproliferative disorder. Indications for surgery included ascites, deteriorating liver function, malnutrition, and wasting. After using an approach with a single thoracoabdominal incision incorporating a median sternotomy, a mesoatrial shunt was constructed using externally supported polytetrafluoroethylene grafts (Fig 23–6).

In each patient satisfactory mesoatrial blood flow was established to-

		Hemodynamic Data in Patients Undergoing Mesoatrial Shunting for Budd-Chiari Syndrome				
Patient	Age (years)	Preoperative IVC gradient (mmHg)	Intraoperative portal vein pressure decrease (mmHg)	Postoperative stay (days)	Patency ±repeat IVC gradient (mmHg)	Follow-up (months)
1	33	Occluded IVC	30→15	42	Patent	16
2	46	17 (20→3)	31→15	15	Patent (4-mm gradient)	15
3	14	25 (25→0)	29→15	17	Patent (4-6-mm gradient)	15
4	25	16 (25→9)	38→16	22	Patent (2-4-mm gradient)	12
5	54	8 (17→9)	18→0	23	Patent	9

IVC, inferior vena cava.
(Courtesy of Stringer MD, Howard ER, Green DW, et al: *Br J Surg* 76:474–478, May 1989.)

gether with a reduction in portal venous pressure (table). Two patients experienced a dramatic rise in cardiac output, and a lesser increase was seen in the other 3 patients. By the time of follow-up at 9−16 months, all patients had made good recoveries. The ascites resolved and liver size diminished. Doppler ultrasound studies and dynamic CT scanning confirmed shunt patency.

Surgical treatment appears to be necessary for long-term recovery in patients with Budd-Chiari syndrome complicated by inferior vena caval occlusion. If the results described here are supported in larger studies, the mesoarterial shunt may be the procedure of choice in these patients.

▶ These are excellent results. Cameron et al. (1) reviewed 7 patients with mesoatrial shunts and found a high incidence of shunt thrombosis. It may well be that the conduit with the external support is what is needed for this situation. McCarthy et al. discussed the medical/surgical management of 30 patients with the Budd-Chiari syndrome and stressed that surgical intervention is usually required (2). The mesoatrial shunt is the more popular procedure for patients with caval obstruction, but Nakao et al. report that radical operation, in which the inferior vena cava is opened to allow removal of the thrombi from the hepatic veins, has proved effective (3).—S.I. Schwartz, M.D.

References

1. Cameron JL, et al: *Ann Surg* 198:335, 1983.
2. McCarthy PM, et al: *Arch Surg* 120:657, 1985.
3. Nakao K, et al: *J Cardiovasc Surg* 25:216, 1984.

Pediatric Wandering Spleen—The Case for Splenopexy: Review of 35 Reported Cases in the Literature
Allen KB, Andrews G (Emory Univ Affiliated Hosps; Egelston Hosp for Children, Atlanta)
J Pediatr Surg 24:432−435, May 1989   23−18

The diagnosis of wandering spleen is rare, especially in children. Only 35 episodes have been reported in children younger than age 10 years. The recommended treatment for wandering spleen has been splenectomy, but increasing knowledge of the importance of the spleen makes removal of the organ, particularly in children, undesirable. Treatment with splenopexy was successful in a young girl.

Girl, 6 years, 6 months, had a history of chronic intermittent abdominal pain. She was hospitalized several times, but the pain resolved spontaneously and her condition was not diagnosed. During the current admission physicians found a left lower quadrant mass. Comparison of the kidney-ureter-bladder examination with a previous intravenous pyelogram established the diagnosis. At surgery the spleen was found to be freely mobile without ligamentous attachments. It was wrapped in a basket of Dexon mesh, placed in the anatomical splenic bed, and tacked to the diaphragm and parietal peritoneum. At 14-month follow-up the girl's spleen was well fixed in the normal anatomical position.

Although most of the adult occurrences of wandering spleen are in young women, males predominate among pediatric cases. The condition appears most often in children younger than age 1 year. Even though a child is not symptomatic, elective splenopexy using the described technique is recommended because of the risk of later having an acute surgical emergency. Replacement of the spleen without fixation almost always results in failure.

▶ This is the first review of the subject that has appeared recently in literature. With refinements in radiographic techniques the diagnosis should be made readily preoperatively. In view of the authors' findings it seems reasonable that if the diagnosis is made, splenopexy should be performed.—S.I. Schwartz, M.D.

Emergency Splenectomy in Adult Idiopathic Thrombocytopenic Purpura: A Report of Seven Cases

Wanachiwanawin W, Piankijagum A, Sindhvananda K, Vathanophas V, Visudhiphan S, Na-Nakorn S (Mahidol Univ, Bangkok, Thailand)
Arch Intern Med 149:217–219, January 1989   23–19

Intracranial hemorrhage is the most serious of the hemorrhagic manifestations of idiopathic thrombocytopenic purpura (ITP). Fortunately, this life-threatening condition develops in less than 1% to 2% of all ITP patients. The therapeutic goal in treating intracranial hemorrhage is to produce a rapid, sustainable increase in the platelet count to a hemostatic level for a considerable period. Platelet transfusion results in an immediate increase in the platelet count, but the hemostatic state does not last long enough to benefit these patients, as transfused platelets are rapidly destroyed. Emergency splenectomy is considered the procedure of choice in the treatment of patients with ITP in whom life-threatening hemorrhage develops.

Between 1962 and 1981, 108 of 567 patients (19%) with newly diagnosed ITP underwent therapeutic splenectomy; 101 splenectomies were performed as elective and the other 7 as emergency procedures. The latter 7 patients (6 females, 1 male aged 16–61 years) had experienced life-threatening events; 6 had progressive intracranial bleeding and 1 had postoperative intra-abdominal bleeding. The interval between the initial symptoms of ITP and emergency splenectomy varied from 6 days to 5 months.

Six of the 7 patients were saved by splenectomy. The 1 patient in whom operation was delayed for 20 days died of progressive cerebral hemorrhage. None of the 6 survivors had postoperative bleeding or surgical complications. Platelet counts increased within a few hours after the operation (table).

Emergency splenectomy is a life-saving therapeutic procedure in pa-

Clinical Data of 7 Patients With Idiopathic Thrombocytopenic Purpura Who Underwent Emergency Splenectomy

Patient No./ Sex/Age, y	Interval Between Onset of Initial Symptoms and Splenectomy, d	Indication for Emergency Splenectomy	Preoperative Platelet Count, × 10⁹/L	Preoperative Platelet Transfusion, U	Postoperative Platelet Count, × 10⁹/L	Immediate Outcome	Follow-up Period	Long-term Outcome
1/F/17	5 mo	Intracerebral and subarachnoid hemorrhage	0	4; immediately PO; 1wk PO; 2 mo PO	100; 10; 150	Good	4 y	Good
2/F/38	9	Suspected intracranial hemorrhage	0	No; 12 h PO; 36 h PO	65; 125	Good	6 mo	One episode of transient thrombocytopenia
3/F/19	4 mo	Suspected intracranial hemorrhage	0	5; immediately PO; 1 wk PO	50; 425	Good	4 y	Good
4/M/22	1 mo	Intracerebral and subarachnoid hemorrhage	0	4; immediately PO; 10 d PO	5; 200	Good	3 y	Relapse after 2 mo, without serious bleeding
5/F/61	6	Suspected intracranial hemorrhage	0	4; 12 h PO; 3 d PO	20; 105	Good	4 mo	Dead, recurrent thrombocytopenia and AIHA
6/F/16	20	Intracerebral and subarachnoid hemorrhage	5	4; immediately PO	10	Died from progressive cerebral hemorrhage	...	...
7/F/45	9	Intra-abdominal bleeding after hysterectomy	0	4; immediately PO; 2 d PO; 1 wk PO	5; 50; 105	Good	6 mo	Good

Abbreviations: PO, postoperative; *AIHA*, autoimmune hemolytic anemia.
(Courtesy of Wanachiwanawin W, Piankijagum A, Sindhvananda K, et al: *Arch Intern Med* 149:217–219, January 1989.)

tients with ITP who experienced life-threatening hemorrhagic complications. Platelet transfusions should be given to maintain a hemostatic platelet level during the critical period before splenectomy.

▶ This is a most unusual series that presents very encouraging results. I have managed 4 such patients operated on in coma; 2 of these patients survived and 2 died. It is important to make a plea for emergent splenectomy rather than plasmapheresis, or any other temporizing medical therapy, in these patients because this is such an urgent situation.—S.I. Schwartz, M.D.

Massive Splenomegaly

Johnson HA, Deterling RA (Tufts Univ)
Surg Gynecol Obstet 168:131–137, February 1989   23–20

Removal of massively enlarged spleens is associated with prohibitively high mortality and morbidity rates. Several authors have defined massive splenomegaly as organs enlarged to more than 1,500 g. However, mortality and morbidity rates increase when any spleen is enlarged to more than 1,000 g. A review of the records of 391 patients who underwent splenectomy during a 16-year period identified 36 with drained splenic weights of more than 1,000 g.

The 20 males and 16 females were aged 17–75 years (average, 55 years). Twenty-one had chronic leukemia or a myeloproliferative disorder. The most common acute indications for operation were pancytopenia and increasing transfusion requirements secondary to symptomatic anemia. The average time between diagnosis and operation was 42 months. Twenty-six patients required an average of 10 units of blood products before operation to correct existing preoperative coagulopathy.

There were no intraoperative deaths. Of the 36 patients, 11 had postoperative complications, fatal in 4. A fifth death occurred 55 days after operation. Of the 21 patients with drainage tubes, 8 had complications, as did 8 of 21 patients with preliminary early splenic arterial ligation. Of all complications, 81% were related to septic events. The average overall survival time was 17.5 months, and that for patients with massive splenomegaly, 28.5 months.

Splenectomy did not increase survival. Preoperative coagulopathy and failure to demonstrate a hematologic response to operation were clear predictors of decreased long-term survival. However, demonstrable hematologic benefit and improved quality of life were achieved in patients with myeloproliferative disorders and non-Hodgkin's lymphoma. Splenectomy in leukemic patients should be performed only for definite surgical indications (e.g., intractability, hemorrhage, or rupture); it should not be performed as a preterminal event, however.

▶ The size of the spleen does not represent a major factor in defining the indications for splenectomy for hematologic disorders. We have found it appropriate to give antiplatelet aggregating drugs prophylactically as well as anticoagulants to patients with myeloproliferative disorders to prevent thrombosis of the splenic vein. I agree that there is no indication to drain these patients routinely. The point that the authors make related to fact that splenectomy should not be performed as a preterminal event merits emphasis (1).—S.I. Schwartz, M.D.

Reference

1. Gordon DH, et al: *Arch Surg* 113:713, 1978.

24 The Biliary Tract

The Surgery of Biliary Atresia
Lilly JR, Karrer FM, Hall RJ, Stellin GP, Vasquez-Estevez JJ, Greenholz SK,
Wanek EA, Schroter GPJ (Univ of Colorado)
Ann Surg 210:289–296, September 1989   24–1

Data were reviewed on the outcome of surgery in 131 consecutive infants with biliary atresia seen between November 1973 and April 1988. Six patients did not have biliary reconstruction because of advanced cirrhosis or a preference for transplantation. The others had excision of all nonpatent extrahepatic bile ducts. Biliary drainage was provided by a Roux-en-Y portoenterostomy in 111 infants and by a gallbladder-common duct conduit in 14. In the past 2 years a conduit intussusception valve has been incorporated (Fig 24–1).

Immediate drainage was achieved in 103 of 125 cases (82%). Reoperation restored bile flow in 14 of 18 infants in the first 6 weeks after operation. Biliary obstruction remained relieved for more than a year in 72 patients (57%). Morbidity, however, was substantial. Twenty-one of 72 infants with sustained bile flow had clinical signs of portal hypertension, and 17 had antibiotic-resistant cholangitis.

Fifty-seven patients were alive at last follow-up, 13 after liver transplantation. Sixty-eight of the 125 patients who had the Kasai operation died within an average of 25 months after surgery. The survivors not given transplants are not "cured," but many have nearly normal or normal liver function, have grown normally, and are active. The average follow-up is 86 months.

When possible, the Kasai procedure should be the initial operative approach to biliary atresia. Grosfeld has obtained the best results in infants younger than age 3 months at operation.

▶ Spokespersons from the pediatric surgical groups strongly support the role of operation as first-line therapy in infants with biliary atresia. They do point out, however, that in patients older than 3 months of age the results are extremely poor, and it might be appropriate to refer such infants for initial transplantation. Grosfeld et al. (1) recently described the treatment outcome of 66 patients with biliary atresia. Hepatoportal enterostomy, performed in 48 cases, was successful in 25% and resulted in improvement in an additional 19%, but it failed in 43%. In patients younger than 98 days the success rate was 31%, and 23% were improved. Ten of 20 patients referred for liver transplantation survived.—S.I. Schwartz, M.D.

Reference

1. Grosfeld JL, et al: *Surgery* 106:692, 1989.

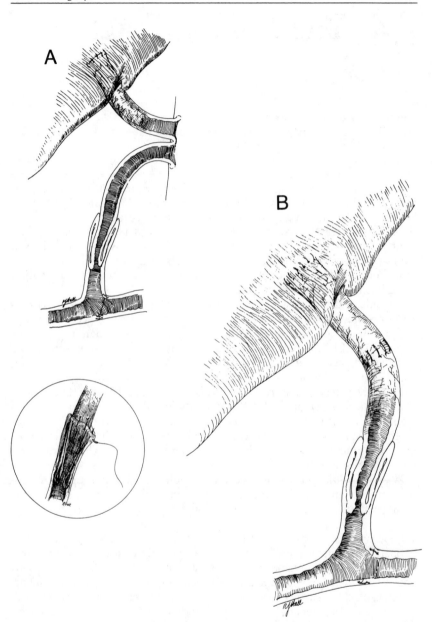

Fig 24–1.—Biliary reconstruction. **A**, initial reconstruction. "Hepatic limb" is as short as possible; "intestinal limb" has incorporated intussusception valve distally. Conduit is exteriorized. **B**, completed reconstruction. Conduit is internalized 6–12 weeks after operation. *Inset* shows details of valve construction, i.e., 3 cm of Roux-en-y jejunostomy has been intussuscepted and affixed with seromuscular interrupted silk sutures. (Courtesy of Lilly JR, Karrer FM, Hall RJ, et al: *Ann Surg* 210:289–296, September 1989.)

Extracorporeal Shock-Wave Lithotripsy of Bile Duct Calculi: An Interim Report of the Dornier U.S. Bile Duct Lithotripsy Prospective Study

Bland KI, Jones RS, Maher JW, Cotton PB, Pennell TC, Amerson JR, Munson JL, Berci G, Fuchs GJ, Way LW, Graham JB, Lindenau BU, Moody FG (Univ of Florida; Univ of Virginia; Univ of Iowa; Duke Univ; Bowman-Gray School of Medicine, Winston-Salem, NC; et al)
Ann Surg 209:743–753, June 1989   24–2

To determine the efficacy and clinical value of extra corporeal shock-wave lithotripsy in the treatment of bile duct stones using the Dornier HM-3 and HM-4 lithotripters, 42 patients with bile duct calculi (most often in the common duct) underwent lithotripsy when conventional nonoperative measures were not feasible. Two thirds of the patients had undergone cholecystectomy, and the same proportion had a history of active biliary colic. The patients had undergone 96 invasive nonsurgical procedures previously. In most patients the shock waves were made to enter the abdomen posteriorly. Nearly one third of the patients had general anesthesia.

A second treatment was required in 15 patients, usually because of inadequate fragmentation of calculi (Fig 24–2). All but 7% of those having only a single stone were stone free at discharge. Half of the patients required adjunctive nonoperative measures for stone removal before discharge, most often transpapillary or percutaneous endoscopic extraction.

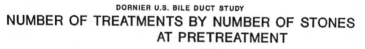

DORNIER U.S. BILE DUCT STUDY
NUMBER OF TREATMENTS BY NUMBER OF STONES AT PRETREATMENT

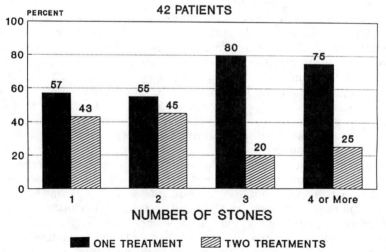

Fig 24–2.—Percentage of patients treated with 1 or 2 extracorporeal shock-wave lithotripsy treatments as a function of number of stones. No correlation is evident for an increasing stone number to necessitate a second treatment. (Courtesy of Bland KI, Jones RS, Maher JW, et al: *Ann Surg* 209–743–753, June 1989.)

No patient had hypotension or syncope as a result of blood loss, and none required transfusion.

Shock-wave lithotripsy reliably leads to fragmentation of bile duct stones and is safe. There were no treatment-related deaths in these predominantly elderly patients. Lithotripsy is a valuable part of a multidisciplinary approach to the management of biliary calculi.

▶ The present study addresses bile duct calculi specifically. A retrospective analysis of shock-wave lithotripsy for the management of gallstone disease (1) reported that, of those patients admitted for treatment of bile duct stones, 27% had surgery and 73% had the calculi removed by endoscopy, at times accompanied by shock-wave fragmentation. Teichmann et al. (2) reported surgical intervention after extracorporeal shock-wave lithotripsy in 5 patients, an incidence of 9% in patients with common duct stones undergoing the latter procedure.—S.I. Schwartz, M.D.

References

1. Paumgartner G: *Ann Surg* 208:274, 1988.
2. Teichmann RK, et al: *World J Surg* 13:317, 1989.

Acute Acalculous Cholecystitis
Frazee RC, Nagorney DM, Mucha P Jr (Mayo Clinic and Found, Rochester, Minn)
Mayo Clin Proc 64:163–167, February 1989   24–3

Acute acalculous cholecystitis (AAC) reportedly accounts for only 5% to 15% of all cases of cholecystitis, but its incidence seems to be increasing. Acute acalculous cholecystitis was diagnosed in 18 men and 2 women aged 22–83 years seen in a 5-year period. Symptoms of AAC developed after an operation in 12 patients, 10 of whom had undergone nonbiliary abdominal surgery; 2 had orthopedic procedures, and 3 were recovering from traumatic injuries. The interval between hospital admission or operation and onset of symptoms of AAC ranged from 8 to 44 days. Ten patients had clinically significant concomitant medical conditions that could have predisposed them to AAC; 9 patients were receiving total parenteral nutrition.

Symptoms included abdominal pain in all 20 patients and fever in 13. Results of laboratory studies showed that 17 patients had leukocytosis; 14 of 17 patients in whom liver function studies were performed had elevated values. The diagnosis in 10 patients was based on clinical findings. The other 10 patients underwent hepatobiliary iminodiacetic acid scanning, which showed nonvisualization of the gallbladder without other hepatobiliary abnormalities. Findings on ultrasonography or CT, performed in 7 patients, were consistent with AAC, including distention of the gallbladder, thickening of the gallbladder wall, pericholecystic collection of fluid, and the absence of stones.

Treatment consisted of cholecystectomy in 18 of the 20 patients; the other 2 initially underwent percutaneous transhepatic cholecystostomy. Six patients died after undergoing cholecystectomy, for a postoperative mortality rate of 30%. However, none of the deaths was directly attributable to hepatobiliary complications of AAC or cholecystectomy.

When compared with a previously reported review of 28 patients treated for AAC during a 16-year study period at the same institution, the findings in this series confirm the high morbidity and mortality associated with AAC and indicate that its incidence is increasing.

▶ The review of ACC by Fox et al. (1) considered 68 patients who had 2.3% of all cholecystectomies performed during the study. Significant cardiovascular disease was found in 50% of the patients and diabetes in 25%. Cholescintigraphy identified the pathology in 14 of 15 patients. Ultrasonography had lower accuracy, and acute pathology of the gallbladder was noted in only about 33%. Cholecystectomy was carried out in all patients. Ternberg (2) has reported a rare variety of acute ACC complicating other illnesses in childhood. In his patients tube cholecystostomy provided adequate treatment.—S.I. Schwartz, M.D.

References

1. Fox MS, et al: *Surg Gynecol Obstet* 159:13, 1984.
2. Ternberg JL: *Arch Surg* 110:543, 1975.

Acute Cholecystitis Occurring as a Complication of Percutaneous Transhepatic Drainage

Lillemoe KD, Pitt HA, Kaufman SL, Cameron JL (Johns Hopkins Med Insts)
Surg Gynecol Obstet 168:348–352, April 1989   24–4

Most complications of transhepatic biliary drainage are relatively minor and can be managed with antibiotics and catheter manipulation. Sepsis, which occurs frequently, is attributed to cholangitis. In some patients, however, acute cholecystitis (ACC) may develop after transhepatic biliary drainage. This complication, previously unreported, causes symptoms similar to those of sepsis but does not respond to antibiotic treatment, external drainage, or catheter change.

During a 42-month period, ACC developed in 9 of 330 patients who underwent percutaneous biliary drainage. Seven of the 9 patients were men, and the mean age was 58 years. The period between drainage and surgery ranged from 3 to 51 days. Various roentgenologic procedures were used in diagnosis (table). Cholecystectomy was successful in 7 patients; they were discharged at an average of 11.7 days postoperatively. The 2 patients who died had unresectable cholangiocarcinoma and severe sepsis.

Acute cholecystitis after transhepatic biliary drainage may result from mechanical obstruction of the cystic duct caused by the catheter itself, inflammation, or edema. Although most patients with cholangitis or sepsis

Patient Work-Up, Management, Pathologic Findings, and Outcome

Patient No.	Radiology	Operation	Pathology	Gallstones	Bile cultures	Outcome
1		Cholecystectomy; pancreatoduodenectomy	Acute cholecystitis	–	Achromobacter xylosoxidaus	Discharged POD 15
2	Ultrasonography	Cholecystectomy; Roux-en-Y; cystojejunostomy	Acute cholecystitis	–	Enterobacter cloacae; Serratia marcescens	Discharged POD 13
3	Computerized tomography cholescintigraphy	Cholecystectomy	Gangrenous cholecystitis	–	Negative	Discharged POD 12
4	Ultrasonography	Cholecystectomy; L hemicolectomy	Acute cholecystitis	–	Enterococcus; Acyetobacter anitratum	Discharged POD 10
5	Cholangiography, ultrasonography	Cholecystectomy	Acute cholecystitis	+	Enterococcus	Discharged POD 8
6		Cholecystectomy, resection of hepatic bifurcation with hepaticojejunostomy	Acute and chronic cholecystitis	+	Enterococcus; Klebsiella pneumoniae	Discharged POD 14
7		Cholecystectomy	Gangrenous cholecystitis	–	Enterobacter cloacae	Discharged POD 10
8	Cholangiography	Cholecystectomy	Perforated gangrenous cholecystitis	–	Enterococcus; Citrobacter freundii	Died POD 18
9		Percutaneous cholecystostomy	Acute cholecystitis*	–	Enterococcus; Pseudomonas aeurginosa	Died POD 25

*From autopsy.
POD, postoperative day.
(Courtesy of Lillemoe KD, Pitt HA, Kaufman SL, et al: Surg Gynecol Obstet 168:348–352, April 1989.)

associated with transhepatic biliary drainage can be managed easily, those not responding to treatment should be evaluated for ACC. Sonography, CT, or radionucleotide scanning are the recommended diagnostic studies. Also, in patients with unresectable malignant conditions who will undergo prolonged hepatic drainage, cholecystectomy should be performed at the time of laparotomy.

▶ The article brings into focus the complications that have not previously been addressed. The authors' suggestion that cholecystectomy be performed at the time drainage is established at an operation is appropriate, particularly as a drain that resides inside the common duct may itself obstruct the cystic duct orifice.—S.I. Schwartz, M.D.

Cholecystectomy and Colorectal Cancer
Moorehead RJ, McKelvey STD (Queen's Univ of Belfast, Ireland)
Br J Surg 76:250–253, March 1989   24–5

A 1983 epidemiologic study first suggested that bile acids are involved etiologically in the development of colorectal cancer. However, the precise action of bile acids in tumor promotion or initiation remains to be determined. Certain surgical procedures such as cholecystectomy can affect the size of the bile acid pool. The proportion of secondary bile acids, mainly deoxycholic acid, in the bile of post-cholecystectomy patients is significantly increased.

In explanation of this phenomenon it has been proposed that whereas before cholecystectomy the bile acid pool circulates 2 or 3 times per meal, after cholecystectomy it circulates even during the fasting state. If this is so, the enhanced circulation could result in increased exposure of bile acids to the degrading action of intestinal bacteria.

A study that reported an association between bowel cancer and cholecystectomy involved the prospective follow-up of 1,681 postcholecystectomy patients. The relative risk of colorectal cancer developing after cholecystectomy was 1.7. Other studies have reported even higher relative risks for right-sided cancer in women, but most of these studies were retrospective case-control studies. A review of the more current papers suggests further support for the proposed association. However, other studies have found no evidence of an association between colorectal cancer and previous cholecystectomy. In 1 of these, follow-up of 16,773 postcholecystectomy cases found no increased risk of large bowel cancer.

Clearly, further retrospective studies will not elucidate the issue. The question will be resolved only by prospective follow-up of postcholecystectomy patients who are screened on a regular basis with colonoscopy or barium enema to determine conclusively whether the incidence of bowel tumors after cholecystectomy actually is increased.

▶ As this excellent review indicates, there is a difference of opinion related to the association between cholecystectomy and colorectal cancer. There are so many factors involved that it would be difficult to come to an irrefutable conclusion. In view of the number of cholecystectomies performed, it is an issue that needs continuous epidemiologic study.—S.I. Schwartz, M.D.

Selective ERCP and Preoperative Stone Removal in Bile Duct Surgery
Heinerman PM, Boeckl O, Pimpl W (Landeskrankenanstalten, Salzburg, Austria)
Ann Surg 209:267–272, March 1989   24–6

New diagnostic and therapeutic modalities have brought about many changes in biliary surgery in the past 15 years. In selected patients, preoperative endoscopic-retrograde cholangiography and stone extraction (ERCP-ST EXTR) lowers morbidity and mortality rates. A total of 728 patients with primary (85.4%) or secondary (14.6%) biliary tract disease were evaluated prospectively.

When pathologies of the bile duct system were suspected in patients scheduled for primary operations, preoperative ERCP was performed; all patients admitted for secondary operations underwent the procedure. Elective cholecystectomy was performed in all patients not excessively at surgical risk.

Overall, the complication rate was 6%. Of 78 patients who underwent common duct stone removal, 21.8% had complications. The ERCP-ST EXTR procedure reduced the incidence of complications to 2.1%. Retained stone rates were reduced from 2.2% to .5% by ERCP-ST EXTR. Patients with secondary stones treated only by ERCP-ST EXTR had a morbidity rate of 2%, with no retained stones and no mortality.

With surgical common bile duct exploration, biliary and nonbiliary complications are at least doubled after elective cholecystectomy. Preoperative stone removal would presumably decrease the risk of complications. Apparently, endoscopic removal of common bile duct stones before elective cholecystectomy is indeed a means of reducing morbidity and mortality in patients having biliary tract surgery.

▶ In those centers with facile gastroenterologists having true expertise in ERCP, this represents a logical and reasonable approach. Certainly, if successful, endoscopic extraction of stones precludes the need for common duct exploration and reduces the morbidity of an operative procedure. It is to be emphasized that this entire thesis is dependent on the capability of performing ERCP and stone extraction in the overwhelming majority of patients and without a significant complication rate. Cotton et al. (1) indicated that there is a subset of patients in whom the common duct stones can be removed and the gallbladder left in situ. Follow-up of these patients has revealed a low incidence of subsequently required cholecystectomy.—S.I. Schwartz, M.D.

Reference

1. Cotton PB, et al: *World J Surg* 12:111, 1988.

Late Results of Immediate Primary End to End Repair in Accidental Section of the Common Bile Duct

Csendes A, Díaz JC, Burdiles P, Maluenda F (Univ of Chile, Santiago)
Surg Gynecol Obstet 168:125–130, February 1989   24–7

The incidence of gallbladder disease in Chile is the highest in the world. Approximately 50% of all women and 25% of all men have gallstones. The immediate and late results of repair of the common bile duct after its accidental section during cholecystectomy were determined in 43 patients, 20 of whom had been operated on at 1 institution.

During a 2-year period, 16,500 patients underwent cholecystectomy for benign disorders of the biliary tract at that institution; 10 patients sustained an accidental injury of the common bile duct during operation, for an incidence of 1/1,600 operations overall. Another 10 patients in whom the common bile duct was accidentally cut during cholecystectomy sustained their injuries before the 2-year study period. Twenty-three patients were referrals from other institutions. The common bile duct was completely severed in 36 patients (84%) and was partially cut in the other 7. Lesions occurred at the hepatic duct 3 times more often than at the choledochus. Thirty-nine patients had an end-to-end repair with distal T tube; 4 patients underwent some type of bilioenteric anastomosis.

During a mean postoperative follow-up of 4 years, a benign structure developed in 29 patients; only 8 patients were free of symptoms and well. Ten of 33 patients who had a benign stricture after primary repair underwent reoperation after a first hepaticojejunostomy. The first reoperation was performed 40 months after the initial operation. Patients with incomplete section had a worse prognosis than those with complete section of the common bile duct. About one third of the patients with benign strictures underwent a second or third hepaticojejunostomy. The late results in these patients were progressively worse, with greater mortality after each procedure. By the time of late follow-up of 42 patients who had undergone primary repair of an accidentally injured common bile duct, 6 had died, 3 of them of postoperative complications after a second or third hepaticojejunostomy.

Accidental section or injury of the common bile duct during cholecystectomy for benign gallbladder disease is a severe complication that often leads to an unfavorable prognosis for the patient.

▶ The article provides further evidence for the dictum that when complete transection of the bile duct occurs, hepaticojejunostomy using a Roux-Y loop generally represents the procedure of choice. It is the unusual circumstance with a knife or scissor transection of the duct in which repair can be effected without tension. The primary anastomosis should be carried out.—S.I. Schwartz, M.D.

Benign Postoperative Biliary Strictures: Operate or Dilate?

Pitt HA, Kaufman SL, Coleman J, White RI, Cameron JL (Johns Hopkins Med Insts)
Ann Surg 210:417–427, October 1989   24–8

Forty-two patients with benign postoperative biliary strictures underwent 45 procedures from 1979 through 1987. Three patients had both surgery and balloon dilatation. Twenty-five had a Roux-Y choledochojejunostomy or hepaticojejunostomy with postoperative transhepatic stenting for a mean of 14 months. Twenty had a mean of 4 balloon dilatations and were stented transhepatically for a mean of 13 months. The mean length of follow-up was 57 months after surgery and 59 months after balloon dilatation.

A successful outcome was achieved in 88% of the surgical patients and in 55% of those managed by balloon dilatation. Three surgical patients had recurrent strictures (12%), as did 9 of those who had balloon dilatation (45%). Significant hemobilia was more frequent after balloon dilatation. The total hospital stay and costs did not differ significantly between the 2 treatment groups. There were no deaths.

Surgical repair of benign postoperative biliary strictures results in fewer problems with cholangitis or jaundice that require further treatment. Balloon dilatation, however, is an alternative for high-risk patients or those who are not willing to have additional surgery.

▶ Most centers would agree that the long-term success rate for balloon dilatation of strictures is approximately 50%. There is general agreement, certainly in the surgical population, that surgical repair results in fewer problems. I would strongly agree with the point made by Professor Myburgh in the Discussion about the use of a transanastomotic "stent." We have found it unnecessary in patients in whom a direct mucosa-to-mucosa anastomosis can be effected, and we, like he, have been impressed with the Hepp procedure of an anastomosis between the left hepatic duct and a Roux-Y limb of jejunum.—S.I. Schwartz, M.D.

Proximal Stenosis of the Bile Ducts: Results With a New Surgical Endoprosthesis

Sezeur A, Kracht M, Fagniez P-L, Rey P, Leandri J, Julien M, Malafosse M (Hôp Rothschild, Paris; Université Paris XII, Créteil; Centre Hospitalier Universitaire Henri Mondor, Créteil, France)
World J Surg 13:100–104, January–February 1989   24–9

A new endoprosthesis was designed for surgical intubation of stenosis of the hilar portion of the biliary tract. Molded according to a patented process (Fig 24–3), the silicone prosthesis has an antiadherent surface. Its length is variable, 5 cm or 7 cm, with a reinforced central portion that resists tumor compression. A system of barbs is incorporated that prevents migration of the endoprosthesis. To facilitate bile drainage, its up-

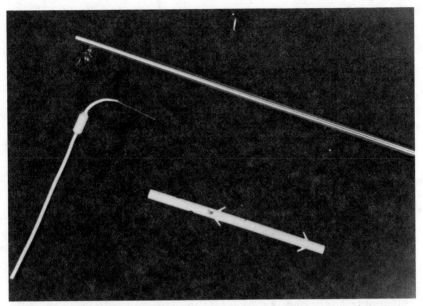

Fig 24–3.—Biliary endoprosthesis (**center**) with its mandrel (**left**) and the insertion device (**top**) on which the mandrel is fixed. (Courtesy of Sezeur A, Kracht M, Fagniez P-L, et al: *World J Surg* 13:100–104, January–February 1989.)

per part is multiperforated. Each endoprosthesis is supplied with a malleable metal mandrel to facilitate intubation. The prostheses are available in 10, 12, 14, 16, and 18 Fr.

Technique.—To perform adequate intubation a complete perioperative cholangiogram is necessary. Between stay sutures the bile duct is opened longitudinally for approximately 1 cm. The tumor is dilated with rigid rubber bougies or malleable dilators having an olive tip. Intubation is performed with an endoprosthesis slightly smaller in diameter than that of the largest bougie used. The mandrel is used only if the endoprosthesis does not pass easily and for intubation of the left hepatic ducts. Both right and left hepatic ducts can be intubated. The bile duct is closed with resorbable sutures.

Of 25 patients with proximal obstruction of the bile ducts operated on, 21 had a malignant tumor of biliary origin. The mean length of hospital stay was 14.4 days. Only 1 patient had obstruction 13 months after placement. Jaundice decreased in all patients except for 1. Migration of the endoprosthesis was not observed. Of 20 patients who died, 18 died of tumor spread. The mean survival time for patients with hilar cholangiocarcinoma was 13.4 months; for those with gallbladder cancer it was 6.5 months, and in the patient with metastatic compression it was 5 months.

The new technique should enable surgical intubation to become more widely used as a palliative biliary bypass in patients with unresectable proximal biliary stenosis. It could favorably replace intrahepatic cholangioenteric anastomosis.

▶ The problem of proximal stenosis of the bile ducts related to tumor at the confluence of the ducts is a significant one, and its incidence is apparently increasing. The results achieved with this prosthesis are encouraging, however; obviating transhepatic passage of a catheter to provide drainage and splinting is a significant achievement.—S.I. Schwartz, M.D.

Malignant Jaundice: Results of Diagnostic and Therapeutic Endoscopy
Soehendra N, Grimm H, Berger B, Nam VC (Univ Hosp Hamburg, West Germany)
World J Surg 13:171–177, March–April 1989   24–10

Ultrasound and direct cholangiography have greatly simplified the diagnosis of malignant obstructive jaundice. Percutaneous transhepatic cholangiography (PTC) is gradually being replaced by endoscopic retrograde cholangiopancreatography (ERCP). Cancer of the head of the pancreas is the most frequent cause of distal choledochus obstruction. A typical appearance of pancreatic cancer can be seen on ERCP; the most frequent types are obstruction and stenosis of the ducts. Most cancers of the pancreas originate in the duct system, and changes are evident on ERCP, which has a sensitivity of between 90% and 95%.

When a lesion is seen in the middle third of the choledochus, the main consideration is carcinoma of the gallbladder and the common bile duct. On ERCP, stenosis seldom appears one-sided; a complete transpapillary examination of the biliary tree is possible only under high-pressure injection with the aid of a balloon catheter or dilator after passing the obstruction. If not successful, PTC can supplement the diagnosis. In the upper third of the choledochus, including the intrahepatic ducts, primary cancer of the bile duct often infiltrating both hepatic ducts is more often seen in this area.

Of 537 patients with obstructive jaundice who underwent ERCP, 208 had malignant obstruction of the bile duct. Cancer of the head of the pancreas was the major cause of obstruction; ERCP was unsuccessful in only 2 cases. The main complication of ERCP was acute pancreatitis, occurring at a rate of 1%. Infection was another complication; the best prevention of septic complications is immediate relief of bile duct obstruction through drainage and clean working conditions.

Endoscopic treatment in malignant obstructive jaundice is palliative. The total rate of complications is 2%, and mortality is 1%. The most frequent complication is cholangitis, usually caused by occlusion of the prosthesis. Even after initial good drainage, the prostheses clog every 3–4 months. Treatment involves early recognition and immediate replacement. Endoscopic placement of the prosthesis has an 85% success rate.

Endoscopic retrograde cholangiopancreatography is being used with increasing success in the diagnosis and for palliative treatment of patients with obstructive jaundice.

▶ Endoscopic drainage of the bile into the intestine certainly is a reasonable method of palliation, particularly as the cure rate for bile duct tumors is so low. Many surgeons have been champions of a more aggressive approach. Iwasaki et al. (1) have reported cures, and Ohto, et al. (2) provided an excellent review of the subject. One of the major issues that requires definition is determination of whether more aggressive excisional therapy affords longer survival and better palliation, as has been suggested by many investigators.—S.I. Schwartz, M.D.

References

1. Iwasaki Y, et al: *Surg Gynecol Obstet* 162:457, 1986.
2. Ohto M, et al: *Surgery* 97:251, 1985.

Transduodenal Sphincteroplasty and Transampullary Septotomy for Primary Sphincter of Oddi Dysfunction

Nussbaum MS, Warner BW, Sax HC, Fischer JE (Univ of Cincinnati)
Am J Surg 157:38–43, January 1989   24–11

Sphincter of Oddi dysfunction has been difficult to define and diagnosis. To determine which patients would most benefit from sphincteroplasty, historical, clinical, diagnostic, and follow-up information was reviewed in a consecutive group of patients who had undergone transduodenal sphincteroplasty with transampullary septotomy for symptoms of biliary colic or recurrent pancreatitis attributed to isolated sphincter of Oddi dysfunction. Of 29 patients seen between October 1979 and November 1987, 24 had undergone endoscopic retrograde cholangiopancreatography (ERCP).

The surgical outcome was excellent in 9, good in 9, fair in 4, and poor in 7 (table). Of 20 patients with sphincter fibrosis, 15 had excellent or good results, and only 3 of 9 patients with inflammation, or neither inflammation nor fibrosis, had an excellent or good outcome. Of 17 patients with underlying pancreatitis, 7 (41%) had an excellent or good outcome. However, sphincteroplasty resulted in an excellent or good outcome in 92% of patients when performed for biliary symptoms. Of 8 postcholecystectomy patients who had pancreatitis, 5 (63%) had an excellent or good outcome. When sphincteroplasty was performed for biliary symptoms, 4 of 5 postcholecystectomy patients had a good or excellent outcome.

Poor results in this series were considered so primarily because of preexisting pancreatitis with continued pain despite adequate sphincteroplasty and transampullary septotomy. When pancreatitis is associated with obvious stenosis and fibrosis of the sphincter of Oddi, the best results occur in postcholecystectomy patients, although a 40% unfavorable

Relationship of Sphincter States, Previous Cholecystectomy,
and Symptoms to Outcome

	n	Excellent	Good	Fair	Poor
			Outcome		
Total	29 (13)	9 (4)	9 (5)	4 (1)	7 (3)
Sphincter status					
Fibrosis	20 (10)	8 (4)	7 (4)	3 (1)	2 (1)
Inflammation	5 (2)	1 (0)	0 (0)	1 (0)	3 (2)
Neither	4 (1)	0 (0)	2 (1)	0 (0)	2 (0)
Preoperative symptoms					
Biliary colic	12 (5)	7 (2)	4 (2)	0 (0)	1 (1)
Pancreatitis	17 (8)	2 (2)	5 (3)	4 (1)	6 (2)
Combination of variables					
Biliary colic with fibrosis	9 (4)	6 (2)	3 (2)	0 (0)	0 (0)
Biliary colic with or without inflammation	3 (1)	1 (0)	1 (0)	0 (0)	1 (1)
Pancreatitis with fibrosis	11 (6)	2 (2)	4 (2)	3 (1)	2 (1)
Pancreatitis with or without inflammation	6 (2)	0 (0)	1 (1)	1 (0)	4 (1)

Values in parentheses represent patients with previous cholecystectomy.
(Courtesy of Nussbuam MS, Warner BW, Sax RC, et al: *Am J Surg* 157:38–43, January 1989.)

outcome can be expected. In contrast to those with pancreatitis, most patients who have symptoms of biliary colic or dyskinesia, and evidence of ampullary fibrosis, can be expected to have a favorable outcome.

▶ It is extremely difficult to define a group of patients with pancreatitis for whom sphincteroplasty would be helpful. Considering the patients reported by Moody et al. (1), it is difficult for me to ascribe a salutary effect to transampullary septotomy in patients who do not have evidence of pancreatic ductal involvement. As Dr. Elliott points out in the Discussion, the real problem is making a preoperative diagnosis of sphincter stenosis. In a series such as this it would be important to do postoperative cholangiopancreatography in both groups of patients (i.e., those with or without a salutary effect) to determine what the status of the sphincter truly is.—S.I. Schwartz, M.D.

Reference

1. Moody FG, et al: *Ann Surg* 197:627, 1983.

Long-Term Survival in Carcinoma of the Biliary Tract: Analysis of Prognostic Factors in 146 Resections
Ouchi K, Matsuno S, Sato T (Tohoku Univ, Sendai, Japan)
Arch Surg 124:248–252, February 1989   24–12

Patients with carcinoma of the extrahepatic biliary tract, including the gallbladder, almost always have a poor prognosis. When possible, aggressive resection is the best approach to such patients. The records of 146 consecutive patients treated with resection of these carcinomas were reviewed in an attempt to identify factors of possible prognostic value.

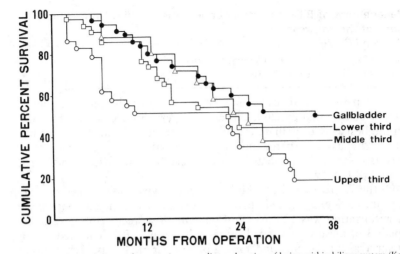

Fig 24–4.—Survival curves after resection according to location of lesion within biliary system (Kaplan-Meier method). (Courtesy of Ouchi K, Matsuno S, Sato T: *Arch Surg* 124:248–252, February 1989.)

Patients with gallbladder carcinoma with tumors that lacked serosal infiltration or vessel invasion, were grossly papillary, or were papillary or well differentiated histologically survived longer than patients without these tumor characteristics. In patients with upper-third lesions, those with tumors having the characteristics described above, or that were treated with hepatic lobectomy, had a greater chance of long-term survival (Fig 24–4). Patients with middle-third tumors whose lesions were grossly papillary or nodular or whose margins were tumor free tended to have a longer survival. In patients with lower-third tumors, long-term survival was obtained most often in those without lymph node metastasis or vessel invasion.

▶ The 5-year survival of about 45%, reported in this article, is not in keeping with most series in which survival associated with carcinoma of the gallbladder is essentially anecdotal. Papillary lesions should be considered separately because they truly have a different biology. In our experience it is unusual to be confronted with a tumor without serosal or vessel invasion. In most series the only survivals recorded are in patients with tumors found incidentally during cholecystectomy for cholelithiasis. As Houry et al. (1) point out, gallbladder carcinoma continues to be a discouraging disease, and they reported 20 patients treated with postoperative radiotherapy. In patients operated on for cure, 1 patient was alive for more than 5 years, and the remainder died. Chemotherapy had no effect.—S.I. Schwartz, M.D.

Reference

1. Houry S, et al: *Br J Surg* 76:448, 1989.

Management of Biliary Obstruction in Patients With Unresectable Carcinoma of the Pancreas

McGrath PC, McNeill PM, Neifeld JP, Bear HD, Parker GA, Turner MA, Horsley JS III, Lawrence W Jr (Med College of Virginia)
Ann Surg 209:284–288, March 1989   24–13

Most patients with carcinoma of the head of the pancreas have advanced disease that precludes curative surgery. Surgeons must then decide on the best way to palliate for biliary obstruction. The efficacy of biliary enteric bypass and percutaneous transhepatic biliary drainage (PTBD) was assessed in 73 patients with unresectable pancreatic cancer treated from 1980 to 1987.

Of the 73 patients, 52 had biliary enteric bypass. None died during operation; 15% experienced operative morbidity. The median postoperative hospitalization was 12 days. In 4 patients (8%) recurrent jaundice developed; 3 of these were treated successfully with PTBD. The median length of survival for patients undergoing biliary enteric bypass was 7 months.

Twenty-one patients had PTBD, with a technical success rate of 81%. This group had a 33% early complication rate and a 33% in-hospital mortality rate. The median length of stay after drainage was 13 days. Of the 14 patients surviving initial hospitalization, 86% had late complications necessitating 16 hospital admissions and 10 emergency room visits, for a total of 155 hospital days. Patients undergoing PTBD had a median survival time of 4 months from diagnosis and 2 months from drainage.

Surgical bypass is an excellent means of palliation for patients with malignant biliary obstruction. This procedure results in low morbidity and mortality in properly selected patients. Alternatively, PTBD is useful for treating patients with extensive disease who are poor surgical candidates or in whom surgical drainage has failed.

▶ A series of articles this past year addressed this specific issue. Rothschild et al. (1) compared the outcome of endoscopic and percutaneous techniques with operative techniques in 157 patients with obstructive jaundice. Of patients undergoing endoscopic papillotomy for stone disease, 56% required either further endoscopic percutaneous or surgical intervention. In patients with malignant disease, cholangitis developed in 40%, and 70% required further transhepatic or surgical intervention. By contrast, in those undergoing surgical intervention primarily, (50% with stone disease and 27% with malignant neoplasms) cholangitis developed in only 7%, and 18% required further intervention. Rosemurgy et al (2) compared choledochoenteric bypass with cholecystoenteric bypass and found the choledochoenteric bypass significantly more effective and reliable.—S.I. Schwartz, M.D.

References

1. Rothschild JG, et al: *Arch Surg* 124:556, 1989.
2. Rosemurgy AS, et al: *Am Surg* 55:55, 1989.

25 The Pancreas

Splanchnic Neural Regulation of Pancreatic Polypeptide Release in the Isolated Perfused Human Pancreas

Brunicardi FC, Druck P, Seymour NE, Sun YS, Gingerich RL, Elahi D, Andersen DK
(State Univ of New York, Brooklyn; Washington Univ; Beth Israel Hosp, Boston)
Am J Surg 157:50–57, January 1989
25–1

The regulation of pancreatic polypeptide (PP) secretion by neurotransmitters within the celiac neural fibers was examined in the isolated perfused human pancreas. Samples were obtained at autopsy from 20 individuals aged 16–71 years without a history of pancreatic disease.

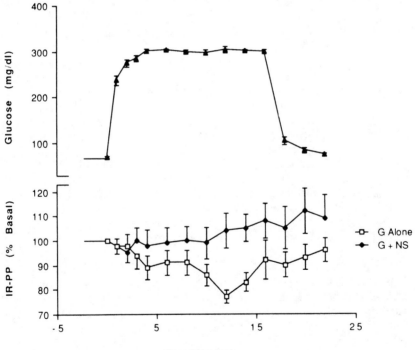

Fig 25–1.—Mean immunoreactive (IR) PP response to 16.7 mM glucose alone (15 test periods) and to 16.7 mM glucose plus bipolar electrical stimulation of the splanchnic neural fibers (17 test periods). *Top graph*, glucose square wave created by increasing the glucose concentration by way of side-arm perfusion. *Bottom graph*, IR-PP response to hyperglycemia and to bipolar electrical stimulation of the splanchnic neural fibers during hyperglycemia. Immunoreactive PP release was inhibited by G alone ($P < .005$) and stimulated by G + NS ($P < .05$). Values expressed as the mean ± SE. G, glucose; NS, nerve stimulation. (Courtesy of Brunicardi FC, Druck P, Seymour NE, et al: *Am J Surg* 157:50–57, January 1989.)

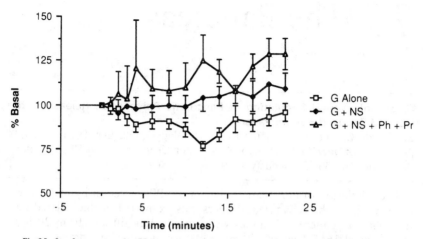

Fig 25–2.—Immunoreactive PP responses to hyperglycemia, combined nerve stimulation, and cholinergic stimulation. The effect of 4 μM phentolamine (Ph) and 6 μM propranolol (Pr) together plus nerve stimulation (NS) plus 16.7mM glucose (G) is shown in comparison to NS plus 16.7mM glucose (G + NS) and 16.7 mM glucose perfusion alone (G alone). The G + NS + Ph + Pr resulted in a significantly greater polypeptide response than G alone ($P < .025$) but was not statistically significantly greater ($P = .056$) than G + NS. Values expressed as the mean ± SE. (Courtesy of Brunicardi FC, Druck P, Seymour NE, et al: *Am J Surg* 157:50–57, January 1989.)

The basal immunoreactive PP secretion of 57 pg/gm/min correlated significantly with age. Pancreatic polypeptide secretion declined in response to hyperglycemia (Fig 25–1). Electrical stimulation of the splanchnic neural fibers reversed the effect of hyperglycemia. α-Adrenergic blockade with phentolamine augmented the effect of nerve stimulation. β-Adrenergic blockade suppressed the PP response. The secretion of PP increased with nerve stimulation during total sympathetic blockade (Fig 25–2), and it increased markedly with combined cholinergic stimulation and infusion of gastric inhibitory polypeptide.

Splanchnic innervation has a prominent role in regulating islet cell secretion in the isolated perfused human pancreas. Linked neural and hormonal mechanisms probably operate to control PP secretion.

▶ These remarkable studies, performed on the isolated human pancreas, confirm previous observations in experimental animals. The greatest stimulation of pancreatic polypeptide was achieved with a combination of β-adrenergic blockade, glucose infusion, and electrical stimulation of the splanchnic nerves. There has been some debate over the role of adrenergic regulation; clearly, in this preparation, α-adrenergic stimulation serves to suppress PP release, a phenomenon that may simply be a reflection of changes in blood flow. This would be an excellent model to test the insulin-releasing properties (so-called incretin effects) of gut hormones such as gastric inhibitory polypeptide, bombesin, and cholecystokinin. The remarkable stability of the preparation suggests that some long-term (i.e., several-hour) observations may be possible.

We should probably note that it may be impossible to repeat or to extend these studies. Every potential organ donor in America is going to have the pancreas taken for transplantation.—J.C. Thompson, M.D.

Surgical Treatment of Acute Necrotizing Pancreatitis

Wilson C, McArdle CS, Carter DC, Imrie CW (Royal Infirmary, Glasgow)
Br J Surg 75:1119–1123, November 1988   25–2

Surgery now is accepted as the proper management of acute necrotizing pancreatitis, but questions remain about the ideal timing, the need to remove uninfected necrotic tissue, and the type of procedure to use. Among 21 patients operated on between January 1980 and June 1986, 14 had necrosectomy with subtotal resection (digital débridement of nonviable pancreatic and peripancreatic tissue) and 7 had resection of less extensive disease (5 resections were distal).

Four patients died after resection and 4 died after necrosectomy. Major complications were frequent. All 3 patients who survived pancreatic resection had a prolonged postoperative course. Half of all survivors required further surgery. No deaths were recorded in the 3 patients who had postoperative pancreatitis, but one third of those with gallstone or alcohol-related pancreatitis died.

Acute necrotizing pancreatitis remains a serious disorder. Most patients can undergo necrosectomy in the second week or later. Although presently the pancreatic bed is packed after necrosectomy, the value of this approach remains to be demonstrated. This is also true of postoperative lavage of the lesser sac.

▶ Is there any way we can truly improve the dismal outlook in patients with necrotizing pancreatitis? Most agree that patients who do not do well should have an operation, but we do not know for sure when to do it, how often to repeat the procedure, and how much to remove. We shy away from any kind of formal resection and try simply to dig out necrotic peripancreatic debris. We have found no good effects of peritoneal lavage. If a major pancreatic abscess is present, the risk of death greatly increases, and it is vital to get out all of the pus. This may require frequent reoperations. Because these patients tend to have serious pulmonary, renal, and other metabolic manifestations of the general fall-apart syndrome, mortality is high. Surgeons initially thought they were débriding the pancreas, but Howard and others have shown that the tissue mass removed serially may amount to 4 or 5 times the mass of the pancreas.

This is one of those instances in which you may decide that a patient is too sick to operate on; the patient then gets much sicker and you do operate. We have the strong belief that patients with alcoholic pancreatitis fare worse than patients with gallstone pancreatitis, although in this series both groups seemed to do equally badly.—J.C. Thompson, M.D.

Colonic Complications of Severe Acute Pancreatitis

Aldridge MC, Francis ND, Glazer G, Dudley HAF (St Mary's Hosp, London)
Br J Surg 76:362–367, April 1989   25–3

Colonic involvement in severe acute pancreatitis is an uncommon but potentially fatal complication. Only 36 patients with colonic necrosis or perforation have been reported in the past 22 years.

Between 1979 and 1987, in one of the largest series, 22 patients with severe acute pancreatitis were treated with intensive supportive therapy. Nineteen patients underwent subtotal pancreatic resection and 3 had peripancreatic débridement. Nine of the 22 patients had colonic involvement to the extent that the bowel was deemed nonviable by the operating surgeon and was resected. An additional patient with severe acute pancreatitis had almost total colonic necrosis at emergency laparotomy for peritonitis.

The 10 patients who underwent bowel resection ranged in age from 26 to 72 years (median, 59 years). Six were thought to have pancreatitis as a consequence of a high intake of alcohol. Two of these 6 also had gallstones. All 10 patients had severe acute pancreatitis with a median of 4 Ranson criteria. In 7 patients colonic involvement was discovered at the time of operation for pancreatitis. Two patients had fecal fistulas within 1–3 weeks after operation. Colonic involvement was diagnosed in 1 patient when abdominal sepsis persisted despite treatment. Seven patients underwent colon resection with exteriorization via a proximal colostomy and 3 had an ileostomy. Six of the 10 patients died within 1–30 days after colonic resection, 5 of overwhelming sepsis and multiple organ failure and 1 of massive retroperitoneal hemorrhage. Three of the 4 survivors have since undergone successful colonic reanastomosis.

On histologic examination only 4 resected colon specimens had evidence of ischemic damage. The other 6 specimens had no evidence of mucosal or submucosal ischemic damage, but showed pericolitis, which had perforated in 4 cases. These findings suggest that colonic damage may oc-

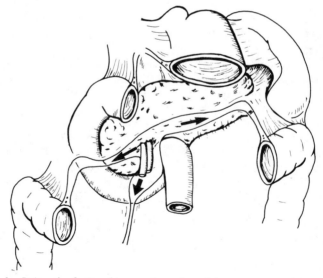

Fig 25–3.—Peritoneal reflections from anterior surface of the pancreas provide a route for the spread of pancreatic enzymes and inflammatory products within the transverse mesocolon and the small bowel mesentery. (Courtesy of Aldridge MC, Francis ND, Glazer G, et al: *Br J Surg* 76:362–367, April 1989.)

cur from 2 separate mechanisms: either through direct spread of pancreatic enzymes and peripancreatic inflammatory tissue involving the serosa of the colon (Fig 25–3), or through thrombosis of mesenteric and submucosal vessels that leads to mucosal infarction.

▶ The close anatomical relationship of the left transverse colon and splenic flexure to the body and tail of the pancreas occasionally results in combined pathology (for example, erosion of the colon in hemorrhagic pancreatitis as chronicled in this paper, or involvement of the pancreas and spleen in abscesses arising from colon perforation caused by either diverticulitis or carcinoma). Osler suggested that if you study syphilis, you would know medicine; the General Surgeon who knows all about the complications of pancreatitis has a good grasp of the huge numbers of possible incarnations of intra-abdominal pathology.—J.C. Thompson, M.D.

Involvement of Cholecystokinin Receptors in the Adverse Effect of Glucocorticoids on Diet-Induced Necrotizing Pancreatitis
Gomez G, Townsend CM Jr, Green D, Rajaraman S, Uchida T, Thompson JC
(Univ of Texas, Galveston)
Surgery 105:230–238, August 1989   25–4

Corticosteroids have long been implicated as a possible cause of acute pancreatitis, but the mechanism by which corticosteroids affect pancreatitis is unknown. Recent in vitro studies suggested that cholecystokinin (CCK) may contribute to the course of acute pancreatitis. In other studies, long-term administration of glucocorticoids increased the secretory response to CCK of the normal rat pancreas.

To assess the effect of long-term glucocorticoid administration on the course of acute pancreatitis caused by a choline-deficient, ethionine-supplemented (CDE) diet, hydrocortisone in a dosage of 10 mg/kg/day was given to mice for 1 week. Acute necrotizing pancreatitis was induced thereafter with a CDE diet for 60 hours. At the start of the CDE diet some of the hydrocortisone-treated mice were also given the CCK-receptor antagonist CR-1409. Control mice were given saline solution. All treatments were continued during and after the CDE diet. Mice were observed for a total of 336 hours, and survival was assessed in each group.

Forty percent of mice in the control group survived. Long-term hydrocortisone administration alone did not produce pancreatitis, but it significantly increased pancreatic necrosis caused by the CDE diet from 40% to 70% and significantly reduced survival from 40% to 9% (Fig 25–4). Administration of CR-1409 to hydrocortisone-treated mice abolished the adverse effect of hydrocortisone on survival: 46% of the CR-1409-treated mice survived.

Administration of hydrocortisone alone for 1 week did not increase serum amylase levels. However, after 60 hours of the CDE diet, serum amylase levels were significantly increased in all treatment groups. Administration of the CCK blocker CR-1409 during acute pancreatitis com-

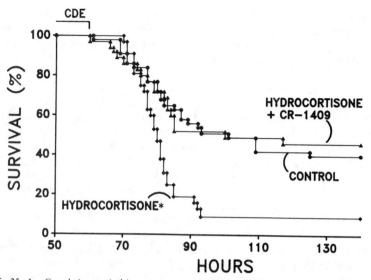

Fig 25-4.—Cumulative survival in acute pancreatitis in mice. Hydrocortisone (10 mg/kg/day) was given for 1 week before pancreatitis. Acute pancreatitis was induced by feeding the mice a CDE diet for 60 hours. At the onset of the CDE diet, a group of hydrocortisone-treated mice received the CCK-receptor antagonist CR-1409 (5 mg/kg, 3 times a day). Control mice received injections of saline solution. All treatments were continued during and after the CDE diet. Survival was observed for up to 336 hours. The increased mortality produced by the chronic treatment of hydrocortisone was abolished by CR-1409 (43 control, 32 hydrocortisone-treated, and 35 hydroscortisone plus CR-1409-treated mice; *asterisk*, different from control). (Courtesy of Gomez G, Townsend CM Jr, Green D, et al: *Surgery* 105:230–238, August 1989.)

pletely abolished the enhancement effect of hydrocortisone on serum amylase levels.

Although chronic glucocorticoid administration per se does not cause pancreatitis, it contributes adversely to the severity of pancreatitis from other causes. The adverse effect appears to be attributable to the CCK receptor-mediated sensitization of the pancreas to endogenous CCK. Thus CCK-receptor blockade may improve survival among patients with necrotizing pancreatitis associated with long-term glucocorticoid administration.

▶ As Dr. Fischer observes in the Discussion of this paper, this finding has clinical relevance. Week in and week out we sit in our Morbidity and Mortality Conference and listen to tales of transplant patients taking steroids in whom pancreatitis develops. These studies in mice suggest that cortisone depends on participation of CCK to bring about pancreatitis, and that if the CCK receptors can be blocked it might be possible to forestall the development of pancreatitis.—J.C. Thompson, M.D.

Treatment of Chronic Alcoholic Pancreatitis by Pancreatic Resection
Keith RG, Saibil FG, Sheppard RH (Univ of Toronto)
Am J Surg 157:156–162, January 1989

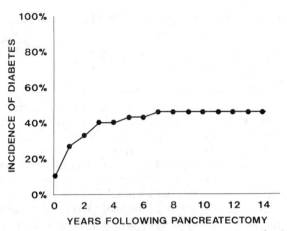

Fig 25−5.—Event sequence graph of insulin-dependent diabetes in patients after 80% pancreatectomy. (Courtesy of Keith RG, Saibil FG, Sheppard RH: *Am J Surg* 157:156−162, January 1989.)

Although pancreatic duct decompression is a widely accepted treatment for painful chronic pancreatitis when the ducts are diffusely dilated, the appropriate surgical management of painful chronic pancreatitis in patients with stenotic pancreatic ducts is controversial. Forty-one selected patients with chronic pancreatitis caused by alcoholism underwent resection when pancreatography demonstrated stenotic pancreatic duct abnormalities precluding decompressive procedures. Five patients had Whipple resections, 32 had 80% resections, and 7 had total pancreatectomies.

Mortality was 10%, with 1 perioperative and 3 late deaths. On long-term follow-up, complete freedom from pain was reported by all of the patients who had total pancreatectomy and half of those who had 80% resection, but by only 1 of 5 patients who had Whipple resection. Diabetes occurred in 1 patient after Whipple resection, in almost half of those after 80% pancreatectomy (Fig 25−5), and in all patients after total resection, in whom it was frequently complicated by recurrent alcoholism. Jaundice was a rare complication of disease progression; none of these patients had cholestasis preoperatively. Recurrent alcoholism, reported in 32% of the patients, contributed to 2 deaths.

Recurrent alcoholism represents a serious risk, having devastating effects on treatment outcome.

▶ We have not been happy with total pancreatectomy for chronic alcoholic pancreatitis because of the unreliability of the patient. Although some talk about post total pancreatectomy diabetes being easy to manage, it is not easy in a third to a half of the patients, and if they are off drinking somewhere they will die. For practical purposes, I am reluctant even to think about this unless the patient is tightly connected to a local Alcoholics Anonymous group. Even then, of course, you cannot tell. I was surprised to see the plateauing of diabetes at nearly 50% after 80% pancreatectomy. This indicates that a good number of β cells are left in the cephalic 20% residual.—J.C. Thompson, M.D.

Insulin Antibodies and Management of Diabetes After Total Pancreatectomy

Ishikawa O, Ohhigashi H, Sasakuma F, Imaoka S, Hasegawa K, Okishio T, Sasaki Y, Koyama H, Iwanaga T (Ctr for Adult Diseases, Osaka, Japan)
Surgery 105:57–64, January 1989   25–6

Diabetes in patients who have undergone total pancreatectomy can be difficult to manage. These patients must depend entirely on exogenous insulin, and they lack pancreatic glucagon, the most effective protection against hypoglycemia. To assess the relationship between formation of insulin antibodies and diabetic stability, postoperative changes in insulin antibody levels were measured in 18 patients after total pancreatectomy.

Eleven patients were treated with animal-derived insulin and 7 received recombinant DNA human insulin. Levels of blood sugar and urinary glucose excretion were measured daily by the patients after hospital discharge. Levels of insulin antibody were checked weekly or biweekly at an outpatient clinic.

No patient who received recombinant DNA human insulin had more than a 50 μU/mL level of immunoreactive insulin bound with insulin antibody (binding IRI) for a mean period of 17 months. However, 6 of 11 patients who received insulin of beef and porcine origin had a plasma-binding who received of beef and porcine origin had a plasma-binding level of IRI that was elevated by more than 500 μU/mL. These 6 began to experience unstable diabetic control and had frequent polyuria, thirst, weight loss, and periods of cold sweat and weakness. Three of the 6 were hospitalized and given human DNA insulin in place of animal-derived insulin; they recovered from unstable diabetic control.

Measurements of high-affinity antibodies (Ab_1) and low-affinity antibodies (Ab_2) led to the conclusion that unstable diabetic control in pancreatectomized patients occurred at very low levels of Ab_1, in contrast to patients with insulin-dependent diabetes.

Because antigenicity is lower in human insulin than in animal-derived insulins, the former is recommended after total pancreatectomy. Human insulin, however, has also shown antibody formation; thus serial determination of insulin antibody, especially of the Ab_1 level, is recommended.

▶ This appears to be an important contribution. Although perhaps the majority of patients after total pancreatectomy have a diabetic state that can be managed fairly well, between 25% and 33% have a brittle diabetes, often characterized by wild swings of glucose levels (1). The instability appears to be caused by the concomitant lack of pancreatic glucagon and insulin (2, 3). The great difference demonstrated in the present study in the response to synthetic human insulin vs. insulin from beef or cattle suggests a way out of the dilemma. If human insulin is used, anti-insulin antibodies can be averted and control greatly enhanced. Total pancreatectomy is often an easier operation than a Whipple resection and would be chosen more often if the risk of difficult diabetes could be averted.—J.C. Thompson, M.D.

References

1. Pliam MB, et al: *Arch Surg* 110:506, 1975.
2. Muller WA, et al: *Diabetes* 23:512, 1974.
3. Bolli G, et al: *Diabetologia* 22:100, 1982.

Intraductal Papillary Neoplasms of the Pancreas: A Clinicopathologic Study of Six Patients
Morohoshi T, Kanda M, Asanuma K, Klöppel G (Showa Univ, Tokyo; Matsudo City Hosp, Chiba, Japan; Free Univ of Brussels)
Cancer 64:1329–1335, Sept 15, 1989   25–7

Intraductal papillary neoplasms of the pancreas are uncommon. In contrast to patients with invasive ductal adenocarcinoma, those with intraductal papillary tumors appear to be curable by total pancreatectomy. The exact clinicopathologic identification of these tumors is therefore extremely important. To describe the clinicopathologic features of intraductal papillary tumors, such tumors were obtained from 3 men and 3 women aged 64–79 years. Two tumors were obtained as incidental autopsy findings from patients who had died of other causes. The other 4 tumors were excised during pancreatectomy. Three patients had long histories of symptoms mimicking chronic pancreatitis. The tumors involved the main pancreatic duct in the head–body region of the pancreas, either diffusely or focally. No enlarged lymph nodes or obvious lymph node metastasis was seen on gross examination.

Histologic examination of the tumors revealed well-differentiated papillary or papillotubular patterns (Fig 25–6). Mitoses were infrequent. Atypical tumor tissue had remained confined within the ducts, and fatty tissue surrounding the pancreas had not been invaded. Most of the tumor cells were mucus-secreting cells that occasionally stained for carcinoembryonic antigen and carbohydrate antigen. Three tumors contained foci of pronounced to severe cellular atypia and carcinoma in situ.

During follow-up ranging from 4 months to 8 years there was no tumor recurrence or metastasis. Because of their favorable prognosis, intraductal papillary neoplasms should be considered uncommon, low-grade malignancies that should not be confused with ductal adenocarcinoma.

▶ Although these tumors do occasionally produce small cystic dilatation of the main pancreatic duct, they differ from the mucinous cystadenocarcinomas of the pancreas in that they rarely evolve into invasive carcinomas. The intraductal papillary cancers will recur if locally excised but the prognosis seems to be excellent after pancreatectomy. Intraductal papillary cancers of the head of the pancreas, treated by Whipple resection, have a nearly uniformly high rate of survival. Although multiple foci have been reported, the vast majority of tumors are localized within a small area in the pancreas. They may be well demonstrated by CT studies, and especially by endoscopic retrograde cholangiopan-

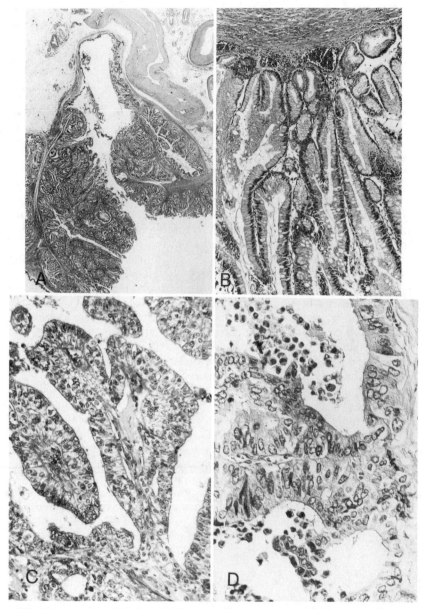

Fig 25–6.—Pancreatic intraductal papillary neoplasm. **A,** intraductal tumor showing papillary projections with fibrovascular tissue stalks [hematoxylin and eosin (H & E); original magnification, ×10]. **B,** papillations with well-differentiated, mucus-producing epithelium (H & E; original magnification, ×100). **C,** papillae with atypical epithelium (H & E; original magnification, ×200). **D,** papilliferous epithelium with severe cellular atypia (H & E; original magnification, ×400). (Courtesy of Morohoshi T, Kanda M, Asanuma K, et al: *Cancer* 64:1329–1335, Sept 15, 1989.)

creatography. Contrary to the series reported here, the majority of our patients have been young women, usually Latin-Americans.—J.C. Thompson, M.D.

Pancreatic Lymphoma: Is Surgery Mandatory for Diagnosis or Treatment?
Webb TH, Lillemoe KD, Pitt HA, Jones RJ, Cameron JL (Johns Hopkins Med Inst)
Ann Surg 209:25–30, January 1989   25–8

The pancreas is the primary site of the disease in only a small percentage of patients with non-Hodgkin's lymphoma. Also, pancreatic non-Hodgkin's lymphoma is found in only a very small number of all patients with pancreatic malignancies. Results of treatment of 9 patients with pancreatic lymphoma over a 5-year period were reviewed.

The median age was 64 years. Weight loss was a common symptom, as were jaundice, abdominal pain, anorexia, and nausea. Five patients had palpable abdominal masses, 7 had elevated levels of liver transaminases, and 8 had an elevated serum level of alkaline phosphatase. In all 9 patients CT revealed a soft-tissue mass in the pancreas; the median diameter of the mass was 7 cm. Diagnosis was established by radiographically guided needle biopsy in 4 patients, at laparotomy in 4, and by peripheral lymph node biopsy in 1. Most patients had disseminated disease; 5 were in stage IV.

All patients underwent combination chemotherapy, and 6 were also treated surgically. No patient was given radiotherapy. Six patients achieved complete remission and had no evidence of disease at a median of 24 months after treatment. One patient died after refusing to complete chemotherapy, and another died of an unrelated malignancy. A third patient, the only 1 with the well-differentiated lymphocytic cell type, survived for only 7 months despite aggressive combination chemotherapy.

Pancreatic lymphoma can mimic ductal adenocarcinoma of the pancreas. Computed tomography is useful in demonstrating the large, rapidly growing masses typical of pancreatic lymphoma. Histologic typing and immunologic subclassification can be obtained by radiographically guided percutaneous needle biopsies. Surgery aids in diagnosis when biopsy is nondiagnostic. Chemotherapy achieved excellent long-term results, even in patients with late-stage disease and diffuse histiocytic lymphoma.

▶ This is another rare pancreatic tumor that differs from the intraductal papillary tumor described in the previous paper in that the lymphomatous involvement of the pancreas usually produces a large tumor that often grows to palpable size and that involves much, if not all, of the gland. The excellent results obtained by chemotherapy are encouraging.—J.C. Thompson, M.D.

Pulmonary Complications of Acute Pancreatitis: Light and Electron Microscopic Changes in an Experimental Model
O'Donohoe MK (Univ College, Dublin)
Surg Res Comm 6:275–281, 1989   25–9

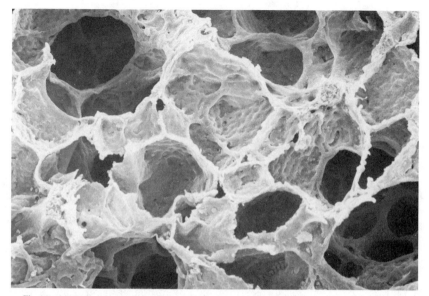

Fig 25–7.—Scanning electron micrograph of normal rat lung. Original magnification as shown. (Courtesy of O'Donohoe MK: *Surg Res Comm* 6:275–281, 1989.)

Previous studies established an association between acute pancreatitis and respiratory dysfunction, but the cause of this association is not fully understood. To assess the changes that occur in the lung after severe acute pancreatitis, light and scanning electron microscopy (SEM) were

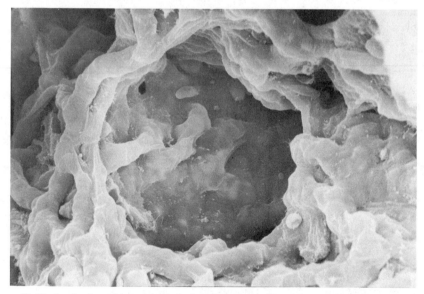

Fig 25–8.—Rat lung 18 hours after induction of pancreatitis. Vascular congestion and crenation of types I and II pneumocytes can be seen. Original magnification as shown. (Courtesy of O'Donohoe MK: *Surg Res Comm* 6:275–281, 1989.)

used to study 32 adult Sprague Dawley rats. Acute pancreatitis was induced in 20 rats via retrograde trypsin infusion into the biliopancreatic duct. Sham laparotomy was performed in the remaining 12 control rats. The animals were killed at 6-hour intervals over 24 hours, and their lungs were examined histologically via light microscopy and SEM.

All animals had hemorrhagic pancreatitis, as confirmed on histologic examination and by a significant rise in serum amylase levels. Changes in the lungs were consistent with atelectasis and pulmonary vascular congestion; a polymorphonuclear infiltrate was observed at 18 hours and 24 hours. Pulmonary changes were scored on a scale of 0 to 3, with 0 indicating no pathology (Fig 25–7) and 3 denoting maximal pathology. The observed changes were confirmed by SEM. After 6 hours and 12 hours there was evidence of increased capillary dilatation. After 18 hours SEM showed crenation of types I and II pneumocytes (Fig 25–8). That the severity of these changes was increased with time was found with both SEM and light microscopy.

The reduction in size and damage to type II pneumocytes as seen with SEM supports the theory that a reduction in surfactant production may be a major cause of atelectasis, and that acute pancreatitis is associated with injury to type II pneumocytes.

▶ I have been telling medical students for years that one of the causes of pulmonary complications in patients with acute pancreatitis is diminished pulmonary surfactant. This is the first clue that I have that may explain why surfactant is diminished. The beautiful morphological demonstration of damage to the type II pneumocytes supports the theory that reduction in surfactant production is the major cause of atelectasis. The author suggests that destruction of surfactant by phospholipase, coupled with damage to the pneumocytes that produce the atelectasis, may synergize to cause great harm. There are obviously other keys to the puzzle, because only a fraction of patients with pancreatitis experience severe respiratory trouble.—J.C. Thompson, M.D.

26 The Endocrine Glands

Functioning Oxyphil Cell Adenomas of the Parathyroid Gland: A Study of 15 Cases

Wolpert HR, Vickery AL Jr, Wang C-A (Massachusetts Gen Hosp, Boston)

Am J Surg Pathol 13:500–504, June 1989   26–1

Parathyroid adenomas composed predominantly of chief cells are the most frequent cause of primary hyperparathyroidism. The rare oxyphil cell parathyroid adenoma was generally considered nonfunctioning until

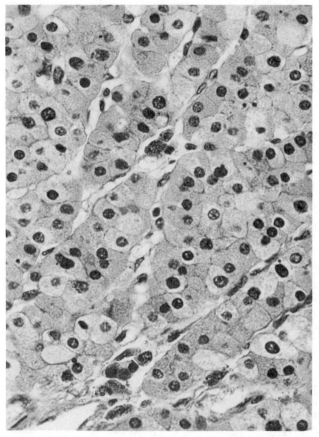

Fig 26–1.—A high-power view of a parathyroid oxyphil cell adenoma illustrating the classic appearance of large polygonal cells arranged in sheets and cords with abundant, brightly eosinophilic cytoplasm and small, central nuclei. (Courtesy of Wolpert HR, Vickery AL JR, Wang C-A: *Am J Surg Pathol* 13:500–504, June 1989.)

1978. A retrospective review of 500 consecutive patients at Massachusetts General Hospital with hyperparathyroidism associated with parathyroid adenoma diagnosed in 1979–1987 yielded 15 (3.0%) oxyphil cell adenomas. Criteria for diagnosis included oxyphil cells constituting at least 90% of the enlarged gland, a normal second parathyroid gland, and a postoperative decrease in serum calcium levels to a normal range. Based on these criteria, 34 of the 65 previously reported patients are excluded.

The 15 patients in the present series included 11 women and 4 men (median age, 58 years). Eight patients were asymptomatic, 6 had probable symptoms related to their disease, and 2 had palpable neck masses; 13 had increased serum parathyroid hormone levels. Postoperative serum calcium levels were normal for a median of 2 years in 8 patients available for follow-up.

The adenomas were soft and encapsulated with a predominance of dark-brown cut surfaces. The median size of the adenoma was 2.5 cm; the median weight of 9 adenomas was 2.8 g. Microscopically, the adenomas were composed of large polygonal cells arranged in solid sheets and anastomosing cords and trabeculae (Fig 26–1). Fibrovascular septae with connections to the fibrous capsule were common.

Among the total of oxyphil cell adenomas the true incidence of functioning tumors is unknown. Although the exact role of the oxyphil cell in parathyroid function has not been determined, there is clear evidence that the oxyphil cell parathyroid adenoma causes primary hyperparathyroidism. As is the case with chief cell adenoma, most patients are women in their fifth and sixth decades.

▶ This article was selected to remind all of us that functioning parathyroid adenomas are not limited to chief cells. The parathyroid oxyphil cell was formerly thought to be a degenerated chief cell that had no secretory function. Many oxyphil adenomas fail to function and do not meet the rigid criteria outlined by the authors.—J.C. Thompson, M.D.

Clarifying the Role of Fine-Needle Aspiration Cytologic Evaluation and Frozen Section Examination in the Operative Management of Thyroid Cancer
Kopald KH, Layfield LJ, Mohrmann R, Foshag LJ, Giuliano AE (Univ of California, Los Angeles)
Arch Surg 124:1201–1205, October 1989   26–2

Preoperative biopsy of thyroid nodules using fine-needle aspiration (FNA) as an aid in planning the extent of excision has been accepted by some centers but not by others. Some surgeons are still reluctant to use FNA and prefer waiting for intraoperative frozen-section analysis to determine the extent of thyroid resection. To compare the accuracy of FNA with that of intraoperative frozen-section analysis in the diagnosis of thyroid cancer data on 486 patients who underwent thyroidectomy between

1975 and 1988 were studied. Of 146 patients with thyroid cancer confirmed on permanent hematoxylin-eosin sections 126 had intraoperative frozen-section analysis, 62 underwent preoperative FNA, and 56 had both studies.

Of the 126 histologically confirmed thyroid cancers examined during operation on frozen section, a carcinoma was correctly diagnosed in 69% of the cases; in the other 31% intraoperative frozen-section analysis failed to identify thyroid cancer. Preoperative cytologic evaluation with FNA, performed in 62 patients, correctly identified thyroid cancer in 71%. In the 56 patients who had both preoperative FNA and intraoperative frozen-section analysis, the malignancies were accurately detected with both methods in 57%. In 18%, FNA was correct, whereas frozen section examination was in error; in 11%, frozen-section analysis was correct and the results of FNA were negative.

Preoperative FNA biopsy, with less morbidity and expense, is at least as accurate as intraoperative frozen section examination in making a definitive diagnosis of thyroid cancer.

▶ The results reported are excellent, but I could not find their false positive rate. Clark, in the Discussion, states that the false positive rate is 1%, which corroborates the authors' statement that if the FNA cytologic examination is positive for cancer, one can go ahead and plan a thyroidectomy.

Every author who writes enthusiastically about FNA cytology is clearly working with a good cytologist, because the whole method is absolutely cytologist dependent. The 2 variables are, of course, the skill of the cytologist and the accuracy of sampling. A small focus of cancer hidden in a huge goiter would probably be missed (by any sampling method, for that matter). Some series have reported a much higher yield than the 71% positive reported here. Nonetheless, the method is not perfect and depends entirely upon the cytologist.— J.C. Thompson, M.D.

Goiters and Airway Problems
Shaha AR, Burnett C, Alfonso A, Jaffe BM (Health Science Ctr, Brooklyn)
Am J Surg 158:378–381, October 1989   26–3

The incidence of goiter in the United States is steadily decreasing because of the routine use of iodized salts. However, large neglected goiters that can compress airways and cause life-threatening acute respiratory distress still occur in endemic goiter belt areas.

During a 7-year period 46 men and 74 women aged 32–89 years were treated for airway compression secondary to large goiters. Most patients had long-standing histories of goiters with chronic symptoms or acute episodes of exacerbation. Twenty-four patients were asymptomatic; airway changes were first noted on routine examination. Sixty-five patients with large goiters had chronic symptoms such as cough, nocturnal dyspnea, or breathing problems. Pulmonary function tests and CT were not performed routinely. Computed tomography was done mostly to examine

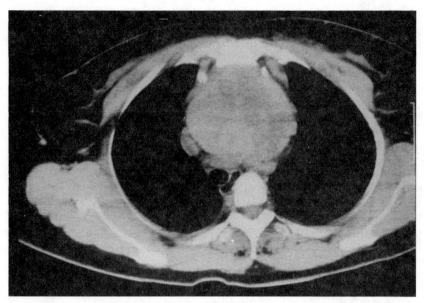

Fig 26–2.—Computed tomograph showing a large substernal goiter with tracheal displacement. (Courtesy of Shaha AR, Burnett C, Alfonso A, et al: *Am J Surg* 158:378–381, October 1989.)

patients with substernal goiters to assess the substernal location and relative position of the trachea (Fig 26–2). Indirect laryngoscopy was most helpful in determining the position of the larynx and condition of the vocal cords. However, the decision to operate was based mainly on physical examination and clinical indications.

Thirty patients had acute airway distress, 12 of whom had emergency intubation and respiratory support. Two of these patients, with diffuse pulmonary metastases and diminished pulmonary reserve, died. One patient refused operation and died after 8 days on mechanical ventilation. Another patient who had lymphoma required tracheostomy for airway distress and radiation therapy. The remaining 116 patients underwent thyroidectomy.

Nodular goiters were discovered histologically in surgical specimens from 101 patients; Hashimoto's thyroiditis was found in 2 patients, and thyrotoxicosis in 1. Twelve patients had well-differentiated papillary or follicular thyroid carcinoma. Ninety patients had substernal goiters, but only 1 required sternal splitting. There were no postoperative deaths. Complications were minor and included temporary hypoparathyroidism, superior laryngeal nerve injury, and temporary recurrent laryngeal nerve palsy in 1 patient each. Three patients had hematomas that required reoperation.

It is important to recognize that long-standing goiters can cause airway compression, which occasionally will lead to life-threatening acute airway distress. Early surgical decompression is recommended, particularly if the patient is symptomatic or if there is mediastinal extension.

▶ There are several important messages to be related regarding large thyroids and airway compression, but I would concentrate on 2 of them. If not yet, some day you may well be called to the emergency room to see a patient with a huge mass in the neck who is thrashing about, obviously hypoxic. Someone may have attempted unsuccessfully to perform endotracheal intubation and may press upon you the idea that a tracheostomy would be helpful. Resist that suggestion and get a skilled person, if not yourself, to put in the endotracheal tube. If the patient is older than age 60, there is a good chance that the compressing thyroid is in fact involved with anaplastic carcinoma, which is almost certainly best treated by radiation and certainly does not respond well to attempts at tracheostomy. The second message is that, as stressed by the authors, many very large substernal goiters can be removed without splitting the sternum. Gentle traction will help to worry the gland out from under the manubrium. Two sterile soup spoons used in manner similar to obstetric forceps can often help in the extrication.—J.C. Thompson, M.D.

Local Recurrence in Papillary Thyroid Carcinoma: Is Extent of Surgical Resection Important?
Grant CS, Hay ID, Gough IR, Bergstralh EJ, Goellner JR, McConahey WM
(Mayo Clinic and Found, Rochester, Minn)
Surgery 104:954–962, December 1988   26–4

Controversy continues about the benefits of total thyroidectomy vs. conservative resection in the treatment of papillary thyroid carcinoma. The records of 963 patients who had complete resection of the cancer with curative intent from 1946 through 1975 were reviewed. Unilateral procedures included subtotal and total lobectomies. Bilateral resection was subdivided into subtotal and total thyroidectomies. Unilateral resections predominated until 1955, when bilateral procedures became more common. The median follow-up was 23 years. Three categories of tumor recurrence were identified: neck nodal metastases, local recurrences, and distant metastases. A scoring system was devised that indicated risk of local recurrence based on 4 factors: *a*ge, tumor *g*rade, *e*xtent, and *s*ize (AGES).

Most of the patients (69%) underwent bilateral subtotal thyroidectomy, and the majority (90%) were in the AGES low-risk category. Local recurrence occurred in 52 patients (5.4%). Age of 60 years or older, extrathyroidal tumor invasion, tumor size 4 cm or larger, unilateral resection, surgery before 1955, and an AGES score of 4.00 or more all were associated significantly with local recurrence by univariate survival analysis. Among low-risk patients, similar rates were found for local recurrence whether bilateral resection was subtotal or total. High-risk patients had a significantly lower risk of local recurrence after bilateral resection, whether subtotal or total. Local recurrence location outside an ipsilateral or contralateral thyroid remnant was associated with a significantly higher risk of subsequent death.

Permanent hypoparathyroidism and damage to recurrent laryngeal nerves are risks of total thyroidectomy, and survival benefits of the procedure are not apparent. The best available option for patients with papillary thyroid carcinoma is bilateral resection, consisting of ipsilateral total lobectomy and contralateral subtotal or near-total lobectomy, preserving the nerves and at least 1 parathyroid gland.

▶ The controversy of whether to do a total or a subtotal resection of the thyroid for papillary cancer is obscured by the experience of the protagonist. Those thyroid surgeons who spend day in and day out operating on the thyroid gland gain vast experience and can surely perform a total thyroidectomy with scant risk to the patient. Surgeons who perform fewer than 15 or 20 thyroidectomies per year (and that must include the majority of general surgeons) may run a significantly higher risk of inadvertent parathyroidectomy or injury to the recurrent laryngeal nerve in doing a total thyroidectomy as opposed to a total lobectomy on one side and a subtotal on the other. The data here from the Mayo Clinic indicating that no patient with tumor recurrence limited to the thyroid remnant died of thyroid cancer provide solace to those surgeons who do not routinely do total thyroidectomies. One of the problems in our business is that masters who recount their experience may suggest courses of action that, when adopted by lesser mortals, may lead to high complication rates. I can certainly understand the abstract beauty of taking out the entire gland in a patient with thyroid carcinoma, but proponents of the routine application of such a course have a difficult brief. They would have to prove that the addition of total removal of all thyroid tissue is more important than the numbers of injured nerves and hypocalcemic patients that would result. Tough brief.—J.C. Thompson, M.D.

Metastatic Papillary Carcinoma of the Thyroid: The Significance of Extranodal Extension

Spires JR, Robbins KT, Luna MA, Byers RM (Univ of Texas MD Anderson Cancer Ctr, Houston)
Head Neck 11:242–246, May–June 1989   26–5

Studies of prognostic indicators in thyroid carcinoma have not considered the significance of extracapsular spread of regional metastatic disease. The importance of cervical nodal metastases in patients with extracapsular invasion was assessed retrospectively.

During a 10-year period, 63 of 88 patients who underwent a planned neck dissection for metastatic thyroid carcinoma had disease limited to the thyroid and lymph node, without soft tissue extension (group I). In 25 patients (group II) there was involvement of perinodal soft tissue, extracapsular invasion. Median ages were 28 years in group I and 29 years in group II. Women comprised 68% of group I and 52% of group II. Both groups had a median follow-up of more than 8 years.

Regional recurrence was discovered in 18 patients (29%) in group I and in 5 in group II (20%) (Fig 26–3). Distant metastases developed in 6 group I patients and in 4 group II patients. Rates of overall survival and

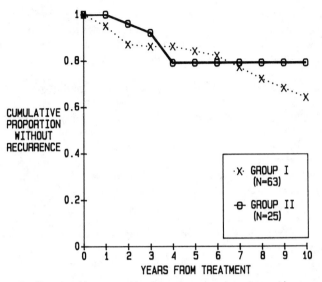

Fig 26–3.—Papillary thyroid cancer; regional recurrence rate in patients without extracapsular nodal disease (group I) and patients with extracapsular nodal disease (group II). (Courtesy of Spires JR, Robbins KT, Luna MA, et al: *Head Neck* 11:242–246, May–June 1989.)

recurrence-free survival were similar whether patients had only extracapsular nodal disease, extension through the thyroid capsule and extracapsular nodal disease, or neither (Fig 26–4).

In contrast to other reports, extension of carcinoma through the cap-

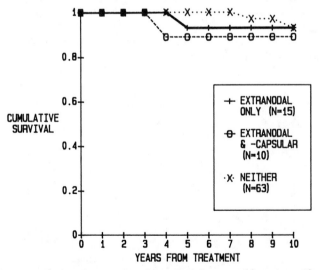

Fig 26–4.—Papillary thyroid cancer; survival rates (death from cancer) for patients with extracapsular nodal disease and extracapsular thyroid disease, for those with extracapsular nodal disease, and for those with neither extracapsular thyroid disease nor extracapsular nodal disease. (Courtesy of Spires JR, Robbins KT, Luna MA, et al: *Head Neck* 11:242–246, May–June 1989.)

sule of the thyroid gland did not adversely affect the outcome and had no prognostic significance. Although previous studies have identified patients of younger age and female sex to have higher rates of survival, those factors were not significant in the present series.

▶ It is difficult to read this abstract without a feeling of therapeutic nihilism regarding papillary cancer of the thyroid. It certainly offers no support to the rigorous suggestion that all patients should have total thyroidectomy (see the comment following Abstract 26–4). It is certainly hard to deny that papillary carcinoma of the thyroid is a unique neoplasm when you read evidence that any extrathyroid extension of the tumor at the primary site that was surgically resectable had no prognostic significance. Examination of the 2 figures confirms the lack of significance of extracapsular nodal disease.—J.C. Thompson, M.D.

Stimulatory Effect of Vasoactive Intestinal Polypeptide on Human Normal and Neoplastic Thyroid Tissue
Siperstein AE, Miller RA, Clark OH (Univ of California, San Francisco)
Surgery 104:985–991, December 1988   26–6

Apart from thyroid-stimulating hormone (TSH), vasoactive intestinal peptide (VIP) is present in nerves that innervate thyroid vessels and follicles, and it has a role in regulating thyroid function. Vasoactive intestinal peptide stimulates adenylate cyclase activity in cultures of normal and hyperplastic thyroid tissue, thereby increasing the intracellular cyclic adenosine monophosphate level. To determine how TSH and VIP signal the interior of the cell to effect their actions, thyroid tissue from 4 follicular adenomas, 3 follicular carcinomas, and 3 papillary carcinomas were studied.

Both normal and neoplastic tissues exhibit patterns of stimulation by VIP that resemble those seen with TSH. Vasoactive intestinal peptide

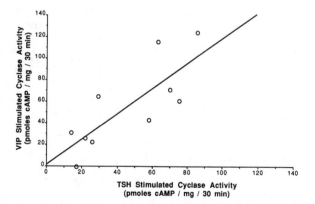

Fig 26–5.—For normal thyroid tissue there is a positive correlation (*P* < .006) between VIP-stimulated cyclase activity *(vertical axis)* and TSH-stimulated cyclase activity *(horizontal axis)* for 10 patients studied. (Courtesy of Siperstein AE, Miller RA, Clark OH: *Surgery* 104:985–991, December 1988.)

stimulated adenylate cyclase activity more than did TSH in normal tissue, and the 2 hormones had an additive effect. The stimulatory effects of the 2 hormones correlated positively (Fig 26–5). In neoplastic tissue TSH was a more potent stimulus than in normal tissue.

Vasoactive intestinal peptide is a potent stimulus of adenylate cyclase in normal and neoplastic human thyroid tissues. The function of VIP in neoplastic tissue remains uncertain. Further studies of this sort may help to elucidate the factors regulating the aberrant growth of thyroid tumors.

▶ Six years ago, VIP was shown to stimulate human thyroid cell function (1). The authors now report that VIP is a less potent stimulator of intracellular adenylate cyclase in thyroid tumor tissues, from which they conclude that neoplastic thyroid cells contain fewer VIP receptors; whereas TSH is more potent in neoplastic than in normal thyroid as an adenylate cyclase stimulant, VIP is less potent. Actually, VIP is a neurotransmitter agent and may not function as a hormone at all. From which nerves (sympathetic or parasympathetic), one wonders, is the VIP released?—J.C. Thompson, M.D.

Reference

1. Toccafondi RS, et al: *J Clin Endocrinol Metab* 58:157, 1984.

Islet Cell Carcinomas of the Pancreas: A Twenty-Year Experience
Thompson GB, van Heerden JA, Grant CS, Carney JA, Ilstrup DM (Mayo Clinic and Found, Rochester, Minn)
Surgery 104:1011–1017, December 1988   26–7

Islet cell carcinoma of the pancreas is an indolent neuroendocrine neoplasm. Most of these tumors are hormonally active. When they are functioning, a number of clinical syndromes may develop. A series of surgically treated patients was reviewed to determine the distribution of functioning and nonfunctioning tumors, and the response to treatment.

From 1965 to 1984, 58 patients were treated for islet cell carcinoma of the pancreas. They were followed for a mean of 7.4 years; 54% had functioning and 46% had nonfunctioning carcinomas (Fig 26–6). The most common functioning tumors were gastrinomas, affecting 19% of the patients. The prevalence of nonfunctioning tumors increased steadily from 25% to 65% during the 15 years studied. Curative resections were done on 26% and noncurative procedures on 74% of the patients. Overall operative mortality was 3%. Symptoms improved after surgery in 90% of those having curative procedures and in 51% having noncurative procedures. The 3-year survival rates in the curative and noncurative groups were 87% and 66%, respectively, with an overall survival of 42% at 5 years. Absence of hepatic metastases was a major predictor of survival 3 years after surgery. Survival at 3 years was better in patients with gastrinomas than in those with nonfunctioning tumors. Although surgical cure was rare, long-term palliation could be achieved in many patients

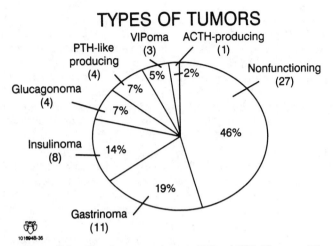

Fig 26–6.—Types of islet cell carcinomas seen between 1965 and 1984. (Courtesy of Thompson GB, van Heerden JA, Grant CS, et al: *Surgery* 104:1011–1017, December 1988.)

with an aggressive surgical approach, occasional total gastrectomy, combination chemotherapy, H_2 blockade when indicated, and the long-acting analogue of somatostatin (Figs 26–7 and 26–8).

Islet cell carcinomas comprise a rare heterogeneous group of tumors that behave in different ways. Generally, they are slow growing, and patients have a long life expectancy from the time of diagnosis. Death is caused by local growth, metastatic disease, and the consequences of uncontrolled hormonal production. Palliative debulking, total gastrectomy,

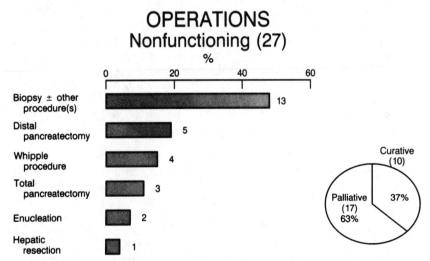

Fig 26–7.—Operations performed on nonfunctioning islet cell carcinomas. Percent curative vs. noncurative. (Courtesy of Thompson GB, van Heerden JA, Grant CS, et al: *Surgery* 104:1011–1017, December 1988.)

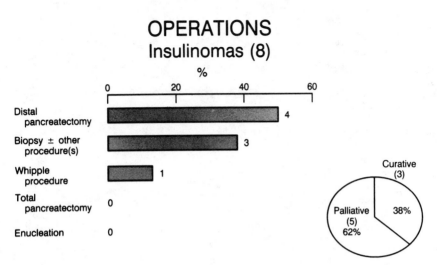

Fig 26–8.—Operations performed on malignant insulinomas. Percent curative vs. noncurative. (Courtesy of Thompson GB, van Heerden JA, Grant CS, et al: *Surgery* 104:1011–1017, December 1988.)

chemotherapy, H$_2$ blockers, and the somatostatin analogue can all play important roles in long-term palliation.

▶ Can any other institution match this 20-year experience? In general, gastrinomas are the most often malignant form of functioning islet cell tumor (usually thought to be about 60% to 70% of non-multiple endocrine neoplasia type I gastrinomas); insulinomas are thought to be the least often malignant of functioning islet cell tumors (the incidence is usually cited as 10% although even this may be high). Of the 58 patients reported here, nearly half (27) had nonfunctioning tumors, and gastrinomas were the most common of the functioning tumors (ACTH-producing being the least common). Only 1 of 11 gastrinomas was treated by curative resection, which corroborates our experience (we have never effected a curative resection in excision of pancreatic gastrinomas in our series of 34 patients with Zollinger-Ellison syndrome). Even though the authors correctly contrast the relatively good survival rate in patients with endocrine tumors of the pancreas to the dismal survival of those with exocrine tissue cancer, the overall 5-year survival rate was 42%. The amazing thing about these patients is how long many of them live with sizeable hepatic metastases, a fact that Dr. Zollinger has repeatedly called to our attention.—J.C. Thompson, M.D.

Normoglycemia After Implantation of Purified Islet Cells in Dogs
Warnock GL, Cattral MS, Rajotte RV (Univ of Alberta, Edmonton)
Can J Surg 31:421–426, November 1988   26–8

A cure for experimentally induced diabetes in rodents by implanting free grafts of insulin-producing tissue was first reported 15 years ago.

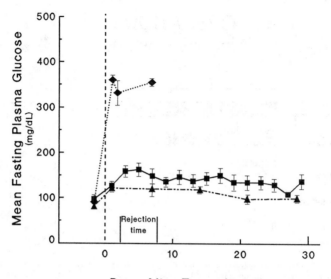

Days After Transplantation

Fig 26–9.—Results of alloimplantation of pure islets into spleen with CsA immunosuppression *(squares,* compared with 3 apancreatic control dogs *(diamonds)* Normoglycemia occurred immediately and was maintained throughout study in 6 recipients of CsA at trough serum levels of more than 300 μg/L. The fasting plasma glucose level after splenic allograft implantation was higher than that after splenic autograft implantation *(triangles).* (Courtesy of Warnock GL, Cattral MS, Rajotte RV: *Can J Surg* 31:421–426, November 1988.)

Further studies showed that islet cell transplantation can prevent or reverse the complications of diabetes mellitus. However, these procedures have been less successful in large mammals and humans. A major problem has been the inability to isolate enough pure, viable islet cells from a single pancreas. This problem was studied using a canine model.

A total of 29 mongrel dogs were rendered diabetic by total pancreatectomy. An average of 123×10^3 highly purified islets were implanted as splenic allografts, splenic autografts, or liver autografts. In autograft recipients fasting normoglycemia was maintained for as long as 10 months. The onset of hyperglycemia was delayed in 3 liver recipients and 1 splenic autograft recipient at 1.5, 2, 8, and 10 months, respectively. The K values during intravenous glucose tolerance testing were higher than 1. Six allograft and cyclosporine (CsA) recipients were normoglycemic when CsA trough serum levels were more than 300 μg/L, although the fasting plasma glucose levels were higher than those in autograft recipients (Fig 26–9).

Purified islets of Langerhans can maintain prolonged fasting normoglycemia in a large mammal. There were some delayed failures of autograft function, which may have been caused by the intraportal site of implantation. Single-donor purified islets induced normoglycemia after alloimplantation into pancreatectomized recipients on CsA immunosuppression with adequate serum CsA levels.

▶ Even though the clinical use of islet transplantation has been halted for the last several years because of lack of effectiveness, and even though pancreatic whole-organ allografts are currently widely and successfully utilized, the great potential attractiveness of islet cell transplantation persists; if the problem of dosage (i.e., the need for more islets) can be overcome, it will almost certainly be the preferred solution. As the islet cell constitutes only a small fraction of the total pancreatic mass, transplantation of the entire pancreas involves allografting the massive excess baggage of all those endocrine cells, which only cause trouble by serving as a huge dose of antigen and by producing potentially dangerous proteolytic enzymes.

Warnock and colleagues have been working for years to improve the yield of functioning islet cells and to improve their "take" when injected. Several other groups in the United States, notably at Washington University in St. Louis, have been working on the same problem. Although progress is slow, results are encouraging, and within a few years we may again be engaged in clinical trials of islet transplantation. One of the beauties of this procedure is that one can potentially transplant a load of islet cells from a donor and, if the dose of cells later proves insufficient to manage the diabetes, another dose from another donor can be given; all this is done through percutaneous catheters, thus avoiding the problems of multiple operations. The ultimate goal is to manage diabetes by percutaneous injections of isolated islet cells. Whether the liver or spleen or some other site (bone marrow?) is the most favorable lodging site for the islet cells is as yet unknown.—J.C. Thompson, M.D.

The Effects of a Somatostatin Analogue, SMS 201–995, on Pancreatic Secretion in the Pig and in Man
Baxter JN, Ellenbogen S, Roberts N, Mackie CR, Jenkins SA (Royal Liverpool Hosp, England)
Surg Res Comm 4:215–228, 1988   26–9

Somatostatin analogues such as SMS 201–995 may be therapeutic in the closure of pancreatic and high-output small bowel fistulas. To study the effects of SMS 201–.995 on exocrine pancreatic secretion, direct cannulation of the pancreatic duct was carried out in the pig and in 1 patient. In 7 healthy volunteers pancreatic function was studied after SMS 201–995 administration using a tubeless pancreatic function test. The analogue, administered intravenously to pigs, significantly inhibited the stimulated volume, electrolytes, and enzyme output of pancreatic juice. Subcutaneous SMS 201–995 produced similar effects in the patient (Fig 26–10). It also inhibited the basal output of amylase, lipase, and total protein, but increased the concentration of amylase. A significant rebound hypersecretion of lipase and total protein occurred in the patient the day after SMS 201–995 administration. In 7 healthy volunteers, subcutaneous SMS 201–995 inhibited pancreatic function.

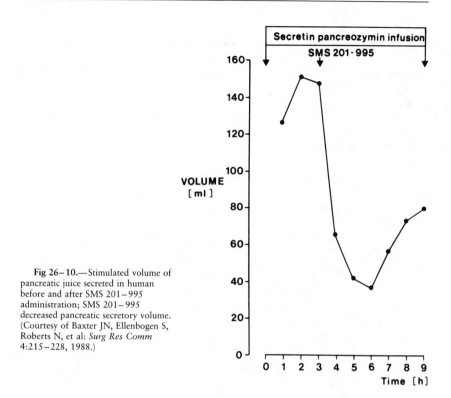

Fig 26–10.—Stimulated volume of pancreatic juice secreted in human before and after SMS 201–995 administration; SMS 201–995 decreased pancreatic secretory volume. (Courtesy of Baxter JN, Ellenbogen S, Roberts N, et al: *Surg Res Comm* 4:215–228, 1988.)

This somatostatin analogue appears to be a potent inhibitor of exocrine pancreatic secretion. Because SMS 201–995 can be given subcutaneously, it has advantages over somatostatin, which must be given intravenously in the treatment of conditions in which pancreatic secretion must be suppressed. Thus SMS 201–995 may be beneficial in treating pancreatic and small bowel fistulas and acute pancreatitis.

▶ Somatostatin appears to be, for practical purposes, the universal "off" switch. It suppresses hormone release, and it suppresses motility and secretion of the gut. Figure 26–10 shows clear suppression of pancreatic secretion in man. The somatostatin analogue (Sandostatin) appears clearly to be the agent of choice in treatment of secretory diarrheas caused by nonresectable tumors, for management of small bowel and pancreatic fistulas, and probably for alleviation of symptoms of the dumping syndrome (1, 2).—J.C. Thompson, M.D.

References

1. Dcruz DP, et al: *Postgrad Med J* 65:116, 1989.
2. Primrose JN, Johnston D: *Br J Surg* 76:140, 1989.

Flow Cytometric Analysis of Deoxyribonucleic Acid Ploidy in Benign and Malignant Aldosterone-Producing Neoplasms of the Adrenal Gland

Rainwater LM, Young WF Jr, Farrow GM, Grant CS, van Heerden JA, Lieber MM (Mayo Clinic and Found, Rochester, Minn)
Surg Gynecol Obstet 168:491–496, June 1989   26–10

More than 50 patients with aldosterone-producing adrenocortical carcinomas have been reported. In the hope that nuclear DNA ploidy could serve as a prognostic marker, specimens of 20 benign and 6 malignant aldosterone-producing neoplasms were examined by flow cytometry to estimate their DNA ploidy. This parameter correlates with the histologic classification of nonfunctional adrenal neoplasms. A method of analyzing nuclei extracted from paraffin-embedded archival pathologic material was used.

The DNA histograms of 17 benign aldosteronomas resembled those of normal adrenal cortical parenchyma from human adults. Adrenal tissue from 3 patients with malignant aldosterone-producing tumors exhibited a tetraploid and polyploid pattern. Tissue from the other 3 patients with malignancies exhibited DNA aneuploid patterns. Three patients with aneuploid patterns died of the disease, which in 2 of them was metastatic.

Flow cytometric analysis of DNA ploidy may be a more important prognostic than diagnostic measure in evaluating patients with aldosterone-producing malignant neoplasms.

▶ Studies of DNA ploidy show that aneuploid tumors have a worse prognosis in the breast, colon, and stomach (see Abstract 20–12). This study adds the adrenal gland to the list. The failure of flow cytometry to differentiate diagnostically between benign and malignant tumors is disappointing.—J.C. Thompson, M.D.

Subject Index

W

X

Z

Author Index